THE FUTURE U.S.
HEALTHCARE SYSTEM
WHO WILL CARE FOR THE
POOR AND UNINSURED?

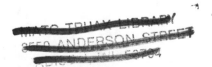

THE FUTURE U.S.
HEALTHCARE SYSTEM
WHO WILL CARE FOR THE
POOR AND UNINSURED?

edited by
Stuart H. Altman
Uwe E. Reinhardt
Alexandra E. Shields

DEVELOPED UNDER THE AUSPICES OF
THE COUNCIL ON THE ECONOMIC IMPACT
OF HEALTH SYSTEM CHANGE

A PROGRAM SUPPORTED BY
THE ROBERT WOOD JOHNSON FOUNDATION

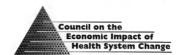

Council on the
Economic Impact of
Health System Change

Health Administration Press
Chicago, Illinois

Waltham, Massachusetts

02   01   00   99   98   5   4   3   2   1

Library of Congress Cataloging-in-Publication Data

The future U.S. healthcare system : who will care for the poor and uninsured?
  / edited by Stuart Altman, Uwe Reinhardt, and Alexandra Shields.
      p.   cm.
    Includes bibliographical references and index.
    ISBN 1-56793-067-0 (alk. paper)
    1. Medically uninsured persons—Medical care—United States—Finance.
  2. Poor—Medical care—United States—Finance.   I. Altman, Stuart H.
  II. Reinhardt, Uwe E.   III. Shields, Alexandra E.
  RA413.7.U53F88   1997
  362.1'086'9420973—dc21   97-23221
                                                                            CIP

The paper used in this publication meets the minimum requirements of
American National Standard for Information Sciences—Permanence of Paper
for Printed Library Materials, ANSI Z39.48-1984. ∞ ™

"The final great issue is this: what do we owe each other, not simply as individuals, but as a community or nation?"

Michael Katz, *In the Shadow of the Poorhouse,* Basic Books, 1996, p. 332.

Contents

Foreword

Having rejected comprehensive national healthcare reform, the United States has now embarked on an experiment that could be called "market solutions as the default national healthcare policy." This experiment has shown some early signs of success in the area of medical cost containment. At least for large employers, health insurance rates are stable—and in some cases actually declining—for the first time in decades. Increases in Medicaid expenditure rates are the lowest in many years. In 1994, physician income declined for the first time in at least two decades, although it crept up again in 1995. Hospitals throughout the country are merging, shrinking, and even closing.

There is no question that the market can efficiently reduce excess capacity, and that seems to be happening to the medical care sector today. But the triumph of the market has unmasked some major problems that the United States has yet to face.

The most pressing of these is the persistent problem of the uninsured and its companion issue—indigent care. Under the old system of laissez-faire, fee-for-service reimbursement, indigent care—as well as much graduate medical education and some clinical research—were subsidized by private payors. These cross-subsidies are now imperiled in a price-competitive, market-driven system.

What are the facts about the medically uninsured? As described in this volume, they are sobering:

- More than 40 million people were without health insurance at any given time during calendar year 1995. This number represents an increase of almost one million Americans over the previous year.

- More than one-fourth of the American population is uninsured for at least a month during any given year.

- There are tremendous differences among the 50 states in the prevalence of the uninsured.

- Medicaid, the program designed to provide poor people with health insurance, varies from state to state in the extent of its penetration. Some states cover far more of the eligible population than do others, and there is also great variation in the extent of the benefits provided.

- The medically uninsured include almost 10 million children.

- Employer-based health insurance, the major coverage for the nonelderly in the United States, continues to erode. Between 1988 and 1994, four million fewer people were covered by employment-based health insurance. In 1995, 23 million workers were not provided health insurance. These tend to be workers with lower incomes.

- Ten million new people received Medicaid during the same period, 1988–94. That expansion has now slowed. It is unclear whether it will continue to recede.

Despite the persistent problem of the medically uninsured, which now appears to be worsening, we have always consoled ourselves that those who *really* need care will somehow receive it. Though there are compelling data that the medically uninsured have less access to care and receive less of it than those who are insured, for the most part the safety net has protected people against outright medical abandonment.

Under the new policy of market reform, however, the safety-net function is threatened from many sides. First, mainstream providers—hospitals and doctors, both private not-for-profit and for-profit providers—who previously did a certain proportion of charity care must now reduce their prices to attract and retain business. It thus becomes increasingly impossible to pad those prices with the costs of providing free care. In addition, as previously independent physicians now join large corporations, those who still wish to provide free care will not have the freedom to do so.

The second threat comes from the eroding of the financial base of traditional safety-net institutions—public hospitals and clinics. In part, this erosion comes from the loss of Medicaid patients. Because of the surge of Medicaid managed care contracts, for the first time many of these patients find private providers anxious to serve them—and competing to do so. In part, the erosion is a function of the declining tax base of state and county services, reflecting the popular themes of reducing the tax burden and privatizing formerly public institutions.

The third threat is manifest mainly in states with high immigrant populations, such as California. There the public hospitals are now told that they will not be paid for the care they give to illegal aliens, of whom there are many millions in this country.

Thus, we have reason to expect a continuing rise in the already high number of people who lack health insurance. That rise should be gradual if the economy stays healthy, but could become much steeper if the economy turns sour. We also have reason to expect that the provision of charity care in mainstream and traditional safety-net institutions will become more difficult for those institutions to sustain.

Does this mean that we will suddenly encounter poor people dying in the streets with ruptured appendixes? No, the reality will be much more subtle and will take some time before we understand it. Analysts concerned about these trends should be careful not to exaggerate the peril. Two recent social experiments illustrate this point. In California, Proposition 13 was passed in 1978 limiting rises in local property taxes. Opponents of the measure predicted immediate, dire consequences for local schools, which are supported by those property taxes. In fact, it took a long time for the schools to feel the adverse effects of Proposition 13, probably more than a decade.

Another example occurred after Medicare Prospective Payment was enacted in 1982. Many instant analyses predicted shorter lengths of hospital stay—a correct prediction—and increasing numbers of hospital admissions. The increase in hospital admissions was predicated on the belief that hospitals would "game" the system by differentially admitting short-stay patients. But that predicted change did not occur. Instead, many simpler types of operations just shifted from hospital to outpatient settings, the most notable example being cataract surgery.

So the changes in indigent care that will result from the new market forces may take some time for us to understand. To the extent that calamitous scenarios are forecast and do not occur, they may distract us from the subtler, potentially more important changes that will evolve over the next decade.

As a nation we have staked our healthcare future on a market-based approach, for better or worse. This development has at least one salutary indirect effect: It has finally unmasked fundamental unresolved dilemmas that we in the United States have ignored for so long. Should everyone have the right to basic healthcare? To what extent should the healthy subsidize the sick? The wealthy, the poor? What is government's role? Is medicine merely a business like any other? Should there be limits on the profits obtained from providing healthcare services? How do we continue to invest in medicine's future, in research and training?

This volume provides important background information on these questions, helps frame the issues, and provides concrete policy recommendations to stimulate further reflection and action.

Steven A. Schroeder, M.D.

Acknowledgments

As with any edited volume, this book reflects the vision, commitment, and effort of many people beyond those listed among the editors and authors. We are particularly indebted to the Robert Wood Johnson Foundation for its financial support of the Council on the Economic Impact of Health System Change and of the Third Princeton Conference, which provided the initial forum for discussion of issues addressed in this volume. Steve Schroeder, M.D., President of the Foundation and a respected leader in the healthcare community, has been a consistent source of inspiration and guidance to the Council and to this project in particular. The Foundation has long maintained a commitment to keeping concerns affecting the poor and medically uninsured in the public eye. As a physician, Steve often reminds us of the social obligation to provide needed medical care to all of our citizens. Nancy Barrand, RWJ Project Officer for the Council, spearheaded the initial planning for the conference and offered valuable direction and support in the process of developing this book. We would also like to thank Rush Russell, RWJ project officer, for his ongoing support of Council activities.

At Princeton, we would like to acknowledge the support of Dean Michael Rothschild of the Woodrow Wilson School for hosting the Princeton Conference on Health Care for the Poor and Uninsured. Ruth Miller and her staff are also to be thanked for the excellent logistical support they provided for that initial event.

The unsung heroes of any successful project are often the editorial, administrative, and research staffs, without whom many books would lack the professional luster we have all come to expect. From Brandeis, we would like to thank Elaine McGarraugh for her superb editing, as well as

Liz Rosenkranz, Betsy Shields Lynch, and Andrea Fishman for research assistance and project support. Mary Flynn and Ann Cummings provided additional administrative support.

Finally, we are indebted to the staff at Health Administration Press for their constructive suggestions and editorial acumen in shepherding this book from manuscript to press. The final product owes much to their efforts.

1

Healthcare for the Poor and Uninsured: An Uncertain Future

Stuart H. Altman
Uwe E. Reinhardt
Alexandra E. Shields

Introduction

One might wonder why we have chosen to tackle once again the issue of healthcare for the poor and uninsured in the United States. Much has been written about this subject over the years, and yet Americans continue to tolerate a sizable percentage of their fellow citizens remaining without a guaranteed source of healthcare coverage. This is not to say that attempts to remedy the problem haven't been made. There have been repeated attempts—by seven presidents since Woodrow Wilson—to legislate a comprehensive plan for national health insurance, and yet all have failed. Perhaps where the chance of success was highest and the experience of failure most devastating was the attempt by the Clinton administration in 1993–1994. Following that failed effort, the momentum and commitment to press toward universal coverage seemed to collapse. It was as if the problem of the uninsured had disappeared. Of course, it did not. In fact, the numbers of uninsured have grown from about 32 million in the early 1990's to more than 40 million today. Nor are we better prepared today to help those without the financial means to pay for needed healthcare. Access to medical care for those without insurance remains an uncertain reality. As documented throughout this volume, the uninsured face more serious challenges today then at any time in the recent past, and changes in the healthcare system promise only to exacerbate the current situation.

It was these concerns that prompted the Council on the Economic Impact of Health System Change to convene a policy meeting in Washington, D.C., and later organize a national conference to examine the deteriorating trends in healthcare coverage and identify potential policy solutions. By all accounts the conference in Princeton, which was co-hosted by Princeton University, was a major success. Participants included many of the leading healthcare analysts in the country as well as senior staff of the Congress and Clinton Administration. Financial support and intellectual guidance on structuring the program was provided by the Robert Wood Johnson Foundation. While the policy debates of that gathering were thoughtful and provocative, much needs to be done if we are to avoid a crisis in the coming years.

This volume represents an effort to disseminate some of the most recent thinking about the problem and possible solutions, and to spur renewed efforts aimed at stemming the rising tide of Americans with no health insurance and uncertain access to needed medical attention. It includes half a dozen papers presented at the Princeton conference, as well as a host of new papers requested by the editors in order to present a complete overview of the problems related to the uninsured, as well as a wide range of perspectives about how we ought to proceed. Several options for incremental reform are presented, while other proposals would require bolder, more sweeping policy changes. A few go further, and again implore us to end the situation where the United States is the only major industrialized country without some form of comprehensive national health financing for all its citizens.

The Number of Uninsured in the United States: What Is the Magnitude of the Problem?

Despite numerous writings on the topic of the uninsured, many myths and misunderstandings persist regarding the reasons why many lose their health coverage and remain uninsured, how this lack of insurance affects their access to care, and the extent to which we can count on the Medicaid program to close the coverage gap for low-income families without insurance. The first several chapters of this volume provide background information on precisely these matters.

The most recent data available as of this writing tell us that more than 15 percent of the total population was uninsured in 1994,[1] and

nearly 24 percent of those interviewed in March 1995 had been uninsured in the week prior to the interview.[2] Among those under age 65,
this number jumps from 24 percent to nearly 27 percent, representing
61.2 million people (Employee Benefit Research Institute 1996). Not
only is the number of uninsured growing, but those without insurance
are remaining so for longer periods of time. During the late 1980s,
for instance, the median length of time an uninsured person remained
uninsured was approximately 4.2 months. By 1993, that figure had risen
to 7.1 months (Bennefield 1993).

Recent projections, based simply on extending the current trend
lines in employer-based coverage and Medicaid and Medicare enrollment forward at a constant rate, estimate that the number of uninsured
will grow to 45.6 million or 16.2 percent of the population by the year
2002 (Sheils and Alecxih 1996). While these numbers are troubling,
they may prove to be conservative. Left out of these projections is the
impact of anticipated reductions in publicly financed programs such as
Medicaid and Medicare, which may significantly restrict both access to
insurance and providers' ability to finance uncompensated care in the
future. There has been a marked shift in our political culture recently;
active interest in solving social problems has been replaced by an emphasis on cutting public spending and balancing the federal budget. At
the same time, competitive pressures within the health system may be
compromising its capacity to respond to the needs of the uninsured.

In the first section of this volume, Rowland, Feder and Seliger provide a comprehensive overview of the problem, tracking the erosion of
employer-sponsored insurance (ESI) and dispelling many myths about
who the uninsured are. As they describe, more than half the uninsured
are in families in which the head of household is a full-time worker.
Another 32 percent are in families headed by either a part-time worker
or one who worked full-time for part of the year. Those in small firms
are more likely to be uninsured, as are children and young adults. The
poor are especially at risk. More than 60 percent of the uninsured are
poor or near poor, with a family income less than $24,000 for a family of
four (Short and Banthin 1995).

As Swartz describes in Chapter 3, those without health insurance
are a very heterogeneous group, representing different regions of the
country, different age groups and different income levels. The number
of uninsured also varies dramatically depending on whether one counts
those lacking health insurance at a given point in time or those who
experience at least some spell of uninsurance during a given year. For
example, while 40 million people were uninsured at a particular point in

time, according to the March 1994 Current Population Surveys, 53.6 million were uninsured for at least some portion of the year. Understanding the diversity of the uninsured population is critical to developing policy responses that can successfully address the needs of these various subpopulations within the monolith of the uninsured.

To a large extent, we have relied on the Medicaid program to close the insurance gap for our nation's low-income children and adults. And yet, as Holahan describes in Chapter 4, expansions in Medicaid coverage have been unable to keep pace with declines in other sources of insurance coverage. Dramatic increases in enrollment, compounded by increased spending per beneficiary, have engendered fierce pressure to control Medicaid spending. This has been largely achieved through a combination of restricting enrollment and controlling costs per beneficiary through Medicaid managed care. In 1992, for instance, Medicaid enrollment among the Aid to Families with Dependent Children population grew 11.7 percent over the previous year; between 1994 and 1995, this figure dropped to a growth rate of 0.8 percent. Holahan anticipates that continued reductions in Medicaid enrollment and persistent pressure to contain spending will undercut Medicaid's ability to offset the numbers of families losing health insurance from other sources.

The growing number of uninsured highlights the cracks appearing in the foundation of our employer-based system. Americans have traditionally depended on the workplace as the primary mechanism through which to access health insurance. Our idiosyncratic system, which encourages employers to offer employees health insurance by providing a tax subsidy worth nearly $100 billion, has up until recently done a fairly decent job of providing coverage to the majority of the population. Changes in the marketplace, however, have led to a slow but steady decline in the number of persons receiving health insurance through their employer. In 1988, 61.5 percent of the population was covered through an employer. By 1995 this number had decreased to 56.6 percent. Analysts have projected the number of persons receiving health insurance through an employer will drop to 52.2 percent of the population by 2002 (Sheils and Alecxih 1996).

One way employers have sought to control healthcare costs at the firm level is to increase the cost-sharing burden for employees, particularly with regard to coverage for dependent children. Decreases in ESI coverage may thus be related to employees choosing not to "take up" an offered insurance benefit because of high cost. It is not surprising, then, that the largest decreases in ESI coverage have been for dependent coverage. In 1989, over 22 percent of our nation's children were covered under a parent's health insurance policy. By 1994, this number had dropped to a low of 19.3 percent (Sheils and Alecxih 1996). Some portion of these children were likely covered by expansions of the Medicaid program. The percentage of children receiving health insurance through Medicaid grew over the same period from a little more than 6 percent to 8 percent. While some recent initiatives to expand coverage target children, this group remains a vulnerable subpopulation.

The Implications of Being Without Health Insurance

To be uninsured in the United States, of course, does not necessarily mean that one goes without healthcare altogether. For one, the uninsured at times purchase needed health services with their own financial resources, even if it commits them to long periods of paying off medical bills with installment payments. Most often, however, the high cost of care and the limited financial means of the uninsured make this impossible. Fortunately, in the past, those who could not pay have been able to obtain critically needed health services on a charity basis from hospital emergency departments and many health clinics throughout the country. Indeed, many of these healthcare providers have done much more, serving as a regular source of care for uninsured patients. As Altman and Guterman report in Chapter 9, hospitals alone provided more than $12 billion in uncompensated care in 1994, mostly to the uninsured.

Important as the health services rendered to the uninsured have become, they are far from enough and they are not close to being equivalent to the healthcare received by equally situated insured Americans. This is true whether we measure the differences on the basis of volume of services provided or on the timeliness of these services. It is known from prior research that, after adjusting for other socio-economic factors such as income, family status, and geographic residence, uninsured Americans receive on average only about 60 percent of the health services received by insured Americans (Congressional Budget Office 1993, viii). This is true even for the subgroup of American adults whose health status was judged to be only fair or poor (Long and Marquis 1994). Studies have shown that uninsured Americans relying on the emergency rooms of heavily crowded public hospitals experience very long waits before being seen by a doctor, sometimes so long that they simply leave because they are too sick to wait any longer (Kellerman 1991; Baker and Stevens 1991). After controlling statistically for the effects of diagnosis, race, hospital type and other relevant variables, a study of a large cohort of about 30,000 newborns in California found that uninsured infants received substantially fewer health services than did otherwise similar but insured newborns, and that infants covered by Medicaid received fewer services than privately insured infants (Braveman et al. 1991).

The Issue of Underinsurance

Not only is the growing number of uninsured cause for concern, but the adequacy of insurance protection among those we count as insured is an additional worry. Given the persistent number of persons with no insurance, it is perhaps understandable that policy discussions have focused largely on those "worst off," leaving interventions aimed at the underinsured for a better day. Yet many of those we count as having health insurance have inadequate protection against the costs of catastrophic illness. Many others face out-of-pocket costs that represent an undue burden on household income, placing the economic stability of the family at risk.

One of the difficulties inherent in discussions of underinsurance is the lack of definition.[3] Any estimate of the number of underinsured derives from some notion of what constitutes adequate protection against costs associated with needed medical care. How are we to define adequate coverage? Health insurance benefit packages reflect products of varying "depths" of coverage, and these products are themselves constantly changing in response to market forces. Depending on the definition of underinsurance used, early research showed that between 8 and 26 percent of the privately insured population under 65 were underinsured[4] (Farley 1985). More recent research found that 18.5 percent of the U.S. population were underinsured in 1994 (Short and Banthin 1995). Persons whose out-of-pocket expenses would exceed 10 percent of family income in the face of catastrophic illness were identified as underinsured.[5] Several of this group had policies limiting payments for hospital care, or had standard cost-sharing provisions that put families at risk of spending a large portion of family income on healthcare. When comparing the actuarial value of an individual's plan with that of the largest federal employee plan[6] as a measure of underinsurance, nearly 16 percent of privately insured Americans qualify as underinsured in 1994 (Short and Banthin 1995).

In assessing adequacy of private insurance coverage, the poor are particularly at risk. Even for those low-income individuals who have insurance, the correlation of poor health with low income leaves those least able to pay facing the greatest risk of extraordinary out-of-pocket expenses for healthcare. More than 60 percent of people with private coverage who have income below 125 percent of poverty face significant financial risk in the event of catastrophic illness (Short and Banthin 1995). Traditional health insurance policies with standard cost-sharing limits often represent an undue financial burden on low-income families. Low-income families may be forced to purchase health insurance plans with inadequate coverage, or may forgo the purchase of health insurance altogether.

Why Has the Problem Persisted?

As Steve Schroeder reminds us in Chapter 5, a constant feature of healthcare in the United States is our willingness to tolerate having a large number of people without health insurance, in stark contrast to virtually every other developed nation. He critiques a host of possible explanations and challenges us to refocus national attention on the needs of the uninsured lest we "find ourselves living in a much meaner America than many of us who entered the healing professions ever imagined."

It is a widely held theory among macroeconomists that reductions in the level of unemployment below a certain level—say 5 percent—could be harmful to the economy because it might trigger inflation. Is there an analogous theory concerning the uninsured? To our knowledge, no one has ever seriously argued that a certain number of Americans without any health insurance is in any way a good thing for the health system or the economy as a whole. On the contrary, one can reasonably claim general agreement on the proposition that universal health insurance coverage—at least catastrophic coverage—is an unquestionably desirable social goal.

And yet we have failed repeatedly to realize this goal. The phenomenon of the uninsured and underinsured in the United States is not new. It has been a permanent feature of the American health system. The number stood at close to one-third of the U.S. population before the introduction of Medicare and Medicaid in the mid-1960s. Thereafter it gradually fell to about 12 percent of the population in the late 1970s. Since that time, it has risen steadily, reaching the current proportion of more than 15 percent. As noted above, current projections suggest that in the absence of public policy to stem the rising tide of uninsured, their number may climb to 50 million—or 20 percent of the population—in the early part of the next century. In many parts of the United States—for example in California—it already exceeds 25 percent.

Our failure to solve this major social problem is even more vexing given the views of most Americans, who repeatedly voice strong support for equal access to healthcare for all individuals. In a cross-national opinion survey conducted in 1991 (Taylor and Reinhardt 1991), for example, respondents in the United States and several other countries were asked whether they agreed or disagreed with the following set of statements:

A. Nobody, however sick and however poor, should be bankrupted by paying for the cost of their medical care.

B. People who are unemployed and poor should be able to get the same amount and quality of medical services as people who have good jobs and are paying substantial taxes.

C. The government should do whatever is necessary, whatever it costs in taxes, to see that *everyone* gets the medical care they need.

As shown in Table 1.1, there did not appear to be a significant difference in the respondents' attitudes toward the distributive ethic that ought to rule the delivery of healthcare services in their respective countries. Overall, the responses evince a strongly egalitarian bent, even in the United States.

It is difficult to reconcile this overwhelming endorsement of an egalitarian ethic for healthcare with the historical fact that the United States has never attained the comprehensive, universal health insurance coverage that citizens of other industrialized countries have long taken for granted. In practice, the American health system fails to live up to the egalitarian sentiments the American public expresses, time after time, in opinion surveys.

Articulated sentiments of egalitarianism often fade away when confronted with the cost estimates and uncertainties of particular reform proposals. Depending upon the generosity of the benefit package and the eligibility criteria, the best estimates of independent healthcare analysts are that a program of universal coverage would require an increase in annual health expenditures of between $50 to $150 billion. This represents an increase in total health expenditures of roughly 5 to 10 percent. The United States' gross domestic product (GDP) currently exceeds $7 trillion (*Economic Report of the President* 1996), of which roughly about a third flows through government budgets in the form of taxes of all kinds levied at all levels of government. Hence,

Table 1.1   Responses to a Cross-National Survey on Attitudes Toward Healthcare

A. Healthcare Should Not Bankrupt the Sick

Nobody, however sick and however poor, should be bankrupted by paying for the cost of their medical care.

	United States	Great Britain	France	Canada	West Germany
Agree strongly	75%	82%	61%	79%	65%
Agree but not strongly	9	10	16	8	18
Disagree but not strongly	5	2	7	3	6
Disagree strongly	11	5	15	9	8
Not sure	—	1	2	1	2

B. Everyone Should Get Equal Care

People who are unemployed and poor should be able to get the same amount and quality of medical services as people who have good jobs and are paying substantial taxes.

	United States	Great Britain	France	Canada	West Germany
Agree strongly	61%	79%	67%	79%	69%
Agree but not strongly	23	16	24	15	19
Disagree but not strongly	8	2	4	3	5
Disagree strongly	6	1	3	2	2
Not sure	2	2	2	1	5

C. Government Should Ensure Accessible Care

The government should do whatever is necessary, whatever it costs in taxes, to see that *everyone* gets the medical care they need.

	United States	Great Britain	France	Canada	West Germany
Agree strongly	55%	62%	48%	56%	63%
Agree but not strongly	21	26	33	20	24
Disagree but not strongly	10	6	9	11	7
Disagree strongly	12	3	7	10	2
Not sure	2	2	3	3	4

Source: Taylor and Reinhardt 1991.

expenditures required to support universal coverage might divert an additional 0.2 to 0.7 percentage points of the GDP through the public budget or, alternatively viewed, would raise the government sector's total tax bite of the GDP by between 0.7 and 2.1 percent. By themselves, these numbers are not trivial; nor are they overwhelming. So why do costs loom so important as an impediment to the passage of universal coverage?

The answer, we believe, lurks in the public's general mistrust of any estimate of what such an entitlement plan would cost. This mistrust allows critics of any such plan, and there are always critics, to present far greater cost estimates and thus undermine public support for the plan in question. To a confused public, repeatedly told about huge cost overruns of government programs, these fictional numbers ring all too true.

There are also those, including the architects of the Clinton health plan, who argue that there is at least as much as the cost of universal coverage currently being "wasted" in the existing health system. Therefore, they argue, we could reform the healthcare system and cover all the uninsured for *no* increase in spending! Even if such claims proved true, there would still remain the dilemma of who should benefit if this waste were eliminated. Those paying the existing healthcare bill, including federal and state government, private employers, and individuals, all believe they pay too much. Each would argue they should be first at the credit window if refunds were being made available. A more realistic view of the cost of passing universal health coverage is that health spending would rise from whatever level by 5 to 10 percent.

Of even greater concern to the public is the fear that in order to provide increased benefits to the uninsured, the care available to the middle class would be restricted, and the dreaded word—"rationing"—would enter the American healthcare system. Opponents effectively capitalized on this fear to destroy the Clinton health reform plan.

When President Clinton entered the White House, a substantial majority of Americans supported the passage of guaranteed comprehensive health insurance coverage for all Americans and also wanted the cost of healthcare to be constrained. Yet as the months progressed following the announcement of the Clinton plan, support for the proposal began to wane, and by the fall of 1993, less than a majority indicated support for such a plan. This lack of public support allowed the critics of the plan to prevent any meaningful debate to take place in the Congress. No vote for universal coverage was ever taken by either branch of the Congress. Even more significantly, those in Congress who prevented passage faced no significant loss of power in the next election. Quite the contrary, the conservative wing of the Republican party, which actively campaigned against the plan, secured a major victory in the 1994 election.

While many explanations have been advanced for why the public turned against a plan they had so strongly backed less than a year earlier, in the end Americans feared the plan developed by the Clinton administration would fundamentally change the healthcare delivery system, leading to both increased rationing and a deterioration of the quality of care they received. Ironically, many of the changes advocated by the Clinton plan were already beginning to occur in the healthcare market, including the shift to managed care and restrictions in the use of certain healthcare services.

Also embodied in this retreat from universal coverage was a shift in sentiment from such an egalitarian plan. This shift was particularly troubling for those who supported complete equality of coverage for all, regardless of income, health, or employment status. Whether such a shift is permanent is unclear, but it is perceived as real by many politicians as well as those in the Clinton administration. Results from a poll of national experts and policymakers at the Princeton conference in May 1996 illustrate this retreat. Only 10 percent of those present believed federal health reform would be a major issue in the 1996 presidential election, compared to 79 percent of the general public similarly surveyed (Shactman and Taylor 1996). The "experts" were right. Asked whether all Americans should receive the same quality healthcare, regardless of ability to pay, only 13 percent of these experts—many of them involved in developing the Clinton plan—agreed, compared with 27 percent of the general public. An acknowledgment of this shift in sentiment away from the same coverage for all underpins many of the incremental reforms advocated in this volume.

A final factor underlying the sudden change in sentiment was the public's belief that, while universal coverage is a worthwhile social goal, failure to pass such a plan would not do serious harm to those without insurance. For a population whose information is overwhelmingly shaped and received by television, there are few, if any, dramatic examples on the evening news of individuals "dying on the streets" because they lacked health insurance. Statistical differences in care described previously are not vivid enough to capture the nation's imagination. But can the American public be so sure that lack of health insurance will not produce more serious consequences in the future?

Increasingly Less Healthcare Available for the Uninsured

Up until this point, a seriously ill person without insurance most likely would not be turned away at the door of a local clinic or hospital. Uncompensated or free care has long been provided by physicians and hospitals, financed by a creative use of excess funds received by private patients. According to Congressional Budget Office (CBO) figures, the amount of uncompensated care provided by physicians and hospitals grew from approximately $20 billion in 1991 to $28 billion in 1995 (Thorpe et al. 1995).

Yet the extent to which an increasingly competitive healthcare market has strained providers' ability to provide free care for the poor and uninsured should not be minimized. There is every indication that current problems will become much more serious in the years ahead. The second group of papers in this volume offers an in-depth look at the impact of recent changes on what we often refer to as the traditional safety-net providers.

In Chapter 6, Hawkins and Rosenbaum present a salient description of the challenges faced by community health centers (CHCs), including increasing poverty and uninsurance among those they serve, stagnating and declining direct federal subsidies, and shrinking support from other third party payors, especially Medicaid. Yet community health centers are a critical part of the healthcare safety net. Nearly 90 percent of all health center patients are poor or near poor. Two-thirds of all health center patients are from racial or ethnic minority groups, nearly half are children, and close to half are uninsured. Despite their successes, CHCs today are able to reach only about one-quarter of the 43 million Americans identified by the federal government as medically underserved. Federal grants and Medicaid combined account for nearly 65 percent of CHC revenues. An explosion in the numbers of uninsured presenting for care, decreasing Medicaid revenues, and the effects of competition and managed care threaten the viability of CHCs in the future. The authors argue for a continued and strengthened commitment to subsidize CHCs at a level commensurate with the number of uninsured they serve. This is critical not only to the survival of these provider organizations, but more directly to protect this important source of care for those who invariably fall through the healthcare safety net.

Three chapters in this volume address the capacity of the hospital sector to respond to the increasing need for health services to the uninsured.

In Chapter 7, Gage elaborates on the current challenges faced by safety-net hospitals. Using the volume of services paid for by Medicaid, one study identified 369 hospitals as "urban safety-net hospitals," while another identified 696 hospitals as providing more than 25 percent of their services to Medicaid beneficiaries or low-income patients. Regardless of particular definitions, it is clear that any hospital serving a large number of poor and uninsured patients will find it hard to compete in the managed care world of capitation and greater patient choice. In addition to protecting and preserving their essential sources of government funding, Gage urges creative strategies to broaden support for safety-net hospitals and to help this important group of providers establish integrated delivery systems and otherwise successfully compete in this new environment, lest an important source of care for the uninsured disappear.

Academic health centers, which at a minimum include a medical school and one or more hospitals, have an explicit mission to provide care for the poor, in addition to providing graduate medical education and conducting basic and applied research. As Rueter and Gaskin point out in Chapter 8, academic health center hospitals (AHCs) provide nearly twice the proportion of uncompensated care provided by other hospitals, with public teaching hospitals providing the largest amounts of free care. To a large extent, AHCs have been financially cushioned by the Medicare indirect medical education adjustment and Medicaid disproportionate share payments.[7] With pressure to cut Medicare spending, much of this financial cushion is being threatened. Similarly, the rapid expansion of Medicaid managed care and reductions in disproportionate-share payments are also reducing AHCs' market share and revenues.

In Chapter 9, Altman and Guterman provide a historical overview of the role of hospitals in providing a healthcare safety net for the uninsured, and demonstrate how gains and losses from Medicaid, Medicare and uncompensated care have changed over time. They emphasize the central role of private patient revenues in underwriting the costs of care for nonpaying patients. Price competition in recent years, however, has led private payors to resist payment increases, and there is reason to believe that the demand for uncompensated care will soon outstrip the capacity of hospitals to subsidize such services. Early evidence of this potential problem is seen in analyses of hospital payment-to-cost ratios between 1992 and 1994, where hospitals experiencing the largest decreases in that ratio reduced the amount of uncompensated care by a similar magnitude. In the absence of major reforms to expand coverage for the uninsured, it will become increasingly important to carefully evaluate and target public subsidies to ensure that the delivery system maintains some capacity to meet the needs of the uninsured.

In addition to the problems faced by the traditional safety-net providers, changes in the ownership status of hospitals may further undermine the capacity and willingness of hospitals to provide care for the uninsured. The third group of papers in this volume analyzes the particular impact that the recent shift of many hospitals from not-for-profit status to for-profit status has had and will have on the provision of health services for the uninsured. Three chapters in this volume explore this phenomenon, and review evidence that might tell us how these changes will impact the provision of care for the poor and uninsured.

Shactman and Altman provide an overview in Chapter 10 of recent research, highlighting possible implications of conversions on the provision of charity care, the availability of local health services, and the price of such services. Evidence on the actual effect of conversions on the provision of charity care is inconclusive. For example, while the weight of the research findings clearly supports the view that not-for-profit hospitals provide more uncompensated care than for-profit institutions, recent conversions have spawned community-based foundations with assets in excess of $5 billion that potentially could finance significant amounts of care for the uninsured. Whether these resources will be used for this purpose remains uncertain.

In Chapter 11, Gray argues that conversions are occurring at a more rapid rate than previously thought if one considers the number of hospital beds represented as opposed to the number of organizations. The number of for-profit hospital beds has doubled from 6 percent to 11 percent over the last three decades. Scully provides an alternative view in Chapter 12, claiming that the narrative of rampant conversions is purely anecdotal; the growth in for-profit hospital ownership has increased only 0.4 percent between 1984 and 1994. Scully also argues that for-profit hospitals may actually be more beneficial than their nonprofit counterparts for at least two reasons. At least one study documents increases in the provision of uncompensated care after conversion to for-profit. Second, he points out that communities benefit by for-profit hospitals paying more than $3 billion in taxes as well as providing $4 billion in uncompensated care. This contribution, he believes, balances and possibly outweighs the community benefits provided by nonprofit hospitals.

Concrete Proposals for Change

The second half of this volume is dedicated to offering concrete propos-als for reform of the U.S. healthcare system, whether those reforms be incremental or comprehensive. Part IV offers suggestions and examples of incremental reforms at the national and state levels, while Part V addresses more comprehensive national reforms. Many would agree with Henry Aaron, who argues in Chapter 13 that the collapse of the Clinton reform effort and subsequent Republican domination "have erased government-led reform of private health insurance from the na-tional agenda for the foreseeable future." Certainly the current political environment does not bode well for comprehensive reform advocates. The unwillingness of most taxpayors to support a large-scale government effort, combined with recent successes in controlling healthcare spend-ing and a spurt of tremendous economic growth, have dissipated the sense of urgency and passion for widespread reform. We may have to rely in the short run on incremental improvements and local efforts to expand health insurance coverage.

Incremental Reforms at the National and State Levels

Davis and Schoen offer a pragmatic plan of multiple incremental re-forms in Chapter 14. Acceptance of an incremental approach implicitly involves making choices about which groups should be targeted by new initiatives as resources become available. Davis and Schoen argue that children should be the nation's first priority. They are dependent on others, represent an investment in the nation's future, and are the least expensive to cover. Moreover, health insurance for children—as well as poor and near-poor families—could be achieved by building on the existing Medicaid program. Targeted subsidies for the unemployed and allowing adults under age 65 to buy into the Medicare program round out the list of incremental reforms. Taken together, this group of expansions could do much to close the coverage gap.

   In Chapter 15 Wilensky examines the recently enacted Health Insurance Portability and Accountability Act as a specific example of incremental reform. The provisions prohibiting the use of preexisting conditions to deny coverage and ensuring that individuals who become sick cannot be denied renewal of an insurance policy are the most well-known aspects of this legislation. While it is not anticipated that this legislation will significantly reduce the number of uninsured, the author focuses on provisions in the legislation that begin to address the unfair tax treatment of the self-employed as laying the future framework for tax-subsidized, individually purchased insurance, whether that be traditional insurance policies, medical savings accounts, or long-term care policies. For the remaining problem of the poor and near-poor uninsured who are not working, Wilensky advocates increased flexibility for states in revamping their existing Medicaid programs, while acknowledging that the current focus on deficit reduction over and against new spending on social programs will make progress slow.

Much has been made of the recent devolution of authority from the federal government to policymakers at the state level. The argument has been made repeatedly that states can do a better job of developing social programs for their residents. In return for a predictable price tag on spending in the form of block grants, states are receiving new flexibility in determining how best to use those funds. The reconstituted welfare program and the Medicaid waiver program are examples of this trend. The extent to which we can count on states to blaze the trail toward universal health insurance coverage or to provide an adequate safety net for those uninsured who need medical care remains to be seen. Riley and Scheppach, in Chapter 16 and Chapter 17, offer alternative views on what we can expect from states in the near future.

Riley, who leads the National Academy for State Health Policy, is fairly optimistic. She points to Medicaid managed care and efforts to expand coverage incrementally as proof that states are making meaningful headway. By 1995, 45 states and the District of Columbia were enrolling at least a portion of the Medicaid population in managed care. At least some states used the 5 to 15 percent savings realized through Medicaid managed care to expand coverage, although this is happening less often given other fiscal demands on state budgets. More than half the states in the union have implemented 1115 waivers, been approved to implement waivers, or have a waiver application pending. Twelve of these explicitly expand coverage. While acknowledging a period of state retrenchment between 1994 and 1997, Riley cites several successes, including initiatives in Minnesota, Washington, Oregon, Hawaii, Florida, Tennessee, and Massachusetts as proof that states will continue to be an important laboratory for policy solutions affecting the uninsured.

In Chapter 17, Scheppach, of the National Governor's Association, is not so optimistic. Although state incremental reforms have increased coverage to approximately one million persons since 1990, he sees little progress in the near future. States' energies will be focused primarily on containing costs and increasing efficiency through consolidating public agencies, implementing performance budgeting, monitoring changes in the new healthcare marketplace, and privatizing services where applicable. Emphasis on reducing the federal deficit has ushered in a new period of austerity at the federal level, which translates into pressure at the state level to do more with less. Any savings garnered from Medicaid managed care, he believes, will likely be funnelled to purposes other than expanding health insurance coverage, at the same time that pressures to reduce Medicare spending will reduce revenues to safety-net providers. As Scheppach points out, even in a more receptive political and fiscal environment, the Employee Retirement Income Security Act (ERISA) and the employer-based model of health insurance remain major obstacles to comprehensive reform at the state level.

Comprehensive National Reforms

While incrementalism may be the dominant policy approach for the next several years, many analysts wonder aloud if we may be at a critical juncture that calls for a radical reassessment of our employer-based system altogether. Enthoven and Reinhardt present critiques of our current employer-based system and propose alternative approaches in Chapters 18 and 19. Enthoven advocates an incremental, moderate approach based on expanding participation in health insurance purchasing cooperatives (HIPCs), offering tax incentives to stimulate growth of HIPCs, and ultimately converting the present tax subsidy for private health insurance into a sort of universal voucher by creating a refundable tax credit usable only for the purchase of approved health plans. He admits this approach will likely need to be augmented by an individual employer mandate as well as special programs and publicly supported direct care to serve those who fall through the healthcare safety net.

Reinhardt also offers a pointed critique of the employer-based system and advocates an end to the pretax healthcare subsidy, but parts ways with Enthoven and suggests it is time we consider scrapping the employer-based system altogether in favor of a more equitable system of providing subsidies directly to individuals, and offering providers preferential tax treatment only to the degree that they can document concrete health services provided to those unable to pay. He argues for a system that increases equity, makes social subsidies explicit, and is economically sound.

In Chapter 20, Pauly also exposes many of the inefficiencies and social inequalities inherent in the current system, and probes the difficult question of who will pay for the healthcare we all say we want to provide to the needy. He analyzes what markets will and will not do, and discusses the problem of delivering care to the uninsured from the perspective of physicians, hospitals and the increasingly important outpatient-service sector. Finally, he addresses the question, "If the problem of the uninsured gets worse and worse, how bad does it have to get before there is some action, and what is that action likely to be?" As Pauly reminds us, real reform will cost real money, but it will also solve real problems.

In Chapter 21, Helms suggests a number of principles reflective of a conservative agenda to guide future healthcare reforms, arguing that a concept of economic efficiency and promoting market competition must guide efforts to subsidize healthcare for those we would like to help. His list of recommendations includes avoiding proposals that increase taxes or budget deficits, reducing the level of benefits within existing programs, further reducing government payments for services, and improving the efficiency of government programs and competition in general through improved incentives and consumer information. Specifically, he advocates the elimination of the employer tax subsidy and a defined contribution for the Medicare program.

In Chapter 22, Rice departs from arguments of economic efficiency to explore arguments for universal healthcare coverage based on the work of Rawls, Sen, and other theorists of distributive justice. He provides an analysis of alternative theories, all of which can be used to make the argument that healthcare is a right. Health is not merely another commodity to be purchased in the market according to one's tastes and preferences, these scholars argue. Rather, one's health determines one's real opportunities and capabilities to achieve other desired goals in life. Classic utilitarian theory, which undergirds economics and most public policy, fails to take into account the important function of health in determining the limits of one's opportunities and achievements in life.

Looking to the Future

The critiques and alternatives presented here represent many of the possible paths and strategies for expanding coverage for the uninsured or for achieving universal health insurance coverage. While most agree generally on the goal of universal health coverage, these is less agreement on the appropriate means of achieving that goal. Persons of different political ideologies will chart very different courses. The extent of coverage we should guarantee all citizens and who should bear the cost of services used remain a point of serious debate. Still, any plan aimed at achieving universal coverage will have to address and resolve a host of critical issues that have—up until now—foiled all efforts at reform.

Future policy debates will almost certainly revolve around competing visions of how to spend similar or reduced budgetary amounts on initiatives aimed at helping a growing numbers of persons without health insurance. At the moment, perhaps, it may appear that the healthcare "crisis" has abated. The rate of growth associated with healthcare costs has substantially slowed in recent years, which many attribute to the positive effects of managed care and increased competition. Simultaneously, we are enjoying a period of sustained economic growth. Some incremental legislative efforts have reduced workers' anxiety about losing their health insurance if they lose or change their current job. History has shown, however, the cyclical nature of economic trends. Within the next several years, a recession is likely to occur, and social problems like the lack of health coverage will surely reemerge. But the problems this time could be far worse than in the past. The slow but steady number of uninsured Americans may dramatically increase at the same time that the unintended consequences of competition will have ensured that less healthcare is available for those without an insurance card.

It may be next year or in five years, but any cursory analysis of current trends belies the prospect that we are on a collision course. The combination of diminishing resources and capacity in the face of growing need ultimately raises questions of an ethical nature that the American public will have to face. To what extent are we our neighbor's keeper? What are the consequences of treating healthcare as any other commodity traded in the open market? How large a gap in quality or access of healthcare received by the poor and that received by the middle and upper classes is acceptable? How low is the "floor" below which no American should be allowed to fall, regardless of ability to pay? What is the right balance between social solidarity and individual responsibility? These are some of the fundamental questions underpinning United States social policy that remain to be addressed. It is our hope that this volume will offer the reader a clearer understanding of the current situation, future prospects and policy options relating to healthcare for the poor and uninsured in the United States. Ultimately, we hope to encourage others to take up the difficult tasks of building consensus and implementing meaningful change to ensure that every one of us—in this, the richest country in the world—has access to the appropriate range of healthcare services, regardless of health status or personal income.

Notes

1. The March 1995 Current Population Survey (CPS) is conducted annually by the Bureau of the Census and is the primary data source for point-in-time

estimates of the number of uninsured Americans. It reports that 15.3 percent of the total population was uninsured in calendar year 1994 and 23.7 percent was uninsured in the week prior to the interview in March 1995. The March 1995 Supplement included questions for the first time asking respondents their health insurance status in the week prior to the survey and the type of coverage they had, as well as whether they had any health coverage in the previous year. This marks the first time that the uninsured numbers are not calculated as a residual from other sources of coverage but are calculated directly. While methodological problems with these new questions make the March 1995 Supplement an unreliable source for longitudinal analyses, the point-in-time estimates should still be reliable.

2. This figure contrasts slightly with estimates generated from Survey of Income and Program Participation data that 20.3 percent of the total population was uninsured at any point in the previous year (EBRI, Health Insurance Portability, 1996).

3. Bashur and colleagues (1993) attempt to provide a conceptual framework for underinsurance, identifying three basic dimensions: (1) structural, which includes both categoric exclusions of certain benefits as well as the relative burdens of cost sharing and deductibles; (2) experiential, encompassing both actual out-of-pocket expenditures as well as what is termed a "temporal" aspect, i.e., spells without insurance; and (3) perceptual/attitudinal, reflecting satisfaction of the insured with coverage they have. The characterization of spells without insurance as underinsurance seems problematic. At least from a policy perspective, the problem of persons uninsured for periods of time and the challenge of ensuring continuity of coverage is an entirely different enterprise than addressing the adequacy ("depth") of coverage reflected by different insurance products.

4. This study was based on the first National Medical Expenditure Survey (NMES) of 1977. When "underinsured" was defined as individuals who stand to face (with a one percent chance) out-of-pocket expenditures exceeding 10 percent of family income, 13 percent of the U.S. population was underinsured. Twenty-six percent faced at least some small chance of incurring unlimited hospital expenses. The number of underinsured increased as catastrophic coverage was emphasized.

5. "Catastrophic" is defined here as that level of expenditures equaling the average expenditures for those in the 99th percentile of expenses in 1987 for individuals in each group. Risk groups were assigned according to the expected value, or the probability-weighted average of all possible values, of each person's health expenditures, with those in the top quartile of expected expenditures assigned to the "high"-risk group. The insurance data from NMES was then used to determine which expenses would be covered. Having arrived at projections for 1987, they then projected to 1994 using the Agency for Health Care Policy and Research's (AHCPR) simulation model that adjusts for population growth, demographic shifts, and changes in insurance status.

6. AHCPR contracted with Actuarial Research Corporation to assign actuarial values to all policies collected as part of the data collection effort. Plans' share of average total expenditures can range from 0 to 1.0, with most plans falling in the .65 to .95 range. These assigned actuarial values were used to make comparisons.
7. For example, Medicare pays an additional 7.7 percent for each 10 percent increase in the number of interns and residents to beds (IRB), even though the most recent estimates place the actual added costs of education at only 4.5 percent.

References

Baker, D. W., and C. D. Stevens. 1991. "Patients Who Leave a Public Hospital Emergency Department Without Being Seen by a Physician." *Journal of the American Medical Association* 266 (8): 1085.

Bashur, R., D. G. Smith, and R. A. Stiles. 1993. "Defining Underinsurance: A Conceptual Framework for Policy and Empirical Analysis" *Medical Care Review* 50: 199–218.

Bennefield, R. 1995. *Dynamics of Economic Well-Being: Health Insurance 1991 to 1993.* U.S. Bureau of the Census, Current Population Reports 70-43. Washington, DC: U.S. Government Printing Office.

Braveman, P. A., S. Egerter, T. Bennett, and J. Showstack. 1991. "Differences in Hospital Resource Allocation Among Sick Newborns According to Insurance Coverage." *Journal of the American Medical Association* 266 (23): 3300–8.

Congressional Budget Office. 1993. *Behavioral Assumptions for Estimating the Effects of Health Care Proposals.* Washington DC: Congressional Budget Office.

Economic Report of the President, Transmitted to the Congress, February 1996.

Employee Benefit Research Institute. 1996. "Health Insurance Portability: Access and Affordability." *Issue Brief* 173.

Farley, P. 1985. "Who Are the Uninsured?" *Milbank Quarterly* 1 (3): 476–505.

Kellerman, A. L. 1991. "Too Sick to Wait." *Journal of the American Medical Association* 266 (8): 1123.

Long, S. H., and M. S. Marquis. 1994. *Universal Health Insurance and Uninsured People: Effects on Use and Costs. Report to Congress.* Washington, DC: Office of Technology Assessment and Congressional Research Service.

Prospective Payment Assessment Commission. 1996. *1996 Report to Congress.* Washington, DC: U.S. Government Printing Office.

Shactman, D., and T. Humphrey. 1996. *The Public Versus the Experts: Current Attitudes Toward Health Care Reform* (unpublished manuscript).

Sheils, J., and L. Alecxih. 1996. "Recent Trends in Employer Health Insurance Coverage and Benefits." Paper for American Hospital Association: October 21.

Short, P., and J. Banthin. 1995. "Caring for the Uninsured and Underinsured." *Journal of the American Medical Association* 274 (113): 1302–6.

Taylor, H., and U. Reinhardt. 1991. "Does the System Fit?" *Health Management Quarterly* 13 (3): 2–10.

Thorpe, K., A. Shields, H. Gold, S. Altman, and D. Shactman. 1995. "Anticipating the Number of Uninsured Americans and the Demand for Uncompensated Care: The Combined Impact of Proposed Medicaid Reductions and Erosion of Employer-Sponsored Insurance." Unpublished report prepared for the Council on the Economic Impact of Health System Change.

Part I

The Problem of the Uninsured—It's Real and Getting Worse

2

Uninsured in America: The Causes and Consequences

Diane Rowland
Judith Feder
Patricia Seliger Keenan

Introduction

In the past few years we have witnessed substantial changes in the health-care marketplace. Employers have become cost-conscious purchasers of insurance, and insurers have become cost-conscious purchasers of care. These changes are having significant and, in some cases, dramatic impacts on the way Americans with health insurance receive medical care. However, attention directed to "reforms" in the way health insurance operates sometimes obscures the fact that too many Americans lack any health insurance at all.

This chapter focuses on this lack of health insurance—describing who lacks coverage and why—and reviewing the evidence on why health insurance matters to people's health. Although the findings are hardly new, their persistence is powerful: Today more than 40 million Americans are without health insurance—most of them working-class families, almost a quarter of them children. Employer-purchased coverage, on which most Americans depend, has eroded in recent years, reaching a smaller proportion of the population. Were it not for the presence and expansion of the Medicaid safety net over the same period, as many as nine million more Americans could be without insurance today.

Stated simply, this lack of insurance matters enormously to people's health. A substantial body of literature demonstrates that people without health insurance are less likely to seek medical care, less likely to get it, and, as a result, are likely to experience worse health and higher death rates than people who have insurance protection. Particularly in light of "reforms" in the marketplace that make it harder to support so-called "charity care," failure to sustain and expand healthcare coverage will increasingly mean ignoring the health of growing numbers of Americans.

Who Are the Uninsured?

Because Medicare covers virtually all elderly Americans, most uninsured people are under age 65. Whether nonelderly Americans have insurance largely reflects whether they obtain private health insurance coverage through employment. Figure 2.1 shows that 69 percent of nonelderly Americans in 1993 were insured by a private health insurance

Figure 2.1 Health Insurance Coverage of the Nonelderly U.S.
Population, 1993

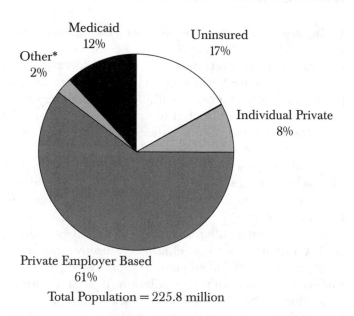

Medicaid
12%

Uninsured
17%

Other*
2%

Individual Private
8%

Private Employer Based
61%

Total Population = 225.8 million

Source: Holahan, Winterbottom, and Rajan 1995.
  Other includes nonelderly, that are covered by Medicare, the Veterans' Administration, CHAMPUS, and military health.

plan—61 percent through employer-sponsored insurance and approximately 8 percent through plans they purchased on their own (Holahan, Winterbottom, and Rajan 1995). Approximately 12 percent of the nonelderly population received coverage through Medicaid, the federal-state health insurance program for low-income families and children and low-income disabled people. Two percent of Americans have health insurance as members of the military, as disabled under Medicare, and through other special programs. This leaves 17 percent of the nonelderly population without public or private insurance—38.4 million people in 1993 (Holahan, Winterbottom, and Rajan 1995). Currently, 40 million Americans are uninsured, virtually all of whom are under age 65 (Bennefield 1996).

Lack of insurance is primarily a problem of working families with modest incomes. Most of the uninsured are not poor; 72 percent of the nonelderly uninsured are from families with incomes above the poverty level ($11,570 for a family of three in 1992). At the same time, most of the uninsured are not rich. Only 13 percent of the uninsured have

Figure 2.2 The Uninsured by Income, 1992

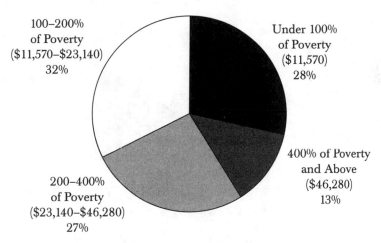

100–200%
of Poverty
($11,570–$23,140)
32%

Under 100%
of Poverty
($11,570)
28%

400% of Poverty
and Above
($46,280)
13%

200–400%
of Poverty
($23,140–$46,280)
27%

Total Uninsured Population* = 37.1 million

Source: Data are from The Urban Institute analysis of the 1993 Current Population Survey.
*Does not include the elderly.

incomes greater than $46,000 for a family of three (Figure 2.2) (Kaiser Family Foundation 1994).

The vast majority of uninsured Americans are workers or live in workers' families. More than half of the uninsured (52 percent) are in families in which the head of household works on a full-time basis for the entire year. Another 32 percent are in families in which the head of the household works either on a part-time basis or works full time for part of the year. Only 16 percent of the uninsured are in families where the head of the household is not employed (Figure 2.3) (Kaiser Family Foundation 1994).

The availability of insurance through employment varies by type of employer, type of employment, and firm size. Employees of manufacturing and unionized firms are most likely to be covered; temporary and part-time workers are most often not covered. Small firms are less likely than large firms to offer health insurance coverage. Less than one-third of firms with fewer than 25 workers offer health benefits, as compared with over 95 percent of firms with 100 or more workers. Forty percent of the uninsured are in families of self-employed workers or

Figure 2.3 The Uninsured by Employment Status, 1992

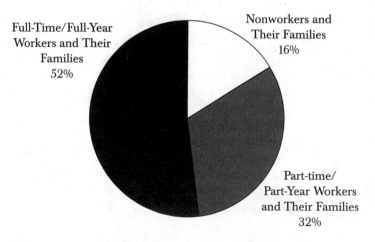

Full-Time/Full-Year
Workers and Their
Families
52%

Nonworkers and
Their Families
16%

Part-time/
Part-Year Workers
and Their Families
32%

Total Uninsured Population* = 37.1 million

Source: Data are from The Urban Institute analysis of the 1993 Current Population Survey.

*Does not include the elderly.

are in families of workers in firms with fewer than 25 employees (Kaiser Family Foundation 1994).

Lack of health insurance appears to be more a reflection of economic barriers than of individual choice. Asked why they did not have health insurance, only 7 percent of uninsured adults reported they were uninsured by choice or because they did not believe in insurance (Figure 2.4) (Davis et al. 1995). In contrast, 59 percent reported they were uninsured because they could not afford health insurance. Another 22 percent cited loss of a job and unemployment, or the lack of health benefits on the job, as the primary reason they lack insurance.

Children under age 18 account for approximately one-fifth of the uninsured population. Despite policy efforts to reduce the number of uninsured children, one in eight American children under age 18 in 1993—8.7 million children—was without insurance (Holahan, Winterbottom, and Rajan 1995). Were it not for the Medicaid program, the number and proportion of uninsured children would be substantially higher. As a result of explicit legislation to improve health insurance

Figure 2.4 Primary Reason Given for Not Having Insurance, 1993

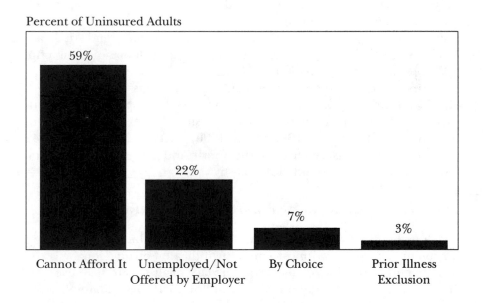

Percent of Uninsured Adults

Source: Davis et al. 1995.

protection for children, Medicaid has become a sizable and critical safety net. Currently, Medicaid provides health insurance for one in four of the nation's children and covers 40 percent of all births (National Governors' Association 1996).

Although Medicaid coverage has assisted a significant number of children, not all low-income people fall within Medicaid's reach. Medicaid coverage entitles states to matching funds from the federal government for certain categories of low-income people, most notably families with dependent children or the disabled. Only childless adults with low incomes who are determined to be permanently and totally disabled can qualify for Medicaid coverage in most states. Over the age of 18, single adults who are not disabled or who do not have children cannot rely on Medicaid as a source of health insurance coverage, even if they are poor.

Adults between the ages of 18 and 24 are one of the groups with the greatest probability of being uninsured. Twenty-eight percent of those in this age group are uninsured (Bennefield 1996). About one in five uninsured Americans are between the ages of 18 and 24 (Kaiser Family Foundation 1994). There is no public safety net aimed at this group, and as young workers, many are not in jobs that offer health insurance as a benefit. Some are in school and remain on their parents' health plan, but others count among uninsured adults.

Although lack of health insurance is a problem throughout the nation, differences in employment patterns, incomes, and Medicaid policies mean that some states and regions have more of their populations uninsured than others. Nationally, 15 percent of Americans are uninsured, but there are tremendous variations by state. Using a 1994 and 1995 average, the percentage of state populations without insurance ranges from 8 percent in Wisconsin to 24 percent in Texas and New Mexico (Figure 2.5) (Bennefield 1996). In 1993, approximately 42 percent of the uninsured lived in the South, and 24 percent lived in the West (Kaiser Family Foundation 1994).

What Is Happening to Health Insurance Coverage?

Inadequate health insurance is not only a large but also a growing problem. The first and most common indicator of inadequacy is the number or proportion of Americans who lack health insurance coverage. That number has increased from 31 million in 1987 to 40.5 million in 1995—from 13 percent to 15.4 percent of the U.S. population (Bureau of the Census 1996).

Figure 2.5 Percent of Total Population Without Health Insurance, by State, 1994–95 Average

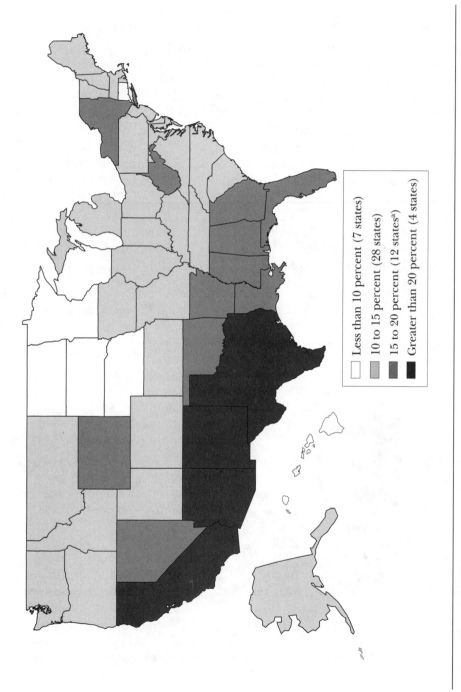

Less than 10 percent (7 states)

10 to 15 percent (28 states)

15 to 20 percent (12 states)[a]

Greater than 20 percent (4 states)

Source: Bennefield 1996.

[a]Includes the District of Columbia.

At the same time that the number of uninsured Americans has increased, so has the number of "underinsured"—that is, people who, despite having insurance protection, are nevertheless exposed to catastrophic financial risks exceeding 10 percent of family income. Recent estimates indicate that 29 million Americans under age 65 (18.5 percent) were underinsured in 1994, as compared with 20 million Americans (12.6 percent) under age 65 in 1977 (Farley-Short and Banthin 1995). The increase in the underinsured population occurred in part because the costs of catastrophic illness grew more rapidly than family incomes and healthcare expenditures overall. Catastrophic coverage in group health insurance plans has deteriorated since 1977, also contributing to the increase in the number of underinsured Americans (Farley-Short and Banthin 1995).

The erosion of empoyer-based health insurance is contributing more broadly to problems with insurance coverage. From 1988 to 1995, the proportion of the U.S. population covered by employer-sponsored

Figure 2.6 Percent of Employer Health Insurance Coverage of U.S. Population, 1988–2002

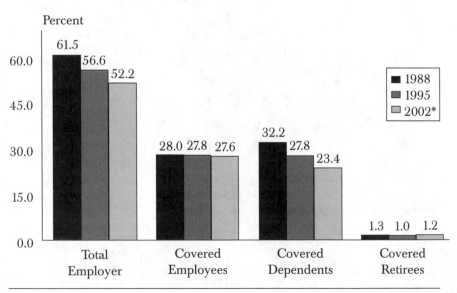

Source: Sheils and Alecxih 1996. Reprinted with permission of the American Hospital Association.
    *Projected.

insurance declined from 61.5 percent of all U.S. residents to 56.6 percent (Sheils and Alecxih 1996). This decline represents the coverage status of three groups who receive employer health insurance coverage: employees, their dependents (including spouses and children), and retirees. The proportion of the U.S. population covered as employees by their own employer has remained relatively constant, at 28.0 percent in 1988 and at 27.8 percent in 1995. However, the proportion of the population covered as dependents has declined, from 32.3 percent in 1988 to 27.8 percent in 1995. The proportion of the U.S. population with employer retiree coverage was 1.3 percent in 1988 and 1.0 percent in 1995 (Figure 2.6).

Employees in the aggregate appear to be retaining their coverage, but they are paying more for it. Employees who keep their coverage are paying higher premiums. In the past year, employee health insurance premiums have increased by 17 percent for indemnity plans and 35 percent for preferred provider organization plans (Sheils and Alecxih 1996). Furthermore, the proportion of workers required to contribute to health insurance premiums increased from 54.8 percent of workers with employer coverage in 1988 to 64 percent in 1995 (Sheils and Alecxih 1996).

Despite the relatively stable proportion of Americans covered by their employer, employees are as likely to lose their employer-based coverage when they stay in a job as they are when they lose or leave their job. Among employees losing employer-based coverage over an 18-month period between 1991 and 1993, 46.2 percent lost coverage while on the same job due to voluntary termination of benefits, employers' dropping coverage, or due to insurance companies canceling the policy or going out of business. That compares with a total of 46.2 percent who lost their health insurance coverage because they changed jobs (23.4 percent) or lost jobs (22.8 percent) (Sheils and Alecxih 1996).

In terms of actual coverage, the erosion of employer-based health insurance coverage has hit dependents of employees the hardest, resulting in a reduction of approximately 4.7 million dependents between 1988 and 1995. If the decline continues at the same rate, 23.4 percent of the U.S. population would be covered as dependents by the year 2002—a further reduction of 7.1 million dependents between 1995 and 2002 (Sheils and Alecxih 1996).

Although there is no discernible trend in the proportion of the U.S. population who are retired and covered primarily by employer health insurance, the proportion of employers offering health insurance to retirees is declining. For early retirees (people who retire before age

65), the proportion of employers offering health insurance coverage declined from 46 percent in 1993 to 41 percent in 1995 (Sheils and Alecxih 1996; Foster Higgins 1996). In addition, the proportion of employers who offer supplemental coverage for retirees on Medicare dropped from 40 percent to 35 percent between 1993 and 1995 (Sheils and Alecxih 1996; Foster Higgins 1996).

The 1988 through 1995 decline in employer-sponsored coverage would have produced a larger number of uninsured Americans had it not been accompanied by an increase in Medicaid coverage (Figure 2.7). Medicaid expansions over that period occurred for several reasons. First, as an entitlement program for low-income people, particularly those on cash assistance, Medicaid's enrollment levels change as the economy changes. Medicaid enrollment consequently increased in the context of the 1990–92 recession (Holahan, Winterbottom, and Rajan 1995). Also, this period reflects the impact of legislation mandating coverage

Figure 2.7 Medicaid Beneficiary Growth by Enrollment Group, 1988–95

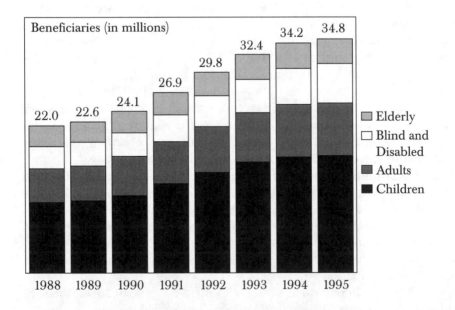

Source: The Urban Institute preliminary estimates based on unedited Health Care Financing Administration 2082 and 64 expenditures data, 1996.

of all pregnant women and children under age six with family income below 133 percent of the poverty level and all children between age 6 and 13 below poverty. Without these expansions to provide broader coverage of poor children and low-income working families, it is estimated that another nine million low-income Americans would have been included in the ranks of the uninsured (Holahan, Winterbottom, and Rajan 1995).

One study examining the effect of expanded Medicaid coverage shows that Medicaid expansions have altered the pattern of uninsured children in Southern states. Children in the South (age 18 and below) are disproportionately uninsured, accounting for 43 percent of uninsured children, but only 36 percent of all children. Between 1988 and 1993, however, in Southern states the proportion of uninsured children up to age 6 declined by 37 percent, and children ages 6 through 12 by 4 percent, largely due to expansions of Medicaid coverage. However, among children ages 13–18, for whom Medicaid has not yet expanded, the proportion of the uninsured increased by 31 percent. Overall, the proportion of uninsured children in Southern states decreased by 3 percent, while increasing by 9 percent in the United States as a whole (Shuptrine and Grant 1996).

There is dispute about whether Medicaid expansions have added new coverage to the uninsured or have replaced coverage employers would have provided with publicly funded Medicaid coverage. In fact, such substitution, or "crowd out," accounts for a relatively small portion of the decline in employer coverage. Between 1988 and 1993, employer coverage declined from 67 to 61 percent of nonelderly Americans. Of the decline, an estimated 13–34 percent was due to Medicaid availability (Holahan 1997). "Crowd out" is least likely to occur among people with incomes below the federal poverty level due to the low rates of employer health insurance coverage for the poor. In the years 1988 through 1993, Medicaid's expansion of coverage to nine million additional poor Americans most likely provided coverage to people who did not have insurance to begin with.

The likelihood that Medicaid expansions will continue to offset deterioration in employer-purchased health insurance coverage is questionable. If employer-provided coverage continues to decline at the rate at which it has been declining, it is estimated that coverage will drop from 56.6 percent in 1995 to 52.2 percent of the U.S. population by 2002 (Sheils and Alecxih 1996). Increasingly, American workers fear they may not be able to retain or afford coverage for their families (*Washington Post*, Kaiser Family Foundation, and Harvard University 1996).

For Medicaid, however, the impetus and ability to expand coverage may well have reached its peak. Due to federal legislation limiting states' expenditures under the disproportionate-share hospital payment program, the fiscal opportunities to expand Medicaid have declined, and fiscal pressure is likely to make further Medicaid expansion more difficult (Holahan and Liska 1996). Medicaid enrollment growth has slowed in recent years, from an average annual growth of 7.9 percent to 5.3 percent in the years 1988 through 1992 and 1993 through 1995, respectively; in 1995, enrollment increased by only 1.8 percent (Holahan and Liska 1996). In the future, erosion of employer coverage and pressure to restrain Medicaid spending and growth at both the federal and the state level portend more substantial growth in the number of uninsured Americans.

What Are the Consequences of Lack of Insurance?

A common perception about the uninsured is that they are able to get care when they need it (Schroeder, in this volume). However, the means by which the uninsured get care, either through uncompensated care provided by mainstream providers, or through safety-net providers such as community health centers and public hospitals, do not guarantee the uninsured access and health outcomes that are comparable to the insured.

Those without insurance have more difficulty accessing the healthcare system than the insured and, as a result, use less care, often suffering adverse consequences due to delayed or postponed care. One-third (36 percent) of the uninsured report they have no usual source of care compared with 17 percent of the privately insured population and 12 percent of the Medicaid population (Rowland 1994). Having a usual source of care is generally identified with better coordination of illness episodes and greater likelihood for provision of preventive care. Lack of a usual care site could result in more fragmented care delivery for uninsured Americans.

Studies have consistently found lower utilization levels for physician care for those without insurance in comparison with the insured population. The utilization differences occur because the uninsured are less likely to seek care, especially for early and preventive care, than their insured counterparts. National survey data show that half of the uninsured did not see a physician in the past year compared with a fourth of the insured population (Figure 2.8).

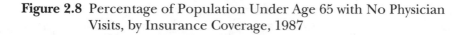

Figure 2.8 Percentage of Population Under Age 65 with No Physician Visits, by Insurance Coverage, 1987

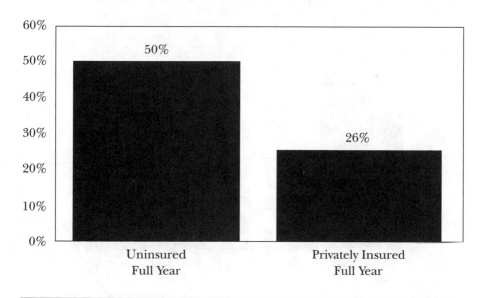

Source: Johns Hopkins University analysis of 1987 National Medical Expenditure Survey.

Due to financial reasons, the uninsured are more likely than the insured to postpone or delay care. Seventy-one percent of the uninsured compared with 23 percent of the privately insured population reported that they had postponed seeking care that they felt they needed over the past year because they could not afford it, and 34 percent of the uninsured compared with 9 percent of the privately insured reported going without needed care in the prior year because of financial reasons (Figure 2.9) (Davis et al. 1995).

Being uninsured results in higher hospitalization rates for health problems that generally do not require hospital care. People with low incomes experience higher rates of preventable hospitalizations than people with higher incomes (Billings, Anderson, and Newman 1996). The uninsured are twice as likely as those with private insurance to be hospitalized for diabetes, hypertension, and immunizable conditions, all health problems that are amenable to treatment and management in a doctor's office (Figure 2.10) (Weissman, Gastonis, and Epstein 1992). Similarly, a recent study of patients with ruptured appendixes found

Figure 2.9 Percentage of Adult Population Postponing or Foregoing
Needed Medical Care in the Prior Year for Financial
Reasons, 1993

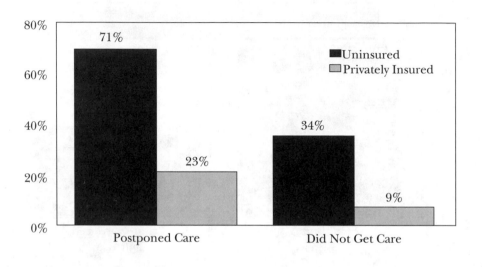

Source: Davis et al. 1995.

that uninsured patients were approximately 1.5 times more likely to
have a ruptured appendix than privately insured patients (Braveman
et al. 1994).

The research on differences in care patterns for uninsured versus
insured individuals increasingly reveals that the uninsured are more
likely to incur adverse health outcomes. One of the consequences of the
lack of insurance is that the uninsured often have higher mortality rates
than the insured. A study of hospitalized patients found that uninsured
patients were up to three times more likely to die in the hospital than
privately insured patients and were less likely to receive procedures
subject to discretion, including total hip replacement and coronary
bypass surgery (Hadley, Steinberg, and Feder 1991). In a study of the
relationship between insurance status and survival rates from 1971 to
1987, the risk of death for uninsured people was 25 percent higher than
that of the privately insured population (Franks, Clancy, and Gold 1993).

The differences in health outcomes by insurance status are particularly striking in the case of women with breast cancer. Early diagnosis
and treatment of breast cancer is important to successful management

Figure 2.10 Ratio of Uninsured to Privately Insured Hospital
Admission Rates, 1987

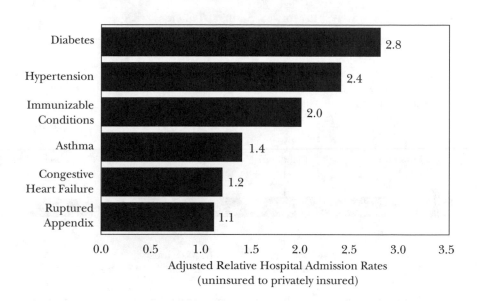

Adjusted Relative Hospital Admission Rates
(uninsured to privately insured)

Source: Weissman, Gastonis, and Epstein. 1992. *Journal of the American Medical Association* 268 (17): 2388–94. Copyright 1992, American Medical Association.

of the disease. However, women without insurance are more likely to be diagnosed at a more advanced stage of the disease than privately insured women. During the four to seven years following their initial diagnosis of breast cancer, uninsured women were 49 percent more likely to die than privately insured women (Ayanian et al. 1993).

In an attempt to get behind these numbers to understand the behavior that produces them, a recent study of adults examined the scope of problems in getting and paying for healthcare faced by the uninsured and the insured. Among those who were uninsured at the time of the survey or over the course of the previous year, a majority (53 percent), translating to 20 million adults, experienced some problem getting and/or paying for healthcare. Just under half (47 percent) reported no problems either getting or paying for healthcare during the previous year (Figure 2.11) (Donelan et al. 1996).

In the study, the uninsured were four times more likely to report an episode of needing but not getting medical care, and three times

Figure 2.11 Distribution of Uninsured Adults by Problem and
Perceived Severity of Problem

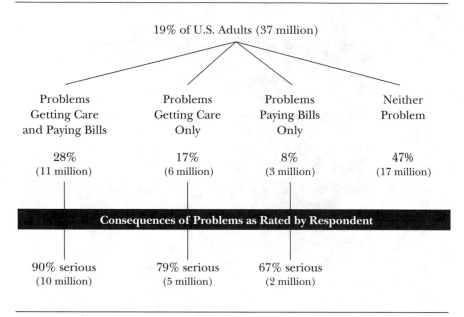

Source: Donelan et al. 1996. *Journal of the American Medical Association* 276 (16): 1346–50.
Copyright 1996, American Medical Association.

more likely to report a problem paying healthcare bills than adults with
insurance. The sickest people surveyed were the most likely to report
problems: Among the uninsured in the poorest health, three out of four
adults (75 percent) reported problems getting care and 67 percent said
they had problems paying for care (Donelan et al. 1996).

Of those who did report problems, the vast majority said they
experienced "serious consequences," in terms of their physical or mental
health, family relationships, employment, and/or household finances,
as a result of their problems getting and/or paying for healthcare. Survey
respondents were asked to describe in their own words the consequences
of problems getting or paying for care:

> Once in awhile I have pains in my eye and my lower back and I
> presume that it's kidney because I've had it before. It was diagnosed
> as a kidney problem. I hear so much about breast exams and I feel
> I should have the test. It affected me mentally because I'm not able
> to pay the bills and I do owe them and they keep calling me. I had

to take the money that was owed for other bills to pay some of the medical bills. I needed boots this winter and didn't get them.

Related to the MS [multiple sclerosis] that I have. I need a specific medicine that lessens the exacerbations of the disease and I can't afford to get it. It's very frustrating and makes me angry because I'm progressing in my disease without the medicine that could possibly slow it up.

My two daughters have a problem with eyesight and I don't have the money to go to the eye doctor, and my children have a toothache and I don't have the money to take them to the dentist. If I pay the doctor I don't have the money to pay the rent and I won't have a roof and it's important to get food. (Donelan et al. 1996)

As explained by the study's principal author, "Most strikingly, the sickest people surveyed are most likely to have problems getting the medical care they need. The vast majority of uninsured adults in poor health had difficulty getting care. This finding directly contradicts the conventional wisdom that truly sick people can always get care when they need it" (Kaiser Family Foundation 1996). Taken together, the findings of the studies illustrate the adverse health consequences faced by the uninsured (Table 2.1).

Conclusion

The combination of private and public mechanisms that provide health insurance to most Americans has always fallen short, leaving millions without adequate protection. But a review of recent experience reveals that matters are growing worse, not better. Employer-based coverage, the source of insurance protection for Americans under age 65, is eroding. Most significant to date has been the decline in employer-based protection of workers' families. At the same time, Medicaid—the public safety net targeted primarily to low-income children and pregnant women—has been expanding, mitigating the impact of private insurance declines on the numbers of uninsured.

However, although the decline of employer coverage is likely to continue, Medicaid expansion is far more questionable. State Medicaid programs, like private employers, are increasingly subject to pressures likely to squeeze, rather than expand, the coverage they provide. Projections of future Medicaid enrollment show a slackening in Medicaid expansion, which when combined with the potential loss of enrollment as welfare reform is implemented, portend a more limited role for

Table 2.1 Studies Examining the Relationship between Health Insurance and Health Outcomes

Citation	Study Population	Major Findings
Ayanian et al. 1993	Matched hospital discharge data and New Jersey State Cancer Registry for 4,675 women followed for up to seven years.	Upon diagnosis, uninsured women had significantly more advanced disease than privately insured women. Adjusted risk of death was 49 percent higher for uninsured women than for privately insured women during the four to seven years following breast cancer diagnosis.
Billings, Anderson, and Newman 1996	Hospital discharge data from 15 U.S. urban areas and 3 urban areas in Ontario, Canada. Data are from 1990 for all areas except New York City, from 1982–1993.	Across all urban areas in the United States, low-income patients experienced higher rates of preventible hospitalizations than patients of higher incomes. Smaller differences in rates were found in the urban areas of Ontario, Canada.
Donelan et al. 1996	Survey interview data from 3,993 interviews of randomly selected adult respondents.	The uninsured were four times more likely than the insured to report an episode of needing and not getting medical care and three times more likely to report a problem in paying for medical bills.
Franks, Clancy, and Gold 1993	National Health and Nutrition Examination Survey Epidemiologic Study that followed 6,913 adults from 1971 through 1987.	Adjusted risk of death was 25 percent higher for uninsured patients than for privately insured.
Hadley, Steinberg, and Feder 1991	National sample of 592,598 hospital discharge abstracts in 1987.	The uninsured were up to three times more likely to die in the hospital than comparable privately insured patients. The uninsured were 29 percent less likely to undergo a coronary artery bypass graft surgery, and 45 percent less likely to undergo a total hip replacement than the privately insured, procedures subject to high physician discretion.
Weissman, Gastonis, and Epstein 1992	Maryland and Massachusetts hospital discharge data from 1987.	In both states, uninsured patients with malignant hypertension had twice the rate of hospitalization than the privately insured. In Massachusetts, uninsured patients with diabetes had nearly three times the rate of hospitalization of the privately insured.

Medicaid in filling coverage gaps. Hence, the number of Americans without insurance coverage—or with inadequate insurance coverage—will likely continue to grow.

Although insurance does not guarantee that our healthcare system will provide appropriate care, it is nevertheless the "key" to that system—without which people's ability to obtain care—and, indeed, people's fundamental health—is seriously compromised. A substantial body of research demonstrates that people without insurance get inadequate or insufficient care and suffer as a result. Direct accounts by the uninsured of the painful choices they face make their suffering palpable.

Changes under way in the healthcare marketplace are likely to worsen the already limited access to care for people without insurance. Aggressive cost consciousness and competition in the insurance marketplace is threatening the surplus earned from insured patients that providers use to finance the care they provide the uninsured. Safety-net providers—the minority of institutions that provide the bulk of uncompensated care—are most at risk in the competitive process. In short, the reforms that are taking place in the marketplace for people who have insurance are eliminating the resources that pay for care to people who lack insurance.

In the absence of measures that secure or expand healthcare coverage for low- and modest-income Americans, the coming years are likely to bring an increase in the number of people without coverage and a decline in the resources devoted to their care. It would be unconscionable to characterize this prospect as a movement toward a more "efficient" healthcare system.

References

Ayanian, J. Z., B. A. Kohler, T. Abe, and A. M. Epstein. 1993. "The Relationship between Health Insurance Coverage and Clinical Outcomes among Women with Breast Cancer." *New England Journal of Medicine* 329 (5): 326–31.

Bennefield, R. L. 1996. "Health Insurance Coverage: 1995." *Current Population Reports.* Washington, DC: U.S. Department of Commerce.

Billings, J., G. M. Anderson, and L. S. Newman. 1996. "Recent Findings on Preventible Hospitalizations." *Health Affairs* 15 (3): 239–49.

Braveman, P., M. V. Schaff, S. Egerter, T. Bennett, and W. Schecter. 1994. "Insurance-Related Differences in the Risk of Ruptured Appendix." *New England Journal of Medicine* 331 (7): 444–49.

Bureau of the Census. 1996. *Health Insurance Coverage. Status and Type of Coverage by Sex, Race, and Hispanic Origin: 1987 to 1995.* Washington, DC: U.S. Department of Commerce.

Davis, K., D. Rowland, D. Altman, K. S. Collins, and C. Morris. 1995. "Health Insurance: The Size and Shape of the Problem." *Inquiry* 32: 196–203.

Donelan, K., R. J. Blendon, C. A. Hill, and C. Hoffman. 1996. "Whatever Happened to the Health Insurance Crisis in the United States?" *Journal of the American Medical Association* 276 (16): 1346–50.

Farley-Short, P., and J. S. Banthin. 1995. "New Estimates of the Underinsured Younger Than 65 Years." *Journal of the American Medical Association* 274 (15): 1302–6.

Foster Higgins. 1996. *National Survey of Employer-Sponsored Health Plans, 1995.* New York: Foster Higgins.

Franks, P., C. M. Clancy, and M. R. Gold. 1993. "Health Insurance and Mortality: Evidence from a National Cohort." *Journal of the American Medical Association* 270 (6): 737–41.

Hadley, J., E. P. Steinberg, and J. Feder. 1991. "Comparison of Uninsured and Privately Insured Hospital Patients: Condition on Admission, Resource Use and Outcomes." *Journal of the American Medical Association* 265 (3): 374–79.

Holahan, J. 1977. "Crowding Out—How Big a Problem." *Health Affairs* 16 (1): 204–6.

Holahan, J., and D. Liska. 1996. *Where Is Medicaid Spending Headed?* Washington, DC: Kaiser Commission on the Future of Medicaid.

Holahan, J., C. Winterbottom, and S. Rajan. 1995. "A Shifting Picture of Health Insurance Coverage." *Health Affairs* 14 (4): 253–64.

Kaiser Family Foundation. 1994. *Uninsured in America: Straight Facts on Health Reform.* Menlo Park, CA: The Foundation.

———. 1996. "The Debate About the Uninsured: How Serious Are Their Problems?" Press release quote of Karen Donelan, 22 October.

National Governors' Association. 1996. *State Medicaid Coverage of Pregnant Women and Children—Summer 1996.* Washington, DC: National Governors' Association.

Rowland, D. 1994. Uninsured in America. Testimony before the Committee on Finance, U.S. Senate, 10 February.

Sheils, J., and L. Alecxih. 1996. *Recent Trends in Employer Health Insurance Coverage and Benefits.* Washington, DC: The Lewin Group, Inc.

Shuptrine, S. C., and V. C. Grant. 1996. *Uninsured Children in the South.* Menlo Park, CA: Kaiser Family Foundation.

Washington Post, Kaiser Family Foundation, and Harvard University. 1996. "Voter Knowledge Post-Election Survey."

Weissman, J. S., C. Gastonis, and A. M. Epstein. 1992. "Rates of Avoidable Hospitalization by Insurance Status in Massachusetts and Maryland." *Journal of the American Medical Association* 268 (17): 2388–94.

3

All Uninsured Are Not the Same

Katherine Swartz

The 40 million nonelderly Americans without health insurance in 1995 have one thing in common—they do not have either private or public health insurance. Beyond this, they are quite diverse with respect to both their observable characteristics and the length of time they remain uninsured. This heterogeneity reflects the variety of reasons that people have for not being able to get or not wanting to obtain health insurance.

If people could easily obtain access to medical care regardless of health insurance status, we would not be as concerned about the uninsured. But various studies of healthcare utilization by health insurance status (e.g., Davis and Rowland 1983) and studies of amounts and types of care provided to people with specific medical conditions but different health insurance (e.g., Wenneker, Weissman, and Epstein 1990; Braverman et al. 1991; Hadley, Steinberg, and Feder 1991) indicate that health insurance is a necessary condition for obtaining most forms of medical care in America today. That 18 percent of the nonelderly population do not have health insurance, despite the fact that healthcare is difficult to obtain without it, implies that there is a public policy problem with health insurance in this nation. The possible roles for government to assist people without health insurance depend on who the uninsured are and why they lack health insurance.

This chapter explores the heterogeneity of the uninsured population and how that heterogeneity drives public policy choices for assisting the uninsured. Because 97 percent of the elderly are covered by Medicare, this chapter focuses exclusively on uninsured people younger than age 65. The discussion of the heterogeneity of the uninsured population begins with a focus on the major characteristics of this population at a specific point in time. Part of the discussion also points out how some characteristics of the uninsured have changed over the past 15 years. Then the uninsured are examined in terms of the distribution of durations of spells without health insurance. The dynamics of people being uninsured imply that the problems of being without health insurance are more widespread within the U.S. population than is implied by the number of uninsured people at a specific point in time (Swartz 1994). Finally, the last section of the chapter, in light of the various known characteristics of the uninsured, looks at possible policy options for helping various subsets of uninsured people gain health insurance.

Characteristics of the Uninsured at a Specific Point in Time

In describing the characteristics of the uninsured at a specific point in time, data from the March 1994 *Current Population Survey* (CPS) are used. The March 1995 *Current Population Survey* is different enough from earlier years of the CPS that it should not be used in the context of a time-series data set created by the examination of different years of the CPS (Swartz 1997). Therefore, 1994 data are used here in order to also note changes in the distributions of characteristics of the uninsured over the past 15 years.

There are four major characteristics that show the differences among people without health insurance: geographic region of residence, age, family income (both in nominal terms and relative to the poverty level), and major activity on which an adult's time is spent. Other characteristics, such as marital status of adults and type of family to which an uninsured person belongs, are also interesting. But such characteristics are less important than the first four in terms of offering "targets" to which public policies might be directed to help people gain health insurance.

Geographic Region of Residence

As can be seen in Table 3.1, more than half (54 percent) of the people without health insurance in 1994 lived in three regions of the United States: the South Atlantic, the West South Central, and the Pacific. By contrast, only 44 percent of the total U.S. population lives in these three regions. The high proportion of people in each region who are uninsured—19.4 to 24.9 percent—accounts for the disproportionate share of the uninsured living in these regions. A high proportion of the Mountain states' population also are without health insurance (18.6

Table 3.1 Region of Residence of Nonelderly People without Health Insurance, 1994

Region	Number (millions)	Percent of Uninsured	Percent of Region
New England	1.491	3.7	12.9
Mid-Atlantic	4.947	12.4	14.9
East North Central	4.981	12.5	13.0
West North Central	2.009	5.0	12.9
South Atlantic	7.704	19.4	19.4
East South Central	2.367	5.9	17.3
West South Central	6.272	15.7	24.9
Mountain	2.474	6.2	18.6
Pacific	7.588	19.1	20.4
Total	39.8	100	17.5

percent), but only 6 percent of the total uninsured population live in the Mountain states because that region is relatively sparsely populated.

The geographical distribution of residences of the uninsured reflects several factors. First, the types of jobs and manufacturing in the Northeast and Midwest have had a long tradition of employer- and union-sponsored health insurance benefits. The local labor markets have evolved such that employers have had to offer health insurance to retain workers more than is the case in similar jobs in the South and Southwest. Second, the states in the Northeast and Midwest have relatively higher income eligibility ceilings for the old Aid to Families with Dependent Children (AFDC) cash assistance program. Because anyone who qualified for AFDC was also eligible for Medicaid, the higher income eligibility ceilings meant that proportionately more people were covered by Medicaid in the Northeast and Midwest than in the South and West. Third, many states in the Northeast have either required the Blue Cross and Blue Shield plans to be the provider of last resort of individual health insurance (i.e., anyone who applies must be covered, with limited preexisting condition exclusions) or have created individual or small group market options that make health insurance more affordable.

Age

As Table 3.2 shows, a quarter of the uninsured population in 1994 were children younger than 18 years of age. This translates to one in seven children (14.5 percent) who have neither private health insurance nor

Table 3.2   Age Distribution of Nonelderly People without Health
Insurance, 1994

Age	Number (millions)	Percent of Uninsured	Percent of Age Cohort
Less than 18	10.137	25.5	14.5
18–24	6.795	17.1	27.0
25–54	20.125	50.1	17.9
55–64	2.776	7.0	13.4
Total	39.8	100	17.5

Medicaid coverage. Seventeen percent of the uninsured were young
adults 18–24 years of age. Although a number of states now require
college students to be covered by health insurance, less than half of 18–
22-year-olds attend college full time (Bureau of the Census 1995). Of
all the age groups, young adults are the most likely to be uninsured—
27 percent are not covered by any type of health insurance. Since
the 1989 recession and subsequent corporate reengineering that has
left many 55–64-year-old people downsized from jobs, a great deal of
attention has focused on the difficulties people near retirement have
in obtaining health insurance when they no longer have employer-
sponsored insurance. Although such difficulties are real, the number of
55–64-year-old people without health insurance in March 1994 was 2.8
million, which is just 7 percent of the uninsured population. Relative to
the other age cohorts, the 55–64-year-old age group is the least likely to
be without health insurance—13 percent are uninsured.

Income

Health insurance coverage is highly correlated with income. Table 3.3
shows that more than half (51 percent) of the uninsured had 1993 annual
family incomes below $20,000. Another 18 percent of the uninsured had
family incomes between $20,000 and $29,999. Thus, almost seven out of
ten of the uninsured live in families with incomes below $30,000. To
put this in perspective, the median family income in 1993 was almost
$38,800.

Thirty percent or more of the people in each of the $5,000 income
groups below $20,000 are uninsured—in spite of the availability of Med-
icaid for low-income individuals who meet the eligibility criteria. People

Table 3.3   Annual 1993 Family Income of Nonelderly People without Health Insurance, 1994

Income	Number (millions)	Percent of Uninsured	Percent of Income Group
Below $5,000	4.742	11.9	35.7
5,000–9,999	4.951	12.4	29.5
10,000–14,999	5.702	14.3	34.7
15,000–19,999	4.912	12.3	30.1
20,000–29,999	7.257	18.2	22.1
30,000–39,999	4.488	11.3	15.1
40,000–49,999	2.499	6.3	9.9
50,000–74,999	3.1	7.8	7.3
75,000–99,999	1.256	3.2	6.8
100,000 and above	0.921	2.3	5.7
Total	39.8	100	17.5

with incomes between $20,000 and $30,000 do not fare much better—22 percent are uninsured. Only when incomes exceed $40,000 do we observe fewer than 10 percent of an income group being without health insurance.

Because a dollar amount of income implies different comfort levels for different family sizes, common practice is to adjust family income by family size and compare that with the federal poverty level to obtain a sense of relative well-being among the population. In 1993, the federal poverty level for a family of four was $15,141; for a single person the poverty level was $7,550; for a two-person family it was $9,661; and for a three-person family it was $11,800. Table 3.4 shows the income distribution relative to the poverty level for people without health insurance in 1994 based on their 1993 annual incomes. Twenty-nine percent of the uninsured had family incomes below the federal poverty level, 32 percent had incomes between one and two times the poverty level, and 39 percent had incomes at or above two times the poverty level.

In spite of the Medicaid eligibility expansions for children and pregnant women, the income distribution of the uninsured has not shifted dramatically since 1987 (Swartz 1989). In 1987, 32 percent of all the uninsured lived in poverty; by 1994, 29 percent of all the uninsured lived in poverty. Where the Medicaid eligibility expansions do seem to have had a positive effect, however, is on the proportion of *people in poverty* without health insurance. In 1987, 38 percent of the people with incomes

Table 3.4 Annual 1993 Family Income Relative to the Poverty Level
for Nonelderly People without Health Insurance, 1994

Relative to Poverty	Number (millions)	Percent of Uninsured	Percent of Income Group
Below poverty	11.53	29.0	32.2
1.0–1.24	3.455	8.7	34.0
1.25–1.49	3.582	9.0	33.7
1.5–1.74	3.19	8.0	28.3
1.75–1.99	2.618	6.6	24.8
2.0–2.49	3.994	10.0	18.8
2.5–2.99	2.744	6.9	13.8
At or above 3	8.721	21.9	8.1
Total	39.8	100	17.5

below the poverty level were uninsured. By 1994, this had improved—32 percent of all people living below the poverty level were uninsured. This trend is encouraging but there are still 11.5 million people with incomes below the poverty level who are without health insurance in the United States.

People who have incomes that we might consider "near poor"— people with incomes between one and two times the poverty level—face a similar high risk of being uninsured. Thirty-four percent of people with incomes between 1.0 and 1.49 times the poverty level, 28 percent of people with incomes between 1.5 and 1.74 times the poverty level, and 25 percent of people with incomes between 1.75 and 1.99 times the poverty level were uninsured. Altogether, 12.8 million people with incomes between one and two times the poverty level were uninsured. Without the expansions of Medicaid eligibility criteria in the 1980s for children with family incomes no greater than 133–185 percent of the poverty level, this number would likely be even greater.

It is only when family incomes exceed three times the poverty level that the proportion of people in an income group who are uninsured falls below 10 percent. Given this, it may be surprising that 22 percent of the uninsured have family incomes above three times the poverty level. However, to be in this group, individuals have to have incomes above $22,650 (in 1993 dollars) if they live as unrelated individuals, above $28,983 if they live in a two-person family, above $35,400 if they live in a three-person family, and so forth. A married couple, for example, with a combined income of $30,000 is in this group. If they each have jobs paying $15,000 but no fringe benefits, they will be uninsured and yet have a family income above three times the poverty level. Similarly, a young adult who is living with his or her parents is considered to have a family income equal to the combined income of all people in the family. If the young adult has a job paying $20,000 but health insurance is not a fringe benefit and the parents earn $35,000, the uninsured young adult is considered to have a family income of $55,000—above three times the poverty level for a family of three. These examples indicate why examining income only in terms of dollars or only in terms of the poverty level can be deceptive if we want to link income and public policies to assist the uninsured.

Major Activity of Adults

As Table 3.5 shows, and has been the case for at least the past 15 years, approximately 60 percent of the adults 18–64 years of age who did not have health insurance were employed in 1993. Another 7 percent were unemployed. The other uninsured adults were in school, worked in the home without pay, were unable to work because they were disabled, or retired.

Perhaps the most telling information about those who work, however, is that the size of the employer has a direct bearing on whether or not the worker has health insurance. Almost 30 percent of workers in firms with fewer than 25 employees were uninsured, compared with 21 percent of workers in firms with 25–99 employees and 11 percent of workers in firms with 100 or more employees. Among self-employed workers, 22.5 percent are uninsured.

Table 3.5   Major Activity of 18- to 64-Year-Old People without Health Insurance, 1993

Major Activity	*Number (millions)*	*Percent of Uninsured*	*Percent of Group*
Working	16.868	58.9	16.0
Unemployed but looking for work	2.008	7.0	44.6
Keeping house	3.996	13.9	19.9
Attending school	2.040	7.1	22.5
Unable to work	0.440	1.5	15.0
Retired/other	3.304	11.5	24.7
Total	28.656	100	18.5

Source: March 1993 *Current Population Survey.*

To summarize, the data on the uninsured at a specific point in time have been remarkably consistent for the past 20 years in terms of portraying a population that consists of many different types of people. However, as the distributions of characteristics in Tables 3.1–3.5 indicate, the uninsured are predominantly younger, have family incomes below two times the poverty level and below the median household income of $32,000 in 1993, and live disproportionately in the southern and western states. Approximately 70 percent of the uninsured adults are in the labor force. Two-thirds of the employed adults without health insurance are either self-employed or work for firms with fewer than 100 employees.

Dynamics of Being Without Health Insurance

A description of the distributions of different characteristics of the uninsured at a specific point in time does not fully capture the diversity of the people without health insurance. People have different reasons for being without health insurance, and not surprisingly the differences in reasons and characteristics mean that the lengths of time that people are uninsured vary. Because people have different durations of spells without health insurance, the total number of people who may experience at least a month without insurance during a year is greater than the number at a specific point in time. Thus, the 40 million people who were uninsured according to the March 1994 *Current Population Survey* represent only the people who were in the midst of an uninsured spell when the survey was conducted. According to the most recent data from the Survey of Income and Program Participation (SIPP), 53.6 million people were uninsured for at least some portion of 1993 (Bennefield 1996).

With data from the 1984 Panel of the SIPP, Swartz, Marcotte, and McBride (1993) estimated the distribution of durations of uninsured spells. Their analyses indicate that the median duration of uninsured spells in the mid-1980s was six months. However, 28 percent of uninsured spells lasted more than a year. Without reestimating the distribution of durations of uninsured spells in the mid-1990s, what can we expect has happened to the median length of an uninsured spell or the proportion of all spells that are longer than one year? The mid-1980s were a time when the economy was in a recovery period with sustained growth and low inflation after a relatively deep recession. The mid-1990s are similar in that the economy is in a sustained period of growth and low inflation after a recession.

Where the mid-1990s do differ from the mid-1980s regarding employment and health insurance is the proportion of employer-sponsored health insurance premiums paid by employees. In the mid-1980s it was the norm for employers to pay all of the premium for an employee and a majority of the additional cost of dependent coverage, but the share of total premiums paid by employees has steadily increased since 1985 (Cowan et al. 1996). KPMG Peat Marwick (1995) reported that in 1994 employers paid between 80 and 88 percent of the premium for an individual policy and between 66 and 77 percent of the premium for a family policy. The shift to employees paying a larger share of a premium is thought to be partially responsible for the decline in employer-sponsored health insurance that occurred during the early 1990s.

Without reestimating the distribution of current uninsured spell durations, it is difficult to know whether the distribution of uninsured spell durations in the mid-1990s is dramatically different from the findings of the 1984 Panel of the SIPP. But we can estimate how the distribution of uninsured spell lengths might or might not be different. Employers requiring employees to pay higher proportions of premiums, especially for dependent coverage, no doubt is causing more people to be uninsured. Such people will increase the proportion of the uninsured spells that last longer than one year. The reengineering of American industries has also caused many people to lose their jobs. In particular, midlevel management positions were eliminated—positions that almost always had health insurance as part of the wage compensation package. However, the unemployment rate of the past four years is lower than the unemployment rate of the mid-1980s, indicating that even with the reengineering layoffs, people have found new jobs relatively quickly. Furthermore, the number of people without health insurance at a specific point in time increased relatively steadily during the 1989–93 period, indicating only a mild effect of the reengineering of American industries on the number of people who became uninsured. Although media stories abound about 55- to 64-year-old managers who have not been able to find employment after being laid off, such stories do not appear to represent most workers who have lost their jobs in recent years. Certainly, younger workers who have been laid off have found new jobs, often with health insurance. Thus, the reengineering of industries and subsequent layoffs do not appear to have increased the proportion of longer spells without health insurance.

There have been very few changes in the individual or small group insurance markets over the last decade that have increased dramatically the number of people with health insurance through these markets. Although some states, such as New Jersey, have implemented legislation to expand access to individual and small-group insurance markets, most of the states seem to be in a wait-and-see stage in terms of intervening in the individual and small-group health insurance markets. Thus, self-employed individuals and workers in small firms today are as much at a disadvantage in terms of obtaining affordable premiums for health insurance as they were in the mid-1980s. Because such individuals are likely to have long uninsured spells because they cannot afford individual or small group market premiums, the lack of significant change in these markets implies that the proportion of spells lasting more than a year is unlikely to have decreased since the mid-1980s.

The analyses by Swartz, Marcotte, and McBride (1993) indicate that the duration of a person's uninsured spell was only affected by family income if the income in the month before losing health insurance was such that it was close to or above the median household income. Monthly income did not have a significant effect on the duration of an uninsured spell if it was below $2,460 (or an annual income of $29,500, all in 1991 dollars). People who do not have a high school diploma are significantly less likely than people with higher levels of education to have shorter uninsured spells. In addition, working part time is more likely to lengthen an uninsured spell. Together these findings imply that people with low educational attainment, who work part time, and have low earnings are more likely to have long spells without health insurance.

In unpublished analyses of uninsured spells among children, Swartz and Marcotte (1993) found that the educational attainment of the primary parent was the most significant factor affecting the duration of children's uninsured spells. Although the distribution of uninsured spell lengths for children was similar to the distribution of adult uninsured spells, anticipating that children's uninsured spells will end for the same reasons as adults is not correct. Sixty-nine percent of the children with an uninsured spell had a primary parent with no more than a high school diploma. Given the finding that adults with low educational attainment who work part time and have low incomes are more likely to have long uninsured spells, the low educational attainment of primary parents of uninsured children makes it unlikely that primary parents will find employment that will provide health insurance coverage for children.

Policy Choices

The diversity that marks the uninsured population is a strong indication that government has a role to play in helping people obtain health insurance coverage. The market for health insurance does not fail just one group of people. Moreover, the fact that one in five nonelderly Americans experiences at least a month without health insurance sometime during a year implies that the problem of being uninsured is widespread. All of this means that a single government policy or program to assist the uninsured will not help everyone who needs health insurance. Instead, a combination of different policies or programs, each targeted to a subset of the uninsured population, will be needed. But *how* the government— federal and state—chooses to implement policies or programs is crucial. As others in this volume argue, government could reform the health insurance markets incrementally so that small subsets of the uninsured are helped in a sequence of measures. Or the government role could be to provide broad-based programs or pass legislation requiring actions that help relatively quickly almost all of the uninsured.

Regardless of whether small incremental reforms or broad-based policies are chosen, the options for assisting people without health insurance are well known. Variations on the options are discussed by others in this volume, but the government role could be one of the following three basic alternatives:

- build on the existing employer-based system of health insurance coverage by requiring all workers and their dependents to be covered by their employer, with government programs for people without a labor force attachment;

- provide a set of programs of health insurance for some types of people, such as poor people or children, and regulate the individual and small-group health insurance markets so that they offer more choices to people who earn too much to be eligible for programs for the poor; or

- act as the financial broker of revenues for health insurance for everyone—thereby breaking the link to employer-sponsored health insurance—and provide everyone with a contribution or voucher for a health insurance plan of their choice.

Build on the Existing Employer-Based System

Requiring all employers to provide health insurance to all their workers and the workers' dependents seems like an easy way of providing health insurance to a great majority of the uninsured—those who work and those who are dependents of workers. Various estimates have suggested that between 75 and 85 percent of the uninsured would be helped by an employer mandate (Employee Benefits Research Institute 1995). The remaining 15–25 percent of the uninsured could then be aided by a government program such as Medicaid. This combination of government policy and government program attempts to match the government's role with the primary reasons that people do not have health insurance. For those who work or are dependents of those who work, lack of health insurance appears to be primarily a function of not having an employer-sponsored health insurance plan. For uninsured people who do not have an attachment to the labor force, lack of health insurance appears to be primarily a function of not having sufficient income to pay the premiums typically found in individual insurance markets.

Requiring employers to provide health insurance to all employees along with providing a government program for anyone who does not have an attachment to the labor force is not as costless or as simple as it may sound. First, requiring employers to provide health insurance to employees may have unintended consequences on employment and on health insurance costs. Second, requiring employers to sponsor health insurance for all employees and their dependents is not a realistic policy without subsidy monies for either some workers or some employers. Finally, a program for people who do not have an attachment to the labor force will be essentially an expansion of Medicaid. As such, it also may have some of the same work incentive problems present in the income assistance and Medicaid programs.

The potential for an employer health insurance mandate to have unintended consequences on employment and health insurance costs must be considered when weighing the advantages and disadvantages of such a policy. In particular, three possible consequences of an employer mandate are (1) increased disparities in what similar people pay for health insurance simply because they work for different firms, (2) family members not able to choose the same set of medical care providers because of different health insurance plans, and (3) production decisions that favor the use of machinery over labor if the costs of health insurance are open-ended for employers.

First, health insurance costs are not equal across firms. Firms with younger, healthier workers face significantly lower healthcare costs than firms with an aging work force. Small firms face higher health insurance premiums than large firms, which typically self-insure. By self-insuring, firms avoid state mandates on the types of benefits that must be covered in a health insurance policy. But small firms usually cannot bear the risk of self-insuring, and therefore have to purchase health insurance in the small-group market in their state. State regulations of small group health insurance differ, particularly as they affect experience rating of premiums and how insurance companies may treat applicants. Because firms face different health insurance costs, workers who work in the same industry and have the same incomes see quite different costs of health insurance. A mandate in employer-provided health insurance would increase horizontal inequities in terms of what neighbors pay for health insurance, and further the current practice of splitting people into groups with predictable costs. People in large and younger work-force firms will face far lower costs of health insurance relative to people in small and older work-force firms.

Second, further reliance on employer-sponsored health insurance will force families to have health insurance from multiple sources if every worker has health insurance from his or her own employer. This splitting of families' health insurance and choices of providers is already occurring and causing confusion. Families should be given the option of which employer's coverage they wish to have and not be forced to have children covered by the insurance of one spouse or the other, simply because one spouse's birth date is earlier in the calendar year.

Third, if an employer mandate is implemented, employers' liability for the costs of health insurance must be limited, perhaps to some percentage of payroll, to avoid creating incentives for employers to shift to production methods that favor using technology over labor. None of the taxes imposed on an employer's payroll (e.g., Medicare Part A, Social Security) by the federal or state governments are open-ended. Contributions to pension funds similarly are limited by either a defined contribution or a known percentage of payroll. If employer contributions to health insurance costs are not limited, employers are exposed to the effects of two forces they cannot control—increases in healthcare costs in general and increases in their own employees' expenditures for healthcare. Without a limit on an employer's financial responsibility for health insurance costs, the cost of labor will increase relative to the cost of equipment. Employers will no doubt look to production methods that substitute machinery for labor, which may particularly affect low-skilled, low-wage workers.

Given the current nominal premium cost sharing between employers and employees for employer-sponsored health insurance, it is unlikely that an employer mandate would require employers to pay all of the health insurance premium for workers and their dependents. More likely, an employer mandate could not require that employers pay more than 50 percent of the health insurance premium for family coverage. As discussed above, however, 70 percent of the people without health insurance at a specific point in time have family incomes below

$30,000. Such people are unlikely to be able to pay more than $50 to $100 per month toward the cost of health insurance. Thus, if an employer mandate is to decrease significantly the number of uninsured workers and their dependents, it will need to lower the cost of health insurance. This could be accomplished by at least two alternatives. One is mandating the employer-sponsored insurance but creating a companion program of subsidies for low-income workers. Alternatively, an employer mandate would be paired with a provision to revise the Employee Retirement and Insurance Security Act so that a minimum benefits package that is a catastrophic health insurance plan could satisfy the mandate. Unless the health insurance costs are lowered for low-income workers, an employer mandate will be ineffective as a policy instrument for decreasing the number of people without health insurance.

If we assume that an employer mandate to sponsor health insurance for all workers and their dependents fixes the problem for the 70–80 percent of the uninsured who have an attachment to the labor force, then government programs would be needed to cover the remaining uninsured who do not have an attachment to the labor force. Most people in this group are children of adults who cannot work and adults who are disabled or unable to work and have low incomes. At a minimum, the government can provide financial access to healthcare for the poor—something the federal and state governments began with the implementation of Medicaid in 1965. Medicaid eligibility could be extended to all people with incomes below the poverty level and to children with incomes up to 200 percent of the poverty level who do not have access to employer-sponsored health insurance. People who are disabled who do not meet the eligibility criteria for Medicare and have incomes above the poverty level could be permitted to have Medicaid coverage by contributing a portion of a Medicaid "premium" on a sliding scale based on their incomes.

In sum, although the uninsured would be helped immediately by government actions requiring employers to sponsor health insurance for all workers and their dependents and a companion program to provide a healthcare program for all people who do not have an attachment to the labor force, such actions are neither cheap nor straightforward.

Provide Government Programs for Groups of Uninsured People

Under this scenario, the government role would be to fill in some holes in the safety net. That role would be one of prioritizing types of people who would be assisted in terms of having financial access to healthcare. Three groups of uninsured people who might be high on such a priority list are children, all people with incomes below the poverty level, and people with extremely high expected medical care costs.

Children might be the first priority for government programs for the uninsured. As discussed above, more than ten million children were uninsured according to the March 1994 CPS, and children account for a quarter of all uninsured people at a specific point in time. Currently, states must provide Medicaid eligibility to children younger than six years of age and living in families with incomes at or below 133 percent of the poverty level. States must also provide Medicaid eligibility to children who were born after September 1983 (i.e., younger than 13 years of age in 1996) and living in families with incomes below the poverty level. By 2002, this latter requirement will cause all children age 18 or younger and living in poverty to be eligible for Medicaid. States may extend Medicaid eligibility to infants (children younger than one year) with incomes up to 185 percent of the poverty level.

One risk of creating government-sponsored health insurance programs for children is that the programs may draw people who might be expected to have private health insurance. This issue has become known as the Medicaid crowd-out effect, but the magnitude of such an effect is the subject of debate (Dubay and Kenney 1995; Cutler and Gruber 1996; Swartz 1996). Unless regulations are in place requiring people to obtain private coverage if they have access to it, the costs of the government programs will be greater than anticipated. As employers have required employees to pay increasing shares of health insurance premiums, particularly for dependents, children are at risk for not being insured through employer-sponsored insurance. For the working poor, especially those in single parent households, the choice between paying for health insurance and other necessities such as clothing or food often is not a realistic choice. Moreover, it is difficult to enforce regulations requiring people to purchase health insurance for their children.

A number of states have implemented programs to subsidize health insurance for children. Some of these programs operate as state-financed programs whereas other programs are part of Section 1115 waiver programs for Medicaid. For example, New York state has had Child Health Plus in place since 1993. Under Child Health Plus, children up to age 15 can be insured for outpatient medical care services. Inpatient care is not included in the benefits package. The justification for this is that it keeps the premiums lower, and hospital costs will be paid by the state through other programs. The insurance is sold through private health insurance companies and managed care organizations, and premiums are set on a sliding scale for people with incomes up to 222 percent of the poverty level. The subsidy money is allocated by the state. In

Massachusetts, legislation to provide health insurance to an estimated 160,000 uninsured children is part of the Section 1115 waiver to the Medicaid program. As in New York, the legislation provides insurance for outpatient care but not inpatient care. Premiums are to be set on a sliding-scale basis, and subsidy money will be raised by an additional 25-cent tax on a pack of cigarettes or tobacco. It is important to note that the programs to provide outpatient health insurance for children require states to create exceptions to the state mandates on benefits that must be covered by health insurance policies sold within the state. Proposals to make such programs national in scope have recently gained a wider audience. Senators Kerry and Kennedy of Massachusetts have proposed legislation to create a health insurance program for all children who are not eligible for Medicaid. The proposal includes sliding-scale premiums and subsidy money for lower-income families.

The sticking points for insurance programs for children is inpatient hospital care and the upper age of "children." By choosing to restrict coverage to outpatient healthcare, the programs are able to predict the medical care costs of children and to keep the premiums low. The choice of 13 as the age ceiling for children's programs is also motivated by the objective of keeping costs per child low. The number of teenage girls who become pregnant begins to rise after age 13, and noncoverage of children older than 13 is driven by a tacit decision to avoid paying for maternity care for teens. Because teenagers get sick, are injured, and need preventive care (particularly booster vaccinations), the programs that stop covering children beyond age 13 are clearly arbitrary. If we want to provide health insurance to children so as to provide them with access to healthcare, outpatient care for teenagers should be covered just as outpatient care for younger children is covered.

A second group of uninsured people that might be high on a priority list are all people with incomes below the poverty level. In 1996, children younger than 13 and pregnant women living in families with incomes below the poverty level were already eligible for Medicaid. However, older children and nonpregnant adults living in poverty who are not eligible for Medicaid under the former AFDC program are likely to be uninsured. As noted above, one-third of all people with incomes below the poverty level are uninsured. People who have incomes below the poverty level are generally the sickest and most disadvantaged of citizens. Many have emotional or physical handicaps that restrict their ability to obtain jobs with wages above the minimum wage, jobs with employer-sponsored health insurance, or to work full time. To expect such people to be able to help pay for health insurance is unrealistic.

Furthermore, when uninsured low-income people need medical care they often obtain it in more expensive settings, such as emergency departments of hospitals. Until recently, such care was cross-subsidized by payments from private insurers and public programs. However, as private insurers, employers, and Medicare and Medicaid are eliminating such cross-subsidies, the necessity for direct payments to hospitals and other providers for care to uninsured people is becoming urgent.

A third group of uninsured people who might be given high priority for a government program of health insurance are those with extremely high expected medical care costs. In effect, the government would be providing reinsurance for people with medical care costs that are expected to be in the top 2 or 3 percent of all individuals' medical care costs. Currently, Medicare does this explicitly for people with end-stage renal disease and implicitly for people who meet the Social Security disability criteria. But not everyone who may have a year or two with extremely high medical care costs will be disabled, and not everyone with extremely high medical care costs in a given year will have the same expenses in the following years. For example, organ transplant recipients can be very expensive in the year or more before transplant and during the year or two after transplant, but then they can resume active lives and not be in the group of people with the top two percent of healthcare expenditures.

Government programs for people expected to have medical care expenses in the top two percent of all people and for people with incomes below the poverty level would also ease the anxieties of insurers in the small group and individual health insurance markets. Insurers' greatest fear in these markets is that people who will apply for coverage are those with the highest probability of using a lot of high-cost medical care. But if people expected to have very high cost medical care and all low-income people are provided with a government-financed program, a large proportion of the people likely to be high-cost users will then be covered and not in the insurers' risk pools. In turn, this should permit those markets to offer health insurance at lower premiums to the younger and healthier people who do not have employer-sponsored health insurance. The expectation is that younger and healthier individuals who currently do not purchase health insurance because they feel the premiums exceed their expected medical care costs will decide that insurance is worth the premiums.

Creating government programs that help different groups of uninsured people requires a mix of setting priorities and consideration of the costs of the programs. For example, a program for children who do not have access to employer-sponsored health insurance will be relatively inexpensive because most children after age two do not use a lot of medical care. But programs to assist those who have difficulty obtaining health insurance in the market will be expensive. On the other hand, if such programs permit individual and small group health insurance markets to have lower premiums for younger and healthy people, the number of people without health insurance may decline by more than just the number of people who would be assisted directly by the government programs.

Government as Financial Broker for Health Insurance for Everyone

An argument can be made that the current system of health insurance provision is inefficient and that it would be more efficient if the federal government were to either provide health insurance to everyone or collect revenues for insurance and provide everyone with a contribution or voucher for purchasing insurance. This argument has been made by Barr (1989) and Kotlikoff (1987) with respect to other social insurance programs. The efficiency argument in favor of government-financed insurance is that the costs of the private system lead to economic inefficiencies. In the case of health insurance, employer-sponsored health insurance leads to inefficiencies in hiring and production decisions by employers.

For decades there have been proposals that the current U.S. system of health insurance should be revamped so that it does not rest on employer-sponsored health insurance. The major arguments for moving away from employer-sponsored health insurance are the wide disparities in premiums faced by similar people employed in firms of different sizes and the age and health work-force profiles (discussed above). In addition, people's health insurance choices and their choices of healthcare providers are increasingly being made by employers. When employers change health insurers or plans, people often have to change healthcare providers, which can be inefficient in terms of lost continuity of healthcare.

The proposals for shifting away from employer-sponsored health insurance generally presume universal health insurance financed by income taxes or payroll taxes. The details of what the health insurance would look like have changed dramatically in the last five years as the surge in enrollment in managed care organizations has altered the landscape of health insurance competition. Prior to 1990, most proposals for an income-tax-based or payroll-tax-based universal health insurance system in the United States were oriented toward a Medicare model of insurance. That is, the federal government would act as a revenue collector and then contract with third-party administrators to process claims for medical care services provided. The government might set fee schedules for services just as Medicare does, but the system would be expected to raise monies and pay claims. It is important to note that this pre-1990 vision of universal health insurance through a federal system of tax premium collection usually assumed that the premiums would be differentiated for four different family types: individual, married couple, married couple with child(ren), and one parent with child(ren). Implicitly, this system of premiums creates a contract with people for their entire lives—they may pay more than their expected medical care costs in their younger years, but they would be subsidized for their health insurance costs in their older years. This life cycle view of health insurance premiums and medical care costs does not exist in the current view of health insurance contracts.

The post-1990 surge in enrollment in managed care organizations and increased use of prospective payments to providers has altered the debate for a government-sponsored universal health insurance. Suddenly the proposals for universal health insurance coverage by way of a government mechanism are faced with calls to permit a choice of plan rather than a third-party administrator processing claims from providers. A prime argument for permitting people to choose plans within a universal health insurance program is that managed care might control healthcare use because of the prospective or capitated payments to providers. If a government-sponsored health insurance program were to include choice of plan—rather than simply choice of medical care provider—the system would operate as a defined contribution system. That is, every person would receive an amount of money or voucher that could be used toward the purchase price of a health insurance plan. If a person wished to spend more on a health insurance plan because it offered services the person wanted, the person could do so. Presumably, a market for catastrophic health insurance would emerge in this type of market.

The benefits of moving to this system of insurance are that we would have universal health insurance, people would have a choice of plans or providers, and many younger people would find health plan choices that suit their needs. The primary disadvantage of the defined contribution plan with a competitive private market is that it would need a mechanism for dealing with high-risk individuals. People who are sicker or expected to have higher medical care costs will face higher premiums in a competitive market. If we are going to pay for this type of health insurance system by way of income or payroll taxes, we need to also limit a person's financial liability for obtaining health insurance. One way of doing this would be to set the defined contribution or voucher at a level sufficient to purchase a minimum package of health benefits. Another outcome of this type of system would be that it permits higher-income individuals to purchase health insurance coverage that may have more services covered than the defined contribution would buy.

Conclusion

People without health insurance are a diverse group of individuals. Although they are predominantly younger, have family incomes below two times the poverty level and below $30,000 in 1993, and live disproportionately in the southern and western states, not all of the uninsured fit this description. Furthermore, it seems unlikely that the distribution of uninsured spell durations has shifted much since the mid-1980s. This means that, although the median length of an uninsured spell is six months, more than a quarter of all uninsured spells last longer than one year. The diversity of types of people who lack health insurance provides evidence of breakdowns in the market for health insurance and indicates a need for government action to assist the uninsured. For the people with short uninsured spells, the need for government assistance seems slight. Such people need to be protected against catastrophic medical events while they are between health insurance plans and against medical bills that may result from illnesses or medical conditions diagnosed while the person was uninsured. But people with longer uninsured spells are most likely to be workers (or their dependents) in jobs that do not provide employer-sponsored health insurance. Thus, the 53 million people who experience at least a month without health insurance during a year need different government programs or policies to assist them while they are uninsured.

Designing appropriate policies to assist the different subsets of uninsured people is not a simple and costless task. Because 70 percent of the uninsured at a specific point in time have family incomes below $30,000 (in 1993 dollars), it is unrealistic to expect that the numbers of uninsured will decline without programs to provide subsidies to purchase insurance or programs that directly provide financial access to medical care, such as Medicaid. It is the details of how government programs might operate with subsidies and how they would be financed that will determine the distributional effects of such programs and how well they might work to reduce the number of people without health insurance. If subsets of the uninsured, such as children, can be assisted incrementally, it may be possible to focus on the uninsured who are likely to have high medical care costs. If the government can be the insurer for people likely to have high medical care costs, the private insurance market may then work for more people who currently do not have health insurance.

The United States is too wealthy a nation to have one-sixth of its nonelderly population uninsured at any specific point in time. If the nation wants to continue to rely on employer-sponsored health insurance, then the government's role must be to provide a combination of government policies and programs to assist those for whom the market does not work.

References

Barr, N. 1989. "Social Insurance as an Efficiency Device." *Journal of Public Policy* 9: 59–82.

Bennefield, R. 1996. "Who Loses Coverage and For How Long? Dynamics of Economic Well-Being: Health Insurance, 1992 to 1993." *Current Population Reports.* Series P70-54. Bureau of the Census. Washington, DC: U.S. Department of Commerce.

Braverman, P., S. Egerter, T. Bennett, and J. Showstack. 1991. "Differences in Hospital Resource Allocation Among Sick Newborns According to Insurance Coverage." *Journal of the American Medical Association* 266 (23): 3300–8.

Bureau of the Census. 1995. "School Enrollment—Social and Economic Characteristics of Students: October 1993." *Current Population Reports.* Series P20-479. Bureau of the Census. Washington, DC: U.S. Department of Commerce.

Cowan, C., B. Braden, P. McDonnell, and L. Sivarajan. 1996. "Business, Households, and Government: Health Spending, 1994." *Health Care Financing Review* 17 (4): 157–78.

Cutler, D., and J. Gruber. 1996. "Does Public Insurance Crowd Out Private Insurance?" *Quarterly Journal of Economics* 111 (2): 391–430.

Davis, K., and D. Rowland. 1983. "Uninsured and Underserved: Inequities in Health Care in the United States." *Milbank Memorial Fund Quarterly/Health and Society* 61 (2): 149–76.

Dubay, L., and G. Kenney. 1995. *Revisiting the Issues: The Evidence of Medicaid Expansions on Insurance Coverage of Children.* Working Paper 6217-010. Washington, DC: The Urban Institute.

Employee Benefits Research Institute. 1995. *Sources of Health Insurance and Characteristics of the Uninsured: Analysis of the March 1994 Current Population Survey.* Special Report SR-28/Issue Brief 158. Washington, DC: Employee Benefits Research Institute.

Hadley, J., E. Steinberg, and J. Feder. 1991. "Comparison of Uninsured and

Privately Insured Hospital Patients." *Journal of the American Medical Association* 265 (3): 374–79.

Kotlikoff, L. 1987. "Justifying Public Provision of Social Security." *Journal of Policy Analysis and Management* 6 (4): 674–89.

KPMG Peat Marwick. 1995. *Health Benefits in 1995*. Newark, NJ: KPMG Peat Marwick.

Swartz, K. 1989. *The Medically Uninsured: Special Focus on Workers*. Washington, DC: The Urban Institute.

———. 1994. "Dynamics of People Without Health Insurance: Don't Let the Numbers Fool You." *Journal of the American Medical Association* 271 (1): 64–66.

———. 1996. "Medicaid Crowd Out and the Inverse Truman Bind." *Inquiry* 33 (1): 5–8.

———. 1997. "Effects of Changes in the 1995 Current Population Survey on Estimates of Health Insurance Coverage." *Inquiry* 34 (1): 70–79.

Swartz, K., and J. Marcotte. 1993. "Children and Spells Without Health Insurance." Working Paper. Washington, DC: The Urban Institute.

Swartz, K., J. Marcotte, and T. McBride. 1993. "Personal Characteristics and Spells Without Health Insurance." *Inquiry* 30 (1): 64–76.

Wenneker, M., J. Weissman, and A. Epstein. 1990. "The Association of Payer with Utilization of Cardiac Procedures in Massachusetts." *Journal of the American Medical Association* 264 (10): 1255–60.

4

The Changing Role of Medicaid

John F. Holahan

This chapter examines the changing role of Medicaid in financing healthcare for low-income Americans. I begin by reviewing much of the recent history of the Medicaid program and then explore reasons why Medicaid grew extremely rapidly between 1988 and 1992 and why this growth decelerated between 1992 and 1995. The suggestion that future growth in Medicaid is also likely to be relatively slow is followed by discussion of the implications of slow Medicaid growth for coverage of low-income Americans and the safety net.

Two alternative scenarios for the future are presented. In the pessimistic scenario, the number of uninsured increases and the ability of the safety net to provide coverage becomes increasingly impaired. In the more optimistic scenario, the federal government and the states respond by expanding insurance coverage, and although some safety-net providers will fail, those that remain will be more efficient and more financially stable and will be able to provide care to low-income people because of the expanded coverage.

Medicaid Growth Explosion, 1988–92

Between 1988 and 1992, Medicaid expenditures grew on average by 22.4 percent per year, increasing from $53.5 billion in 1988 to $119.9 billion in 1992. As shown in Table 4.1, expenditures on the elderly and disabled grew each year by an average of 14.7 percent and 17.0 percent, respectively. Spending on adults and children grew from $13.1 billion to

This work was supported by a grant from the Henry J. Kaiser Family Foundation, Menlo Park, California.

Table 4.1   Total Medicaid Expenditures, 1988–95

	Spending (billions $)			Average Annual Growth (%)	
Expenditures	1988	1992	1995	1988–1992	1992–1995
Total	53.5	119.9	157.3	22.4	9.5
Benefits					
Benefits by service	50.6	98.5	132.8	18.1	10.5
Acute care	25.4	55.5	80.4	21.6	13.1
Long-term care	25.1	42.9	52.3	14.3	6.8
Benefits by group	50.6	98.5	132.8	18.1	10.5
Elderly	18.1	31.4	39.4	14.7	7.9
Blind and disabled	19.3	36.2	49.9	17.0	11.3
Families	13.1	30.9	43.5	23.9	12.1
DSH	0.4	17.5	19.0	149.9	2.7
Administration	2.4	3.9	5.5	12.2	12.6

Source: Holahan and Liska 1997, based on Health Care Financing Administration 2082 and 64 data.

$30.9 billion, an average annual increase of 23.9 percent. Spending on adults and children grew more rapidly than did spending on the elderly and disabled; however, two-thirds of Medicaid spending was on behalf of the elderly and disabled.

Table 4.2 shows that Medicaid enrollment increased from 22.0 million to 29.8 million Americans during this period. Increases in the enrollment of the elderly were relatively small, increasing from 3.1 to 3.5 million, or 3.2 percent per year. There was, however, substantial growth in coverage of the disabled, with enrollment increasing from 3.4 to 4.5 million, or by 6.7 percent per year. The high annual cost of covering the disabled means that this expansion has been extremely important to the cost of the program. The number of adults and children increased from 15.4 to 21.8 million, an average annual increase of 9.0 percent.

There are many reasons for the growth in Medicaid during 1988–92. The most prominent reason was the increase in enrollment. A series of legislative mandates extended Medicaid coverage to pregnant women and children and to the elderly and disabled. In the late 1980s, Medicaid ended the link between participation in the Aid to Families with Dependent Children (AFDC) program and Medicaid coverage. By 1990, federal law required coverage of all pregnant women and infants and children under age six with incomes below 133 percent of the federal poverty

Table 4.2   Medicaid Beneficiaries and Expenditures per Beneficiary, 1988–95

	Beneficiaries (millions)			Average Annual Growth (%)	
	1988	*1992*	*1995*	*1988–1992*	*1992–1995*
Beneficiaries (in Millions)					
Total	22.0	29.8	34.8	7.9	5.3
By Group					
Elderly	3.1	3.5	3.9	3.2	3.0
Blind and disabled	3.4	4.5	5.7	6.7	8.7
Families	15.4	21.8	25.2	9.0	4.9
Benefits per Beneficiary (federal and state) ($)					
Total	2,298	3,303	3,816	9.5	4.9
By group					
Elderly	5,794	8,848	10,166	11.2	4.7
Blind and disabled	5,619	8,099	8,685	9.6	2.4
Families	848	1,416	1,728	13.7	6.8

Source: Holahan and Liska 1997, based on Health Care Financing Administration 2082 and 64 data.

level. States were given the option to extend coverage to pregnant women and infants up to 185 percent of the poverty level with federal matching payments. States are now required to cover children aged 6–13 up to the federal poverty level. Poor children aged 14–18 are scheduled to be phased in by the year 2002. Between 1988 and 1992, 4.5 million pregnant women and children were covered through these mandates.[1] These new eligible groups composed approximately 50 percent of the total increase in enrollment, although they accounted for a substantially lower share of total spending growth.

Congress also extended Medicaid eligibility to elderly and disabled Medicare beneficiaries. The Omnibus Budget Reconciliation Act of 1990 required Medicaid programs to cover Medicare costs for low-income elderly people not eligible for cash assistance. This coverage had been established previously with the passage of the Medicare Catastrophic Coverage Act of 1988, but this legislation was revoked in 1990. This law, involving qualified Medicare beneficiaries (QMBs), required states to cover Medicare premiums and cost sharing for all Medicare-eligible persons with incomes below the federal poverty level. This requirement was expanded in 1995 to require states to provide the Part B premiums for Medicare eligibles between 100 and 120 percent of poverty. Because of poor data, it is difficult to know how many enrollees have been covered by these provisions; one estimate is that there were 1.3 million low-income elderly and disabled in 1995 who received coverage of Medicare through this so-called QMB legislation.[2]

Medicaid also expanded during these years because of the recession, as did other related programs. For example, between 1988 and 1991, AFDC enrollment increased by 15.6 percent and food stamp enrollment by approximately 20 percent. States also took a number of steps to simplify the eligibility and enrollment processes during this period, which further increased Medicaid enrollment.

Supplemental Security Income (SSI) enrollment also rose because of court decisions, principally the *Zebley v. Sullivan* case, which increased coverage for learning disabled children. At the same time, a broadening of the list of qualifying medical conditions affecting disabled children, as mandated by Congress, also expanded SSI enrollment. During these years, many states and localities also intensified efforts to enroll individuals, who would have otherwise been covered by state or local general assistance programs, in SSI to obtain the federal cash contributions as well as Medicaid coverage. Another cause of Medicaid enrollment growth during this period was SSI coverage of many individuals with acquired immunodeficiency syndrome (AIDS), substance abuse, and other social and medical problems.

Furthermore, while the number of Medicaid beneficiaries in nursing homes grew only modestly, the role of Medicaid financing increased because of newly enacted protections against spousal impoverishment, which reduced the out-of-pocket cost for nursing home residents whose spouses continued to live in the community. Medicaid expenditures during this period also grew because of more widespread divestiture of assets so as to become eligible for nursing home benefits and because of greater availability of Medicaid-financed long-term care in the community and at home.

Increases in healthcare prices have been an important determinant of Medicaid expenditure growth and are largely outside the control of Medicaid. Although states did not strictly have to increase provider payment rates with inflation, it has proved difficult over the long term to diverge widely. The Boren Amendment requires states to pay the cost of efficiently and economically operated facilities (e.g., hospitals and nursing homes). The expenses of such facilities typically increase with inflation because of wage costs.

Yet another factor explaining Medicaid expenditure increases during this period was the growth in utilization, in part due to changes in the health status of enrollees. Average Medicaid utilization rates increased because of changes in the population gaining coverage. For example, expansions to cover pregnant women would automatically bring in a group that would incur relatively significant healthcare expenditures. Increased coverage of AIDS patients and substance abusers also adds high-cost groups. The 1989 amendments to the Early and Periodic Screening Diagnosis and Treatment program for children, which required additional screening services plus Medicaid coverage of all needed services irrespective of their coverage under a particular state benefit package, also increased costs to states.

Moreover, states became increasingly aggressive during this period in shifting services to Medicaid that had previously been financed by state dollars alone (Coughlin, Ku, and Holahan 1994). This practice, known as "Medicaid maximization," was adopted so as to take advantage of federal matching funds. Such shifts have occurred in state-funded institutional services for the developmentally disabled, mentally ill, and Title XX recipients (state-funded home- and community-based services for the disabled).

The final cause of the large increase in Medicaid spending during this period was the aggressive use of provider taxes and donations as well as disproportionate-share hospital (DSH) payments (Ku and Coughlin 1995). These arrangements brought federal dollars to the states, with the funds largely distributed to hospitals providing disproportionate amounts of care to low-income individuals. The typical practice was for states to require provider contributions or to impose taxes on providers. Medicaid programs would increase payments to the same providers through DSH payments. Such payments included federal matching funds as well as a return of much, if not all, of the hospital's donation or tax payment. In many cases, these funds were used to assist hospitals in supporting indigent care for low-income individuals. In other cases, federal funds substituted for expenditures that states would have otherwise made, and little new net expenditures for healthcare resulted. However these funds were used, it had a major impact on Medicaid expenditure growth during this period. Disproportionate-share hospital payments accounted for approximately $400 million in 1988 and grew to more than $17 billion by 1992.

One of the effects of the rapid Medicaid growth during this period, particularly in enrollment, was that the percentage of the U.S. population lacking health insurance increased only slightly (Holahan, Winterbottom, and Rajan 1995), even though employer-sponsored coverage declined from 67.0 to 61.1 percent of the U.S. population between 1988 and 1993 (see Table 4.3). At the same time, Medicaid increased from 8.5 to 12.4 percent, and there was a slight increase in nongroup coverage

Table 4.3   Trends in Health Insurance Coverage, 1988–93, by Income, Pregnancy Status, and Age (in percent^a)

Health Coverage	Total	Income below 200 Percent of Poverty			Income 200 Percent of Poverty and Greater		
		Pregnant Women and Children	Adults 18–34	Adults 35–64	Pregnant Women and Children	Adults 18–34	Adults 35–64
1988							
Total	211,584	27,954	19,886	17,728	38,131	44,717	63,167
Employer	67	37	31	32	87	76	83
Medicaid^b	9	38	18	17	1	1	0
Other^c	2	1	2	8	1	1	2
Nongroup	7	4	11	11	5	9	7
Uninsured	15	20	39	32	7	14	7
1993							
Total	225,764	32,627	22,147	20,868	39,309	41,135	69,678
Employer	61	30	26	29	82	70	79
Medicaid^b	12	50	25	20	3	1	1
Other^c	2	1	2	6	1	1	2
Nongroup	8	3	10	9	5	11	8
Uninsured	17	16	39	35	9	16	9
Change in Coverage, 1988–93							
Employer	−6*	−7*	−6*	−3*	−5*	−6*	−4*
Medicaid^b	4*	12*	7*	4*	1*	0*	0*
Other^c	0	0	0	−2*	0	0	0
Nongroup	0*	−1*	−1*	−2*	0	3*	1*
Uninsured	2*	−4*	0	3*	3*	3*	3*

Source: Urban Institute tabulations from the March 1989 and 1994 *Current Population Survey;* also cited in Holahan, Winterbottom, and Rajan 1995.

Note: The population excludes the elderly, the institutionalized, and families with an active military member.
^aPercentages may not sum to 100 percent due to rounding.
^bMedicaid enrollment reflects corrections by The Urban Institute's TRIM2 model.
^cIncludes nonelderly covered through Medicare, CHAMPUS, VA, and military health.

(0.3 percent). The result was that the percent uninsured increased by only 1.8 percent. If Medicaid had not expanded, the percent uninsured would have increased by a substantially greater margin.

The effects of the Medicaid expansions were most noticeable for pregnant women and children below 200 percent of the poverty level. This group experienced a 6.7 percent drop in employer-sponsored coverage, but Medicaid coverage increased by 12.0 percent. As a result, the proportion of low-income pregnant women and children who were uninsured declined by 3.8 percent. For low-income adults between ages 18 and 34, the drop in employer-sponsored coverage was offset by increases in Medicaid, with the result that there was virtually no change in the percentage lacking health insurance. For other groups, there were statistically significant increases in the uninsured rate of slightly under three percentage points—the expansions of Medicaid did not offset the decline in employer-sponsored coverage. The result is that the Medicaid growth during this period had important effects on insurance coverage of the U.S. population, particularly for low-income pregnant women and children.

Some of the reduction in employer-sponsored coverage may have, in fact, been caused by the expansion of Medicaid coverage. This issue is now a matter of serious academic debate. Cutler and Gruber (1995) estimate that between 20 and 50 percent of the expansion in Medicaid represents a crowding out of private coverage. Dubay and Kenney (1995a,b) estimate that the crowd-out effect is approximately 17 percent of the increase in Medicaid enrollment. The difference in Cutler and Gruber's two estimates is that the first represents the percentage of those covered by the expansions who dropped private coverage and enrolled in Medicaid. The latter, and higher, estimate includes a spillover effect whereby individuals who were not Medicaid eligible dropped coverage either because their family members were eligible or because of employer response to the expansions. The lower estimate seems more plausible and is more consistent with the Dubay and Kenney results. If approximately 20 percent of the expansion of Medicaid represents a displacing of private insurance, then 1.8 million individuals dropped employer-sponsored coverage because of Medicaid expanding coverage between 1988 and 1993.

Slowdown in Medicaid Expenditure Growth, 1992–95

Following four years of rapid expansion in the Medicaid program, growth slowed precipitously after 1992. After four years with an average annual growth rate of 22.4 percent, Medicaid spending grew on average by 9.5 percent per year between 1992 and 1995 (see Table 4.1). Spending increased from $119.9 billion in 1992 to $157.3 billion in 1995. Annual increases in spending remained higher for families (12.1 percent) than for the disabled (11.3 percent) or for the elderly (7.9 percent). This slowdown in expenditure growth appears to have continued. Preliminary data suggest that Medicaid expenditures grew by less than 3 percent in 1996.

There are several reasons for the decline in Medicaid spending growth. The first is that increases in Medicaid enrollment slowed substantially. After increasing by 7.9 percent annually between 1988 and 1992, enrollment growth fell to 5.3 percent per year in the following three years (see Table 4.2). Table 4.4 shows that the rate of growth in enrollment of Medicaid beneficiaries declined between 1991 and 1995. Enrollment growth increased by 11 percent in 1992 but by only 1.8 percent in 1995. Enrollment growth among the elderly fell from 7.2 percent in 1992 to 1.2 percent in 1995. In 1995 enrollment of the blind and disabled grew by 6.8 percent, a substantial decrease from the 10.7 percent seen in 1992. Finally, among adults and children, Medicaid growth increased by 11.7 percent in 1992 and 9.1 percent in 1993, but by only 0.8 percent in 1995 (Social Security Administration 1996).

Enrollment growth fell for a number of reasons. First, there has been a decline in AFDC enrollment in recent years because of the improved economy, as well as efforts in many states to reduce welfare program participation, primarily through tougher work requirements. Second, the growth in coverage for children and pregnant women has

Table 4.4 Medicaid Beneficiaries, 1991–95

	1991	1992	1993	1994	1995
Total (millions)	26.9	29.8	32.4	34.2	34.8
Elderly	3.3	3.5	3.7	3.8	3.9
Blind and disabled	4.0	4.5	5.0	5.4	5.7
Families	19.5	21.8	23.8	25.0	25.2
Annual Growth (%)		11.0	8.8	5.4	1.8
Elderly		7.2	3.7	4.0	1.2
Blind and disabled		10.7	11.6	7.8	6.8
Families		11.7	9.1	5.1	0.8

Source: Based on unedited Health Care Financing Administration 2082 data.

also declined. One reason for the faster growth in the early 1990s was the new coverage mandates affecting children and pregnant women. This program now has relatively high participation, so growth has slowed considerably, as would be expected.

Third, the growth in enrollment of the blind and disabled population has also begun to slow down. Much of the growth in the early 1990s was due to court decisions that resulted in dramatic increases in enrollment of disabled children. Since the initial burst of new enrollment, growth rates in enrollment of the disabled has slowed in the last three years. Program data reveal that the early 1990s growth rate of more than 10 percent per year in the SSI disabled fell to approximately 5.8 percent in 1995.

Finally, there has also been a slowdown in enrollment growth among the elderly. Much of the rapid growth among the elderly was due to the introduction of the QMB program. The program experienced rapid growth initially, but, again, as would be expected in any new program, increases in participation have slowed. Moreover, the number of elderly receiving cash assistance through SSI continues to decline.

Another cause in the slowdown of Medicaid growth rates is reduced spending per enrollee. Spending per enrollee in Medicaid fell to 4.9 percent between 1992 and 1995, in contrast with an average annual growth rate of 9.5 percent between 1988 and 1992 (see Table 4.2). There are at least three major reasons for this slowdown. The first is the rapid growth in managed care. Initially, participation in Medicaid managed care was voluntary on the part of the enrollee. The evidence on the success of these voluntary programs in containing costs is mixed, largely because the favorable selection into managed care plans makes it difficult to measure savings (Hurley, Freund, and Paul 1993). In the last few years there has also been a rapid expansion of mandatory Medicaid managed care through Section 1915(b) and Section 1115 waiver programs. The 1915(b) waivers are more limited and are typically restricted to a geographic area within a state. Although enrollment is often mandatory under these programs, health maintenance organizations must still have no more than 75 percent Medicaid or Medicare enrollment. Thirty-three states now have 1915(b) waivers for some type of managed care.

The Section 1115 waivers permit states to move substantially further in enrolling Medicaid beneficiaries in managed care (Wooldridge et al., forthcoming; Rotwein et al. 1995). The most prominent of the early Section 1115 waiver programs have been in Hawaii, Oregon, and Tennessee. These programs typically extend coverage to uninsured people in the state up to higher income levels than typically included in

Medicaid. Hawaii essentially extended coverage to all uninsured persons (excluding the disabled) below 300 percent of the federal poverty level. Oregon extended coverage to all nondisabled people below 100 percent of poverty. Tennessee embarked on a major expansion with the intent of covering all of the uninsured below 400 percent of the poverty level. Expansions were financed largely through the savings derived from the enrollment of people in capitated managed care plans. Other financing came from funds that would have been spent on other state programs and the use of the state's DSH payments.

Currently, 17 states have had Section 1115 waiver programs approved, and 11 have implemented these programs (Health Care Financing Administration 1996). One major change in the evolution of Section 1115 waiver programs is that they have moved away from expansion of eligibility and consolidation of existing non-Medicaid programs that finance healthcare for the poor. Instead, in later waiver programs the major emphasis is on achieving savings through managed care.

The second reason Medicaid expenditures have declined is because of 1991 and 1993 legislation affecting the use of DSH payments (Holahan, Coughlin, Lia, Ku, Kuntz, Wade, Wall 1995). As shown in Table 4.1, DSH payments increased by only 2.7 percent per year between 1992 and 1995, after several years of explosive growth. In 1991, legislation banned the use of provider donations and severely restricted the types of provider taxes that states could employ. In effect, states could no longer make a guarantee that a hospital could be "made whole" for a donation or tax payment through reciprocal DSH payments. The 1991 legislation also capped DSH payments to 12 percent of program expenditures. Any state whose DSH payments exceeded 12 percent would be frozen until DSH payments were at 12 percent of Medicaid expenditures. The states whose DSH payments were below 12 percent were allowed to grow at the same rate as program spending. Because program spending has slowed, the allowed rate of growth in DSH payments has also slowed. The 1993 legislation restricted the level of DSH payments to hospitals. States could no longer pay a hospital more than that facility was losing through low Medicaid reimbursement rates or through the provision of uncompensated care. This severely restricted states' ability to pay large amounts of money to specific, often state-supported, hospitals and significantly reduced Medicaid expenditures in some of these states.

The growth of managed care and the changes in federal DSH policy cannot explain all or even most of the slowdown in Medicaid spending growth. For example, the growth in spending per enrollee fell more for the elderly, and blind and disabled than for families (see

Table 4.2), the population most affected by the growth in managed care. One explanation is the drop in average annual medical price inflation from 8.2 percent during 1988 to 1992, to 5.1 percent from 1992 to 1995. States also appear to have successfully adopted other policies to limit expenditure growth, particularly for long-term care (see Table 4.1). Many states also seem less willing to use Medicaid as the vehicle through which to funnel state spending for a wide range of social service programs. Although the basic financial incentives in Medicaid have not been changed and a return to Medicaid maximization efforts could reappear, for the moment these efforts appear to have stalled.

Medicaid Spending in the Near Future

In the near future, there are strong reasons to believe that Medicaid expenditure growth could well be even slower than it has been in 1992 through 1995. First, the decline in AFDC enrollment in recent years is likely to continue. Because of welfare reform, many of those who have been historically on Medicaid through AFDC will now be enrolled in the Temporary Assistance for Needy Families (TANF) program where they will face tougher work requirements and time limits on benefits.[3] States are required to retain current (July 1996) rules for Medicaid coverage. But some of those who find work are likely to have sufficiently higher earnings so that they would become ineligible for Medicaid under current rules. Many of these families will be eligible for transitional Medicaid coverage for up to 12 months, but past experience indicates very low use of these transitional benefits (Wooldridge 1996); therefore, many who do find employment are likely to cease having Medicaid coverage. Welfare reform may also result in states' maintaining two eligibility administration systems, one for TANF participants and the other for individuals not eligible for TANF who would have been eligible for Medicaid under current rules. The latter group may have lower participation because they are no longer eligible for cash benefits. Currently, participation in Medicaid by those who do not simultaneously receive cash benefits is much lower than for those who do.

Second, the slow rate of increase in coverage of children and pregnant women should continue. Significant growth within this group should not be expected apart from incremental inclusion of poor children under age 18.

Third, slower growth in coverage among the blind and disabled is also likely. As noted above, coverage in the disabled category has declined continually since 1991. Welfare reform legislation will eliminate coverage of some SSI children, though many of these may remain eligible because of provisions covering poor children below poverty. Coverage of immigrants now receiving Medicaid is also likely to decline. Although many states may continue to cover legal immigrants, some may choose not to do so. As a result, SSI and, hence, Medicaid enrollment should decline.

Finally, enrollment of the elderly should continue to experience only modest growth. The number of elderly receiving cash assistance through SSI will most likely continue to decline, and growth in the QMB program should continue to be modest.

The 1991 and 1993 legislation affecting DSH payments should continue to hinder the states' ability to use this mechanism. Legislation enacted in 1993, which restricts states' payments to specific hospitals to cover their losses on Medicaid patients and the amount of uncompensated care they provide, has even made it difficult for some states to spend their current DSH allotments.

Medicaid managed care is also likely to continue to expand substantially. More states have applied for Section 1115 waivers, and most envision enrolling the majority of their adults and children in some form of managed care. Many states are also now exploring enrolling the disabled into managed care plans, although these expansions are more problematic. The key question for the future is whether states can continue to implement managed care successfully. More specifically, can they develop the capacity to serve large numbers of Medicaid enrollees (e.g., almost 3 million in New York)? Can they successfully address (1) problems of enrollment in managed care, providing information to beneficiaries to allow them to make choices among plans effectively; (2) the establishment of capitation rates including risk adjustments; and (3) the monitoring and oversight of the quality of care?

States have been very successful in obtaining early savings from managed care. Savings have come from reducing the use of emergency rooms, inpatient hospital care, and specialists and from limiting provider payment rates. Although this is likely to continue, some caution is in order. Medicaid managed care has been able to exercise market power in part because of excess supply in the hospital and physician markets. When this excess supply is reduced, Medicaid managed care will have substantially less leverage.

In addition, the movement to managed care is occurring at the same time that there is increasing concern over the quality of care provided by managed care organizations. The federal government and states are likely to move in the direction of increased regulation of managed care. The problem is that it is not possible to have low capitation rates and higher minimum standards and still continue to attract managed care plans to compete for Medicaid business. Without enough competitors, states are in a relatively weak negotiating position to contain low capitation rates and to sanction providers who have problems with enrollment practices or with quality of care.

The future growth of Medicaid also depends on whether there is major legislation affecting the program in the 105th Congress. In 1995, congressional Republicans proposed replacing Medicaid with a block grant that would have given states less funding in exchange for much more flexibility.[4] The legislation would have specified federal payments in 1996 to each state and increased federal payments each year by a set amount until the year 2002. The original Republican proposal was intended to yield $183 billion in savings relative to the Congressional Budget Office (CBO) February 1996 baseline. This represented a cut in federal spending of approximately 15 percent over seven years.

The proposal would have given states considerable flexibility to allow them to adjust to lower federal payments. States could decide whom to cover and what benefits to provide. The Boren Amendment that restricted states' flexibility in reducing reimbursements to hospitals and nursing homes would be eliminated. States would be given much more freedom to enroll beneficiaries in managed care plans without federal waivers. Matching requirements for most states would have been reduced; that is, states would have had to spend less of their own money to draw down the full federal payments.

The Clinton administration also made proposals to restrain Medicaid spending by limiting the growth in spending per beneficiary. The Clinton proposal was designed to save approximately $54 billion over seven years. The 1997 Clinton budget contained the same proposal; because of significant reductions in the CBO's baseline projections for Medicaid spending growth, proposed cuts now amounted to only about $6.3 billion. In contrast to the Republican proposals, the Clinton proposal would retain the entitlement for current Medicaid beneficiaries, including AFDC and SSI recipients, currently covered children and pregnant women, and those children who would be phased in by the year 2002.

The proposal would retain the current mandatory benefit package. Under the proposal's requirements, states would have much the same flexibility as they would under block grants. The Boren Amendment would be eliminated, and other restrictions on provider payments would be relaxed. States could more freely enroll individuals in managed care.

The key difference between the Clinton administration and the Republican congressional plans is that the entitlement to a specific benefit package would remain for current beneficiaries. The federal government would share in the cost if enrollment grew for those entitled groups, for example, because of a recession or natural disaster. The congressional block grant proposal would have made it very difficult for states to avoid reducing enrollment. States would have had to hold growth in expenditures per enrollee to extremely low levels to avoid enrollment reductions. The Clinton administration proposal also presented challenges for states, but they could not have stayed below their expenditure caps by cutting enrollment.

As of this writing, the proposals for caps on growth have been rejected by Congress. The proposals for incresed flexibility as well as cuts in disproportionate share payments remain under serious consideration.

Implications

The recent decline in the growth of Medicaid expenditures and enrollment and the likely continuation of these trends suggest that a number of serious problems could develop in the near future. In this section two possible scenarios are presented, one pessimistic and one optimistic. The pessimistic scenario suggests that Medicaid enrollment will level off, if not decline. There should continue to be some growth in coverage of SSI recipients, QMBs, and children and pregnant women, but at a much more modest level than experienced in the past.

More important, there is likely to be less coverage of those who have been enrolled previously in Medicaid through AFDC or related provisions. Although current rules for Medicaid eligibility largely remain after welfare reform, the establishment of separate enrollment procedures for the TANF program and for Medicaid are likely to result in lower participation rates. In addition, individuals who successfully leave TANF for work are likely to have earnings that render them ineligible for Medicaid. Although transitional Medicaid coverage is available, recent evidence suggests that few individuals have taken advantage of these benefits. Finally, Medicaid programs will be less likely to cover legal immigrants. Although many states will continue this coverage, some states may not. For these reasons it is likely that there will be less Medicaid coverage of adults and children.

At the same time, continued declines in employer-sponsored insurance are quite possible. The primary reasons for the decline in employer-sponsored coverage seem to be corporate downsizing and increased employment in small businesses that are less likely to provide health insurance. More corporations are moving toward defined contributions, giving employees more flexibility in how they structure their fringe benefit packages. This is likely to result in some individuals choosing not to purchase health insurance. Other employers are requiring employees to pay a greater share of the premiums. As a result, it appears that many employers and employees are reducing coverage.

The combination of reduced coverage under Medicaid and reduced employer-sponsored insurance could result in a dramatic increase in the percentage of the population that is uninsured. For example, a decline in Medicaid coverage of two percentage points coupled with a three percentage point decline in employer-sponsored coverage would result in (assuming no increase in private nongroup coverage) an increase of the proportion of Americans without health insurance to approximately 22 percent, or approximately 53 million Americans by the year 2000. Both assumptions are realistic given (1) the enactment of welfare reform and (2) recent changes in employer-sponsored coverage.

At the same time, the large inner-city public and nonprofit teaching hospitals and community health centers that have always provided the safety net for the uninsured are likely to come under increasing financial pressures. These pressures will stem from a number of causes, including the reductions in DSH payments due to the 1991 and 1993 legislation described above, as well as the DSH reductions currently being considered by Congress. These DSH payments have played an important role in ensuring the viability of many of these hospitals. Medicaid managed care also will increase pressure on these same institutions. Managed care plans will likely lower Medicaid payment rates to these facilities and probably provide them with fewer patients. Because of their high costs, which are in part related to their role in providing care to the uninsured, these facilities are often not attractive to managed care plans. To the extent managed care plans move Medicaid patients to other facilities, the long-term viability of these safety-net institutions is imperiled.

Finally, these same institutions will be affected by Medicare policy changes and by developments in the private market. Both the Republican Congress and the Clinton administration have called for major reductions in payments to Medicare providers. For example, the Clinton administration has called for reductions in basic hospital reimbursement rates, teaching and DSH payment adjustments, and capital payments (Gage et al. 1997). Many of these reductions will affect the same hospitals that are being affected by the loss of Medicaid DSH payments and Medicaid managed care. Finally, private sector managed care plans are succeeding by obtaining discounts from hospitals and other providers and by steering patients away from more expensive nonprofit and public hospitals to other community facilities. The private sector efforts clearly do not bode well for safety-net hospitals.

Other developments in the market also could cause problems for safety-net institutions. Hospital mergers often result in dominant for-profit or nonprofit hospitals with strong commercially insured patient bases taking over weaker, typically nonprofit institutions. The combined facilities become a stronger entity, more able to compete successfully for privately insured patients. Public and some remaining nonprofit hospitals are left with fewer private patients and a large Medicaid and uninsured patient base. These hospitals consequently have higher costs and even more problems competing for managed care contracts.

Hospital closures or downsizing intensify these problems. Clearly, there is excess capacity in the hospital systems of most urban areas. But as some critical hospitals fail, the burden of uncompensated care will shift to others in the community. For example, loss of emergency room capacity because of a hospital closure shifts the emergency care burden to other hospitals, increasing the number of nonpaying high-cost cases that they are required to treat. If these costs are distributed evenly among the remaining hospitals, there would be no serious problems. But the reality is that no hospital can afford to provide significantly more uncompensated care than its competitors in an increasingly competitive market. A possible exception includes prestigious teaching hospitals whose value to managed care plans allows them to earn a surplus that they may then allocate to pay for uncompensated care.

In the more optimistic scenario, federal and state policymakers will recognize the kinds of problems suggested above. The federal government could enact legislation expanding coverage for children or the working poor through expanding mandated coverage by Medicaid, providing new subsidy arrangements to encourage families to purchase private insurance or extending Medicare for children or early retirees. Alternatively, the federal government could target subsidies to low-income individuals regardless of age. In addition, the federal government could expand and restructure the DSH payments. The federal government has recognized the important role that safety-net institutions play in the healthcare market through its DSH payments, but in this scenario it could also recognize that the current distribution of DSH payments is skewed toward states that have successfully taken advantage of this financing mechanism. Federal funds could be redistributed where they are most needed. Better criteria could be established to ensure that funds were well targeted to hospitals that provide large amounts of care to indigent Americans and, hence, need additional funding.

States on their own could expand Medicaid coverage. They could currently use Section 1902(r)(2) to expand coverage to pregnant women and all children under age 18 to higher income levels. States could use the Section 1115 waiver process to expand coverage. The savings from managed care as well as funds from other state programs and from DSH payments could help finance the expansion. States could do more to publicize transitional benefits to provide health insurance coverage to those who leave welfare and Medicaid for work. States could also extend insurance reforms in individual and small group markets beyond the current requirements of the Kassebaum-Kennedy bill to ensure access to health insurance in the private market for those who seek it.

Under the more optimistic scenario, any legislation that would restrict federal Medicaid expenditures would be based on a per capita cap approach that would give states stronger incentives to control utilization and costs than they do today. At the same time, states would not gain from restricting coverage and could actually gain federal funds if they expanded Medicaid enrollment. Although some safety-net hospitals and community health centers would fail, others would become more financially stable and would have greater access to capital markets. The best safety-net institutions would form their own managed care plans and compete successfully for Medicaid clients.

Unfortunately, it is hard to imagine the optimistic scenario playing out without an expansion of coverage to many of those who are currently uninsured. As stated above, hospitals cannot afford to provide uncompensated care in an increasingly competitive market. The uninsured need public sponsorship to make them attractive to managed care plans. States must not only expand coverage to these individuals but provide for adequate capitation rates. In a world of expanded health insurance and adequate capitation rates, the market should find ways to provide care to most individuals.

Safety-net hospitals include many of the best and most highly respected hospitals in the country. With an expansion of insurance coverage, these institutions are highly likely to be successful in competing for their share of this market. In the absence of universal coverage, safety-net hospitals will require additional direct support from either the federal government through a restructured DSH program or directly from state and local governments to be able to continue to provide care for the uninsured. The bottom line is that, without an expansion of coverage, competition will make it more difficult for safety-net providers to continue to carry out their mission to serve the poor and uninsured.

Acknowledgments

The author thanks Len Nichols and Susan Wall who provided many valuable suggestions.

Notes

1. Urban Institute tabulations based on Health Care Financing Administration 2082 data.
2. Urban Institute calculations from the Health Care Financing Administration 1995 Buy-In File.
3. The Personal Responsibility and Work Opportunity Reconciliation Act of 1996.
4. The Medicaid Transformation Act of 1995.

References

Coughlin, T. A., L. Ku, and J. Holahan. 1994. *Medicaid Since 1980: Costs, Coverage and the Shifting Alliance between the Federal Government and the States.* Washington DC: The Urban Institute Press.

Cutler, D. M., and J. Gruber. 1995. *Does Public Insurance Crowd Out Private Insurance?* Working Paper 5082. Washington, DC: National Bureau of Economic Research.

Dubay, L., and G. Kenney. 1995a. *Did the Medicaid Expansions for Pregnant Women Crowd Out Private Coverage?* Working Paper 6217-010. Washington, DC: The Urban Institute.

———. 1995b. *Revisiting the Issue: The Evidence of Medicaid Expansions on Insurance Coverage of Children.* Working Paper 6422-04. Washington, DC: The Urban Institute.

Gage, B., L. Nichols, K. Liu, G. Kenney, M. Sulvetta, S. Zuckerman, and L. Pounder. 1997. *Medicare Savings: Options and Opportunities.* Washington, DC: The Urban Institute.

Health Care Financing Administration. 1996. *The Status of 1115 Waiver Health Reform Demonstrations.* Washington, DC: U.S. Department of Health and Human Services.

Holahan, J., and D. Liska. 1995. *The Impact of the Medigrant Plan on Federal Payments to States.* Washington, DC: Kaiser Commission on the Future of Medicaid.

———. 1997. "The Slowdown in Medicaid Spending Growth: Will It Continue?" *Health Affairs* 16 (2): 157–63.

Holahan, J., C. Winterbottom, and S. Rajan. 1995. "A Shifting Picture of Health Insurance Coverage." *Health Affairs* 14 (4): 253–64.

Holahan, J., T. A. Coughlin, K. Liu, L. Ku, C. Kuntz, M. Wade, and S. Wall. 1995. *Cutting Medicaid Spending in Response to Budget Caps.* Washington, DC: Kaiser Commission on the Future of Medicaid.

Hurley, R. E., D. A. Freund, and J. E. Paul. 1993. *Managed Care in Medicaid: Lessons for Policy and Program Design.* Chicago: Health Administration Press.

Ku, L., and T. A. Coughlin. 1995. "Medicaid Disproportionate Share and Other Special Financing Programs. *Health Care Financing Review* 16 (3): 27–54.

Rotwein, S., M. Boulmetis, P. J. Boben, H. I. Fingold, J. P. Hadley, K. L. Rama, and D. Van Hoven. 1995. "Medicaid and State Healthcare Reform: Process, Programs, and Policy Options." *Health Care Financing Review* 16 (3): 105–20.

Social Security Administration. 1996. *Children Receiving SSI.* Office of Research, Evaluation and Statistics. Washington, DC: Social Security Administration.

Wooldridge, J. 1996. *Medicaid's Role in Encouraging Transition from Welfare to Work.* Princeton, NJ: Mathematica Policy Research.

Wooldridge, J., L. Ku, T. A. Coughlin, L. Dubay, M. Ellwood, and S. Rajan. Forthcoming. *Implementing State Health Care Reform: What Have We Learned from the First Year?* Washington, DC: U.S. Department of Health and Human Services.

5

The Medically Uninsured—Will They Always Be With Us?

Steven A. Schroeder

A constant feature of health care in the United States is our national willingness to tolerate having large numbers of people without health insurance. This is in stark contrast to the situation in virtually every other developed country, where guaranteed health insurance is provided either by the state or through employers, with government backup for the unemployed. In our country from time to time, the issue of expanded health insurance coverage, or even universal coverage, erupts onto the national scene—as it did in 1948, 1965, 1973, and 1993—usually propelled by public demands for greater security in obtaining medical care. Except in 1965, when Medicare and Medicaid were enacted, achieving both national and political consensus has proved impossible, and the issue has gone back underground, only to reemerge later.

Today about 40 million Americans lack health insurance at any given time,[1] and as many as 50 or 60 million are without it at some time during a calendar year.[2, 3] Between 1991 and 1993, 27 percent of the population was uninsured for at least one month.[4] Most of the uninsured do not qualify for Medicaid either because they are not eligible to receive state welfare or Aid to Families with Dependent Children or because they do not meet other financial or categorical standards. Because the states set their own standards for Medicaid eligibility, there is great variation in the number of poor people—defined as those with incomes below

---

the federal poverty level—who are covered by Medicaid, ranging from a high of 60 percent in Washington, D.C., to a low of 29 percent in Nevada.[5] In addition, an estimated 29 million people under the age of 65 are underinsured for catastrophic illnesses.[6]

Why We Tolerate Having So Many Uninsured

In my role as president of a large philanthropic organization in the area of health, I encounter many people who are extraordinarily knowledge-able about the U.S. health care system. From our informal discussions I have gleaned at least seven explanations—varying in persuasiveness—for our country's tolerance of such a large number of people who are medically uninsured.

The number of uninsured people is exaggerated. This explanation de-rives from suspicion of the murky science of estimating the number of uninsured people on the basis of periodic surveys. Although we must rely on these surveys to gauge the size of this population, their inherent differences in sampling strategies, validity of responses, time periods, and definitions of insurance coverage necessarily generate estimates that vary from one survey to another. But whatever the exact number may be, the approximate number is known, and the trend is clearly in the direction of increasing numbers of people without insurance (Fig. 1).[7, 8]

In addition, some experts feel that the term "uninsured"is mislead-ing. For example, I often hear that many of the uninsured are young, healthy, middle-class people who are just out of college or between jobs. These are people who either do not need health care because they are fundamentally healthy or will soon be in situations in which health insurance will be provided. Surveys reveal a somewhat different picture. They show that the age distribution of the uninsured is quite similar to that of the general population under age 65 years of age (55 percent of the uninsured are under the age of 30, as compared with 50 percent of the general population).[9] The uninsured tend to be poorer than the general population, with 60 percent[2] having incomes either below the federal poverty level or less than twice that level, compared with 35 percent[9] of the general population. Although the uninsured report themselves in better health than do people receiving Medicaid, their reported health is worse than that of people with private insurance.[10] Thus, there is not much support for the explanation that the uninsured are disproportionately young, middle-class, and healthy.

Figure 1 Estimates of the Uninsured Population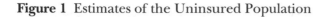

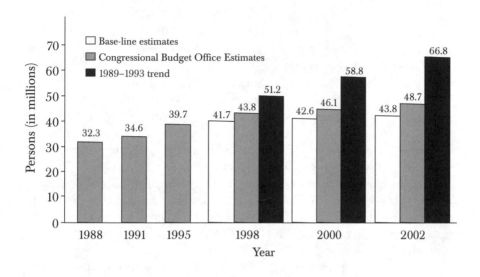

Being uninsured is a temporary situation for most people. Another explanation stems from the great variations in published estimates of how many people go without health insurance for long periods of time, such as 12 months. For example, estimates of the number of people who fall into this category have varied by as much as 12 percent.[9, 11] In the face of such disagreement, the reasoning goes, perhaps the number is being inflated for political reasons, and the problem is not as serious as it seems at first glance.

Many people choose to be uninsured. A variant of the preceding hypotheses is that people in a free society have the right not to be covered by health insurance and that some—or many—make that choice. Though it is not clear how many of the 40 million who are currently uninsured are in this category voluntarily, this argument tacitly assumes that urgent care will be provided when needed and that the decision to spend money on goods other than health insurance represents a rational choice that should be respected. Surveys show, however, that only 2 percent of employed people refuse health insurance coverage when it is offered to them.[12] The reason most uninsured workers do not have health insurance is that they work for firms that do not offer it or they are ineligible.

In addition, there are several difficulties with the notion that people should be able to choose to be uninsured: Should children be put at risk by their parents' decisions? Who is obligated to provide—and pay for—urgent care for the "self-uninsured"? How is urgently needed care defined? Few people who argue for the right to remain uninsured appear willing to countenance denying medical care to people who have voluntarily chosen not to be insured yet are unable to pay out of pocket for, say, treatment for leukemia or automobile injuries.

The uninsured get care anyway. Care for the uninsured in the United States has traditionally been provided in one of two ways. In some instances, it is given as uncompensated care by mainstream providers, who then pass on the costs to people who have insurance. In other instances, it is obtained at institutions that have traditionally provided a safety net, such as public clinics and hospitals financed largely by tax dollars. Do the delays that people commonly experience when receiving such charity care impair their health? Do the uninsured get the care they need?

Recent reports reviewing the importance of health insurance coverage conclude that, as compared with people with private insurance, the uninsured have less access to care, use less care, cannot obtain specific health care services, are twice as likely to be hospitalized for conditions that can be averted by outpatient care (such as acute asthma attacks), and have a higher risk of death when they go into the hospital.[10, 13–17]

My best sense of this issue is that much charity care is currently being provided but that the barriers associated with charity care exact a price in terms of health. More alarming is evidence that in the future charity care will be much more difficult to obtain.

Providing universal health insurance coverage is the right thing to do, but we cannot afford it at this time. I find this argument unpersuasive. If the uninsured were insured today, national health expenditures would increase by only $20 billion[18] out of a total annual expenditure of $1 trillion.[19] This estimate counts only what the net addition to costs would be if the uninsured were covered, however, and does not address such questions as program design; the fate of existing programs, particularly Medicaid; whether private insurance premiums would decrease if cost-shifting ended; or the effect of new coverage on price and resource use. Thus the questions become who would bear the costs and what the effect on other patterns of care would be, rather than whether the $20 billion is affordable.

For specific segments of the population, such as children under 18, the cost of universal coverage is estimated to be quite low—$5.7

billion for 1998—reflecting the twin realities that children have low medical expenditures and that most chronically ill children from low-income families already are covered by Medicaid.[20] By contrast, in 1993 the tobacco industry spent $6.2 billion on advertising and promotion of its products in the United States.[21, 22] So it is hard to argue that the absolute dollar amount is an insuperable barrier.

Government is untrustworthy. Every other country that has achieved broad health insurance coverage has involved its national or provincial government in a meaningful way, either as the primary payer or as guarantor for those unable to obtain insurance by other means. But Americans do not trust government. That is hardly new; evidence of this distrust is ingrained in our Constitution and is on display at Ellis Island in the documents our forebears brought with them as immigrants. Only recently, however, have politicians run for national office on the platform that if elected, they would protect citizens from their own government. Examples before 1996 include George Wallace, Jimmy Carter, Ronald Reagan, and George Bush. Perhaps apocryphal is the story that spread like wildfire during the recent debate on national health care reform in which an elderly Louisiana citizen pleaded with Senator John Breaux to "please keep government's hands off my Medicare."

Polling data reflect the reality. In 1993, only 18 percent of Americans believed they received excellent or good value from their federal tax dollars and only 23 percent generally trusted the government in Washington to "do the right thing."[23] Thus, there exists widespread concern that governmental attempts to expand health insurance coverage will make things worse, rather than better.

The American political system is a barrier to sweeping national changes. A corollary to the distrust of government is the reality that by both design and practice, the way our federal and state governments function is almost incompatible with the leap required to provide all citizens with health insurance. Many factors have been proposed to explain this impasse: the bitterness of partisan politics, unmasked by the demise of the common enemy, global Communism; the influence of the myriad special-interest groups—representing both providers and consumers—that are fearful of losing ground under new legislation; the reluctance of voters to accept the possibility of true cost increases or sacrifices affecting them personally, linked with the reluctance of politicians to confront and explain hard choices; sloganeering ("waste, fraud, and abuse") and superficial press and television coverage of complicated issues; and perhaps most important, the inherent difficulty of making substantial financing and organizational changes in a trillion-dollar industry at a time of relative economic stagnation.

What Lies Ahead?

Taken together, these explanations seem to predict that the large number of medically uninsured people, like the poor, will be with us for some time—whether because we choose not to recognize the problem or because we choose not to solve it. Indeed, their numbers may increase substantially in the next few years, as will the difficulty they will have in obtaining charity care. Several trends support these predictions.

First, the link between employment and health insurance has eroded. Between 1988 and 1994, 4 million fewer people were covered by employment-based health insurance.[11] This trend will probably continue and possibly accelerate. Many firms have dropped health insurance coverage because of its growing cost relative to wages. Other trends—such as the restructuring of the economy—may also be contributing to this erosion.

The expansion of Medicaid enrollment will probably not continue to compensate for the loss of employment-based insurance, as it did during the period from 1988 to 1994, when the states added 10 million new Medicaid enrollees.[11] Constraints on Medicaid financing, anticipated soon from Congress, will certainly slow this expansion and may even reverse it.

In the new era of price competition, we will find doctors and hospitals less financially able to provide charity care. To be able to respond to the market pressure being exerted by insurance companies, managed-care organizations, and employers, health care providers feel they must cut costs to the bone. At the same time, Medicare and Medicaid reimbursement rates are threatened, and even these programs are enrolling people in managed-care programs that look for providers with competitive rates. Academic health centers, which currently provide two-thirds of all charity care, are among the most seriously affected by the changes (Williams O, American Hospital Association: personal communication). They enter today's price competition with higher costs because of their teaching function, the many high-technology, specialized services they offer, and the seriously ill—and costly—patients they serve. Of all providers, they are the ones most likely to have to stop cross-subsidizing care for indigent patients by charging other payers more.

Finally, the traditional providers of last resort—public hospitals and clinics—are also seriously threatened by evaporating income streams,

streams not likely to be replenished by politicians chary of raising taxes. The supplanting of nonprofit hospitals by for-profit facilities will also reduce the system's capacity for charity care, since the for-profit sector claims that it makes its social contributions by paying taxes. The net result will be a diminution of charity care both overall and through the selective reduction of such services as emergency and trauma care.

These trends seriously threaten the security of health coverage and the accessibility of medical care for a large and increasing number of Americans. At least three responses are possible.

The most likely response is business as usual—simply accepting that the uninsured will always be with us and assuming that somehow they will receive medical care when it is really needed, even if it takes a little longer and occurs in bare-bones settings with less-than-optimal outcomes. Another response, which now seems quite unlikely, would be a renewed national determination to provide health insurance for every American, spurred both by moral revulsion at the thought of so many citizens having to rely on uncertain charity for basic medical care and by the political realization that even the middle class is at risk of losing its grip on health insurance.

A middle path, not yet being discussed widely, would be a bipartisan, incremental approach to whittling down the number of uninsured people over, say, a 10-year period. Examples of such experiments already under way in individual states include expanding Medicaid coverage to people with low incomes (Tennessee and Oregon) or to more children (Minnesota); expanding coverage to low-income people (Washington) or children (Florida) through state-subsidized insurance; identifying new sources of taxes—such as tobacco products—to be earmarked to subsidize care for the uninsured (Arizona, California, Massachusetts, Minnesota, Vermont, and Washington); creating all-payer pools for the uninsured (Maryland, New York, and New Jersey); and creating incentives for small businesses to expand their health insurance coverage (California and Florida), since most of the uninsured come from families where at least one member works.

To care for the uninsured, we first need a broad-based agreement on the overall goal. Only then can we begin work on the specific details. Otherwise, the inevitable splintering of potential supporters over issues of implementation will doom any chance for consensus.

Whatever the number of uninsured people, we put the values of the entire health care system at risk by accepting their condition as inevitable. At present, most of the attention in health care is focused on the many changes resulting from market forces—the mergers and consolidations of hospital systems and the new organizational and ethical questions raised by managed care. But meanwhile, the problem of the uninsured continues to grow quietly; in the long run, its effects will be so pervasive that it is bound to reemerge as a major national issue. If it does not, then we will find ourselves living in a much meaner America than many of us who entered the healing professions ever imagined.

Notes

1. Employee Benefits Research Institute. Notes: a monthly newsletter. Washington, D.C.: EBRI Education and Research Fund, 1996; 17(1): 1–7.
2. Rowland D, Lyons B, Salganicoff A, Long P. Profile of the uninsured in America. Health Aff (Millwood) 1994; 13(2): 283–7.
3. Swartz K. Dynamics of people without health insurance: don't let the numbers fool you. JAMA 1994; 271: 64–6.
4. Department of Commerce. Health insurance coverage—who had a lapse between 1991 and 1993? Statistical Brief 95–21. Washington, D.C.: Bureau of the Census. August 1995.
5. Winterbottom C, Liska DW, Obermaier KM. State-level data book on health care access and financing. 2nd ed. Washington, D.C.: Urban Institute. 1995.
6. Short PF, Banthin JS. New estimates of the underinsured younger than 65 years. JAMA 1995; 274: 1302–6.
7. Winterbottom C. Trends in health insurance coverage: 1988–1991. Washington, D.C.: Urban Institute. July 1993.
8. Thorpe KE, Shields AE, Gold H, Altman S, Shactman D. Anticipating the number of uninsured Americans and the demand for uncompensated care: the combined impact of proposed Medicaid reductions and erosion of employer-sponsored insurance. Paper presented to the Council on the Economic Impact of Health Care Reform. Washington, D.C., November 8, 1995.
9. Employee Benefits Research Institute Issue Brief 158, Sources of health insurance and characteristics of the uninsured: analysis of the March 1994 Current Population Survey. Washington, D.C.: Employer Benefits Research Institute. 1995; 1–47.
10. Does health insurance make a difference? Background paper. Washington, D.C.: Office of Technology Assessment. September 1992.
11. Holahan J, Winterbottom C, Rajan S. The changing composition of health insurance coverage in the United States. Washington D.C.: Urban Institute. February 1995.
12. Long SH, Marquis MS. Gaps in employer coverage: lack of supply or lack of demand? Health Aff (Millwood) 1993; 12: Suppl: 282–93.
13. Berk ML, Schur CL, Cantor JC. Ability to obtain health care: recent estimates from the Robert Wood Johnson Foundation National Access to Care Survey. Health Aff (Millwood) 1995; 14(3): 139–46.
14. Weissman JS, Gastonis C, Epstein AM. Rates of avoidable hospitalization by insurance status in Massachusetts and Maryland. JAMA 1992; 268: 2388–94.

15. Hadley J, Steinberg EP, Feder J. Comparison of uninsured and privately insured hospital patients: condition on admission, resource use, and outcome. JAMA 1991; 265: 374–9.
16. Franks P, Clancy CM, Gold MR. Health insurance and mortality: evidence from a national cohort. JAMA 1993; 270: 737–41.
17. Ayanian JZ, Kohler BA, Abe T, Epstein AM. The relation between health insurance coverage and clinical outcomes among women with breast cancer. N Engl J Med 1993; 329: 326–31.
18. Long SH, Marquis MS. The uninsured "access gap" and the cost of universal coverage. Health Aff (Millwood) 1994; 13(2): 211–20.
19. Burner ST, Waldo DR. National health expenditure projections. 1994–2005. Health Care Finance Rev 1995; 16(4): 221–42.
20. Hughes RG, Davis TL, Reynolds RC. Assuring children's health as the basis for health care reform. Health Aff (Millwood) 1995; 14(2): 158–67.
21. Federal Trade Commission. Report to Congress for 1993: pursuant to the Federal Cigarette Labeling and Advertising Act. Washington, D.C.: Federal Trade Commission. 1993.
22. Federal Trade Commission. Report to Congress: pursuant to the Comprehensive Smokeless Tobacco Health Education Act of 1986. Washington, D.C.: Federal Trade Commission. 1995.
23. Blendon RJ, Brodie M, Benson J. What happened to Americans' support for the Clinton health plan? Health Aff (Millwood) 1995; 14(2): 7–23.

II

Traditional Safety Net Providers: Showing Signs of Strain

6

The Challenges Facing Health Centers in a Changing Healthcare System

Daniel R. Hawkins, Jr.
Sara Rosenbaum

Introduction

This chapter focuses on federally recognized health centers[1] and the challenges that face them in a changing healthcare system. Many of the issues raised here are applicable to other types of publicly assisted providers of ambulatory care for the poor. In a transformed healthcare environment, the survival of at least some of these programs[2] may be in doubt, not because publicly subsidized ambulatory healthcare is no longer necessary (ironically it may be more necessary than ever), but because of the cumulative effects of the transformation now taking place in this part of the safety net. Thus, the issues facing health centers can be viewed as indicative of the problems that confront publicly subsidized ambulatory care programs in general.

We begin this chapter with an overview of health centers—what they are, how they are structured, whom they serve, and their principal sources of funding. We also explore health center patient and revenue trends between 1980 and 1995, because these data powerfully illustrate the problems that the program must overcome in the years ahead. The second part of the chapter considers the major trends that will affect the future operation and ultimately the survival of health centers and their response to these trends: high poverty, a widespread lack of health insurance, stagnating and declining direct federal subsidies, and shrinking support from other third party payors, most notably Medicaid. The conclusion offers an assessment of the continued need for publicly supported sources of comprehensive primary healthcare as well as a series of policy recommendations.

Background and Overview

A Brief History of the Establishment and Growth of Health Centers

Begun as a series of demonstration projects in 1965 by the federal Office of Economic Opportunity (the lead agency in the Johnson administration's War on Poverty), the Neighborhood Health Centers Program (as it was then known) was envisioned as a complement to the newly enacted Medicaid program. Medicaid was to provide health insurance coverage for the eligible poor. However, policymakers understood at the time that despite its goal of "mainstreaming" the poor into the private healthcare system (Stevens and Stevens 1975), Medicaid alone could not guarantee access to care (Davis and Schoen 1977). The health centers program was viewed as a vehicle for bringing both newly insured low-income people and those who remained uninsured into the healthcare system; educating patients on how to gain access to and utilize care; and as a means of addressing the myriad social, demographic, and poverty-related problems that are commonly associated with (and, indeed, which in some cases can give rise to) poor health.

The health centers demonstration was designed to accomplish these broad health and social goals through several key design features. First, the program was structured to offer comprehensive primary medical care (including treatment for acute and chronic health conditions), not merely the preventive array of nonmedical health services (such as well-child exams, immunizations, and screening for disease) typically offered by other publicly subsidized providers such as local health agencies, which were far more politically sensitive to private physician resistance to government-sponsored medicine (Rosenblatt, Law, and Rosenbaum 1997). Second, health centers were required to offer other services not traditionally found in private medical care practices, such as services designed to facilitate access (such as family and community outreach, transportation, and multilingual services) and services intended to improve the effectiveness of care (such as health and nutrition education, parenting classes, and referral to other social services).

Third, health centers received not only start-up funding but also operating subsidies. These subsidies effectively took the place of the out-of-pocket payments that underwrite a significant proportion of primary medical care practices but that are lacking in communities with high poverty and a pervasive lack of health insurance. It was these deeply impoverished communities, which historically have collectively lacked the resources necessary to support virtually any form of commerce, including primary medical care practices (Fossett and Perloff 1995) that were targeted for health center subsidies and that health centers must serve as a condition of receiving operating support (Hawkins and Rosenbaum 1993; Kindig and Yan 1993; Kindig 1994). These operating subsidies permitted the centers to survive economically in low-income communities and to discount their charges for care in accordance with a public, prospective, income-adjusted schedule of charges (as opposed to the type of ad hoc charitable debt forgiveness that one might find in a private medical care practice) (Rosenblatt, Law, and Rosenbaum 1997).

Fourth, consistent with the overall goals of their founding agency, the early health centers were also meant to be a source of both economic development and meaningful employment in the low-income inner-city neighborhoods and isolated rural areas where they were located. Early organizers believed that, in this way, the health centers would fulfill a dual purpose of being both agents of care and agents of community change.

Finally, health centers were to be governed by boards of community individuals, a majority of whose members were to be center patients and that were empowered to hire and fire staff and establish operational policies. This lay power over medical professionals that was granted to health center boards was unprecedented in modern American medicine.[3]

Initially the health centers program grew slowly because of its demonstration status, the limited funding provided by Congress, and the program's departure from the medical care "norm." In 1975, when the first legislation authorizing health centers was enacted,[4] health centers served approximately 1.7 million people in both urban neighborhoods and rural agricultural communities. Virtually all health center patients had family incomes below twice the federal poverty level, and most of those served were uninsured (U.S. Senate Labor Committee 1975). As expected, the preponderance of insured patients were covered by Medicaid—although the slow growth of that program in the area of ambulatory healthcare (as a result of limited eligibility standards and low provider payment levels) resulted in coverage of fewer than one-third of poor Americans (Stevens and Stevens 1975; U.S. Congressional Research Service 1995). Although initial estimates assumed that 80 percent of health center operational funds would be derived from Medicaid, as of

1980 Medicaid payments constituted only approximately 14 percent of health center operating revenues.

A "rural health initiative" undertaken by the Carter administration in the late 1970s led to the development of hundreds of new health centers, mostly in southern and western states. Following a brief period of federal funding reductions during the early years of the Reagan administration, federal appropriations were slowly but steadily increased during the mid-1980s to permit centers to provide care for the growing number of uninsured Americans.

Beginning in the late 1980s the health center program began to grow rapidly, following a series of pivotal Medicaid expansions. The first of these expansions was the coverage improvements for children and pregnant women (two major health center patient groups) that were enacted between 1984 and 1990 (Rosenbaum 1992). The second expansion was the establishment of the Medicare and Medicaid federally qualified health centers (FQHC) program in 1989.[5] The FQHC program added coverage of "federally qualified health center services" as a required service for both Medicare and Medicaid. The program also mandated reimbursement for all "FQHC" services,[6] as well as for other Medicaid-covered ambulatory services furnished by health centers in accordance with the same cost-based reimbursement methodology used for rural health clinics since 1977 (and employed by the Department of Health and Human Services (HHS) for federally funded health centers serving Medicare patients since 1966) (Rosenbaum 1992).

Finally, at least some of the growth in health centers' Medicaid revenues can be traced to the fact that, beginning in the mid-1980s and prior to the enactment of the eligibility expansions, health centers began furnishing a greater level of care to patients generally as a result of expansion by the program into sicker patient groups, and as a result of the declining health status of the poor, particularly in inner cities (Rosenbaum and Zuvekas 1993).

In 1995 almost 900 FQHCs operated nearly 3,000 local health center service sites in urban and rural underserved communities across the nation, providing comprehensive preventive and primary healthcare to 9.3 million people, including 3.5 million Medicaid recipients, 1 million Medicare beneficiaries, and 3.8 million uninsured people. The number of patients served reached 10 million in 1996 (U.S. Bureau of Primary Health Care 1996b).

Numerous studies over the past 30 years (including a recent series of studies examining the performance of health centers and other providers under Medicaid) underscore the effectiveness of health centers in furnishing services of good quality and in a cost-effective fashion.[7] Among other matters, these studies have found that health centers furnish higher rates of preventive care, and care of better overall quality, than other providers (Weiner and Engel 1991; Stuart et al. 1995).[8] Centers have been able to achieve reduced rates of hospital admissions and specialty referrals, as well as emergency room use, for their patients and have been shown to improve health outcomes and lower the incidence of chronic disease and disability (Freeman, Kiecolt, and Allen 1982; Grossman and Goldman 1982; Schwartz and Poppen 1982; Gorman and Nelson 1984; De Prez, Pennell, and Libby 1987; Stuart and Steinwachs 1993).[9]

In addition, several studies have evaluated the costs of care (especially to state Medicaid programs) for insured people who use health centers for their primary care, as compared with the costs of care for those who use other Medicaid providers. In general, these studies have found that the costs of *primary and preventive* healthcare services for those using health centers have been comparable to, and in some cases slightly higher, than for those using other providers—although a number of such studies have also cited a greater range and frequency of such services received by the health center users. Most notably, however, virtually all such studies have found that the *total* healthcare costs are much lower—from 22 to 67 percent lower—due to significantly reduced rates of specialty referrals, hospital admission rates, and lengths of stay for people using the health centers compared with those who use other providers (JRB Associates 1981; Braddock 1994; Center for Health Policy Studies/SysteMetrics 1994; Starfield et al. 1994).[10]

A Profile of Health Center Patients and Revenues

Health center patients reflect both the mission of the program and the communities that centers serve. Two-thirds of all health center patients have family incomes below the federal poverty level; 86 percent have incomes below twice that level. Two-thirds of all health center patients are members of racial or ethnic minority groups who face higher health risks and who generally are in poorer health. Almost four million patients are uninsured, accounting for nearly 1 in 10 uninsured Americans. Health centers care for 3.6 million Medicaid recipients, more than 10 percent of all beneficiaries nationally. In 1994 the 400,000 births to health center patients accounted for 10 percent of all live births (and one of every five low-income births) in the United States that year. Forty-five percent of health center patients are children and another

31 percent are women of childbearing age (U.S. Bureau of Primary Health Care 1996a).

Figures 6.1 through 6.3 show the magnitude of the changes that have taken place in the health centers over time. Figure 6.1 presents information on real-dollar appropriation levels and patients served between 1980 and 1995. In 1980 the total federal health center appropriation was $360 million and the program served 5 million people. By 1995 the program had nearly doubled in size (to 9.3 million patients served, with most of the increase occurring between 1990 and 1996); at the same time, despite nominal growth, real-dollar appropriated funding levels had fallen by one-third, to $247 million.

Figure 6.2, which sets forth health center funding levels over time by payor source, answers the obvious question of how this growth was achieved, given the real-dollar decline in appropriated funding levels. In 1980 total health center operating budgets were $690 million. Of this amount, federal grants represented 52 percent of all revenues, whereas Medicaid accounted for 14 percent ($100 million). Other revenue sources (patient fees, private insurance, Medicare, and other funding) comprised 34 percent of health center budgets. By 1995 total health

Figure 6.1 Health Center Grant Funds and Patients

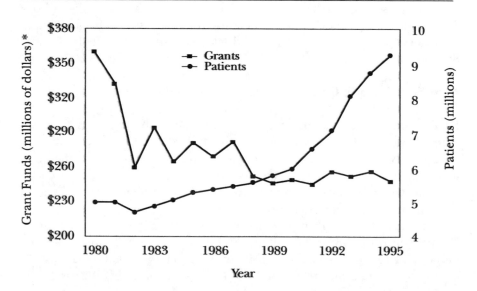

*Adjusted to reflect changes in medical care consumer price index since 1980.

Figure 6.2 Health Center Revenues by Source

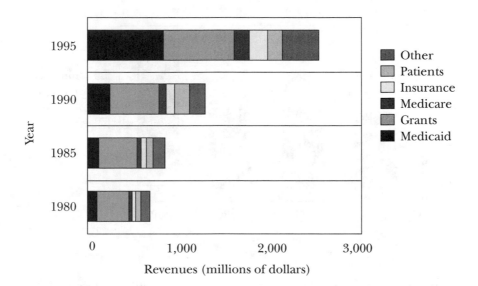

center budgets had nearly quadrupled to approximately $2.6 billion. Of this amount, federal grants accounted for 30 percent, whereas Medicaid revenues amounted to 33 percent ($850 million). Thus, Figure 6.2 indicates that escalating Medicaid revenues drove the increase in overall health center operating budgets, virtually all of which occurred between 1990 and 1995.

Figure 6.3, which displays the composition of health center patients by payor source over time, shows that the growth in health center revenues attributable to Medicaid has benefited not only Medicaid patients, but the uninsured as well. Fifty percent of the 5 million patients served by health centers in 1980 (2.5 million persons) were uninsured. In 1995, the uninsured accounted for 41 percent of the 9.3 million patients served by health centers (3.8 million uninsured patients). Thus, over this 15-year time period, the uninsured remained the single largest group of health center patients, growing by 1.3 million persons over that period.

These figures strongly suggest that health centers used their expanding Medicaid revenues not only to serve Medicaid patients but also to free the centers' grant funding to be used as originally intended: to support the cost of healthcare provided to uninsured and underinsured people. In the absence of a growing discretionary appropriation or other sources of revenue, Medicaid became the engine that allowed

Figure 6.3 Health Center Patients by Payor Source

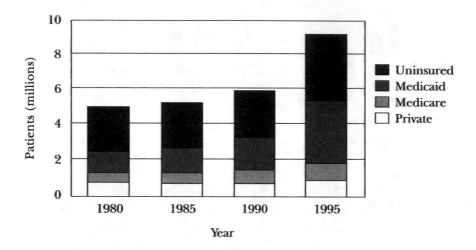

health centers to expand their services and reach millions of additional uninsured people. These trends in patients and revenues underscore the extent of health center reliance on Medicaid in ways that affect their ability to serve both Medicaid beneficiaries and uninsured patients. The statistics also underscore the vulnerability of health centers to major shifts in Medicaid funding as a result of policy and systemic change.

Trends Affecting Health Centers

Despite their success over the years, health centers today are able to reach only about one-fourth of the 43 million Americans who are identified as medically underserved; and more than half of the 2,091 U.S. counties identified as having primary care access problems remain unserved by a health center or equivalent provider (U.S. Bureau of Primary Health Care 1996b). Moreover, recent studies point to persistent disparities in health status between low-income, minority, and underserved Americans and their respective counterparts (Blendon et al. 1989; Wennecker and Epstein 1989; Fossett and Perloff 1995; Grumbach et al. 1995; Kohrs and Mainous 1995). Finally, growing numbers of Americans are experiencing serious health and related social problems that require ever more complex and costly interventions. More than two-thirds of the 345 health centers responding to a 1996 survey of health centers conducted by the

National Association of Community Health Centers (NACHC) reported recent increases in patients who are pregnant teenagers, homeless, people with HIV or AIDS, newly unemployed, or recent immigrants. Most health centers cited teenage pregnancy, substance abuse, domestic and community violence, vaccine-preventable diseases, and infant mortality and infant low birthweight as the most urgent local health needs.

However, the most formidable challenge that confronts health centers today may well be that of maintaining their mission—and indeed, surviving—in the face of the dramatic changes now taking place in the healthcare system against a backdrop of growing income disparities and an eroding health insurance base, particularly among lower-income people. It is probably safe to predict that, despite the need for more subsidized ambulatory care in underserved communities, unless the Medicaid-driven financing base for health centers is significantly restructured, the 1996 patient care figures noted above will become a high-water mark rather than a point of progress. As Medicaid revenues begin declining under the combined pressures of eligibility changes and the effects of managed care on health centers, the numbers of centers and patients served—both insured and uninsured—can be expected to fall.

Moreover, the market-driven changes may have an effect that goes beyond simply the number of patients served: Highly competitive markets favor low cost and high efficiency. Many health center patients have complex health and social problems, and treating such patients may be "inefficient" (i.e., they may consume far more time and resources than the average patient profiled in the actuarial estimates that drive a competitive healthcare environment). Not only may competition cost the centers the resources that they need to subsidize care for the uninsured, but the changes may also force centers to revamp the way in which they practice medicine for the poor—the very thing that has made health centers unique for 30 years.

We identify three major trends affecting health centers: the continued growth in the number of people who lack health insurance, especially among low-income people; the actual and potential loss of Medicaid coverage among key groups of health center patients; and the effects of a competitive market on both health centers' third-party revenues and their uninsured patient demand levels.

The Uninsured

The significant recent growth in the number of uninsured Americans and the disturbing trends regarding health insurance coverage are detailed elsewhere in this volume and by other sources (Employee Benefit Research Institute 1996). Among low-income Americans, the number and percentage who are uninsured is the highest since Medicare and Medicaid were enacted, with the deepest losses in coverage occurring among those in employed families (The Lewin Group, Inc. 1996). More than one-third of low-income people are completely uninsured; and, together with the underinsured (people whose insurance coverage leaves them at risk for out-of-pocket expenses exceeding 10 percent of their incomes), nearly 60 percent of working-age low-income Americans are uninsured for all or most of their healthcare costs (Farley-Short and Banthin 1995). A similar percentage (59 percent) of uninsured people report that they cannot afford health insurance; and nearly half of all uninsured people (and 18 percent of those *with* insurance) report that they have had difficulty getting needed care, with most suffering serious' health or economic consequences as a result (Donelan et al. 1996).

Medicaid Eligibility Reductions

The coming years can be expected to bring significant reductions in the number of people with Medicaid coverage. These changes are the result of several trends. First, even prior to the 1996 enactment of welfare reform legislation, the number of families with children who received welfare had been declining as a result of both improved work opportunities for low-income people and state-initiated reductions under various Section 1115 welfare demonstration programs under way since 1993 (Guyer, Mann, and Super 1996). The second source of expected Medicaid reductions are the many changes that can be anticipated from the enactment of the Personal Responsibility and Work Opportunity Reconciliation Act of 1996 (PRA, P.L. 104-193). The centerpiece of the landmark legislation is the elimination of Aid to Families with Dependent Children (AFDC), the principal source of cash welfare assistance since 1935 to families with children, and its replacement with the Temporary Aid to Needy Families (TANF) block grant. It also eliminates cash-assistance payments to children with "functional" disabilities, such as learning disabilities or emotional disorders. The Congressional Budget Office projected at the time of enactment that the TANF program could reduce welfare rolls by 30–40 percent over five years (Congressional Budget Office 1996).

To prevent the widespread loss of Medicaid among poor women and children who may lose welfare assistance under the new law, the

PRA requires states to continue Medicaid coverage for all people who continue to meet the old AFDC rules in place as of July 16, 1996.[11]

In effect, therefore, the PRA bifurcates Medicaid and welfare eligibility, just as the Section 1115 welfare demonstrations have done. Although theoretically neither the federally sanctioned welfare demonstrations nor the new welfare programs established under the PRA include revisions in Medicaid eligibility, as a practical matter it is extremely difficult for states to separate complex Medicaid eligibility standards from those used to determine welfare eligibility. As a result, people terminated from or denied cash assistance may also lose Medicaid, even though this result was not intended under either the demonstrations or the new law.

If Medicaid were governed by simple poverty-level standards, the dilemma might not be as severe. But the new welfare rules are every bit as complicated as the old ones, and many people can be expected to be incorrectly terminated from the program or denied coverage. Some groups (such as poverty-level children and pregnant women) who lose cash assistance will continue to qualify for Medicaid, but may face a temporary loss of coverage while eligibility under an alternative standard is redetermined, costing them several months of coverage. Others, such as the four million nonpregnant women who depend on Medicaid and welfare, may remain unaware or uninformed of their continued Medicaid eligibility even if they lose cash assistance, leaving them vulnerable to a complete loss of coverage.

Families with children that receive cash assistance comprise the majority of all Medicaid beneficiaries (Rosenbaum and Darnell 1996). Moreover, families with children constitute the majority of health center patients. All health centers, and especially those located in inner cities with high concentrations of poor people, can expect to feel the serious effects of these reductions in the number of welfare (and potentially Medicaid) recipients.

In addition, beginning August 22, 1996 (the date of enactment), the PRA also bars otherwise eligible new legal residents from Medicaid for all but emergency care for five years following entry into the United States and gives states the option to deny Medicaid to most legal residents living in the United States at the time of enactment. The PRA is expected to affect hundreds of thousands of current legal residents, many of whom depend on health centers for linguistically appropriate care, thus adding further to the new law's substantial impact on health centers (Rosenbaum 1996).

Medicaid Funding Reductions Resulting from a Competitive Healthcare Market

At the end of 1995, more than 12 million Medicaid beneficiaries were enrolled in managed care arrangements (Kaiser Commission on the Future of Medicaid 1996). Most enrollees were members of plans operating on a financial risk basis and offering their services to state Medicaid agencies on a discounted basis. Because these organizations contract with their member providers on an "at will" basis, healthcare providers must either accept discounted payments themselves or risk exclusion from the network (Rosenblatt, Law, and Rosenbaum 1997). The overwhelming majority of all Medicaid managed care enrollees are women and children, the principal health center patient groups.

For the most part, the transformation to managed care has been accomplished through the federal demonstration process. Both Section 1115 and Section 1915 of the Social Security Act authorize the Secretary of HHS to allow states to eliminate beneficiaries' freedom of choice and require beneficiary enrollment in managed care as a condition of eligibility (Rosenbaum and Darnell 1996; Kaiser Commission on the Future of Medicaid 1996). As part of the Section 1115 demonstrations (which allow the Secretary to waive virtually all federal Medicaid requirements in addition to freedom of choice), the Secretary has waived FQHC coverage and payment rules in all Section 1115 demonstration states.[12]

In some states, agencies and health centers have developed supplemental payment methods to prevent a precipitous loss of financial support. However, these alternative payment arrangements (such as supplemental payments directly to health centers, in addition to or as part of their payments, as managed care subcontractors) are not required as a condition of federal approval.

In the case of Section 1915 waivers, which do not give the Secretary the power to waive the FQHC payment requirements, the Secretary has nonetheless effectively waived the statute by interpreting the FQHC coverage and payment provisions out of existence. Specifically, the Secretary interprets federal law as permitting states to allow plans to offer FQHC services without having to contract with the FQHC.[13] Moreover, the Secretary has also ruled that FQHC services furnished by non-network centers to beneficiaries are "out of plan" and therefore nonreimbursable if members have access to "FQHC services" through their health plan. This interpretation of the law by the Secretary has effectively eviscerated the FQHC program in virtually all section 1915 states.

Although most health centers are able to participate successfully in Medicaid managed care plans and indeed are frequently offered contracts, most are facing a substantial loss in Medicaid income as a result of the discounted payment system that is the hallmark of managed care relationships between plans and providers. On average, payments under managed care arrangements—in some instances less than $6 per member per month for all ambulatory primary care covered under the center's contract with the plan—amount to less than 60 percent of the health centers' reasonable cost rates (National Association of Community Health Centers 1995). Because health centers have few privately insured or financially secure patients, and thus no ability to shift costs to other paying sources, these deep discounts can be expected to have several effects, including reductions in both the scope of care offered and in the centers' ability to care for uninsured patients. Two recent reviews of contracts between managed care plans and health centers found inadequate payment-rate methodologies in at least half the contracts reviewed and excessive levels of financial risk (for services beyond their control) in at least one-third of the contracts reviewed (Rosenbaum, Serrano, and Wehr, forthcoming; U.S. Bureau of Primary Health Care 1996b).

Managed care also can affect health centers by costing them "market share." Members who either select or are "default assigned" to health plans may or may not have the right to select their primary care provider.[14] Under default assignment, when a Medicaid recipient fails, after a certain period of time (usually 30 days), to choose a managed care plan from among those offered, he is automatically and involuntarily assigned to a single plan by the state agency. Such default assignments, which rarely take into account a patient's previous provider of choice, typically account for 50 percent—and in some states are as high as nearly 100 percent—of all Medicaid managed care enrollments.

Health Center Responses to These Trends

Health centers have, for the most part, recognized or anticipated the managed care changes and have taken steps to achieve high levels of participation in the restructured Medicaid programs. In a 1996 article, Lipson and Naierman (p. 41) state that

> Health centers are positioned well in the current environment because they [offer] primary care services—a valuable commodity in today's health care market . . . [H]ealth centers are actively

marketing their capacity to state Medicaid agencies, health plans, and hospitals. In some communities, . . . health centers are regarded as extremely attractive contractors because of their experience in serving Medicaid enrollees and because of their locations in neighborhoods where many Medicaid recipients live.

The 1996 NACHC survey of health centers found that nearly 85 percent of respondents have increased the number of Medicaid recipients they serve since January 1, 1994. The most notable increases, both proportionally and numerically, occurred in southern and western states, although centers in New Jersey and Massachusetts recorded above-average growth as well. Nearly three-fourths of responding centers reported that they are participating in some form of Medicaid managed care, and in many states health centers have formed networks or full managed care plans, often in concert with other safety-net providers. According to the federal government, at least one-third of all health centers are participating in prepaid managed care arrangements, including virtually all health centers located in the 20 states with either Section 1115 or significant Section 1915 waiver activity (U.S. Bureau of Primary Health Care 1996b). Almost 60 percent of all new Medicaid patients reported by health centers in the NACHC survey were recorded in these 20 states.

At the same time, however, many of the health centers with increased Medicaid-patient populations are reporting losses in Medicaid income as a result of low payment rates from managed care plans. Despite efforts at increased efficiencies, centers have been unable to offset their revenue losses and report that they have, of necessity, resorted to reducing staff, eliminating services, or diverting other revenues (including federal and other funds intended to support care to the uninsured) to cover their losses. In these cases, uninsured and underinsured patients may well be the most profoundly affected.

In addition to dollar losses from managed care, more than 15 percent of respondents to the NACHC survey reported that their Medicaid-patient population has fallen over the past three years, triggering significant losses in Medicaid revenues. These losses averaged more than 1,000 patients per center, or almost one-fourth of their Medicaid patient population. Although some centers pointed to statewide reductions in Medicaid caseload (notably terminations of state "general assistance" programs in Michigan and Ohio) as the main cause of their declines, 73 percent of centers reporting losses of Medicaid patients said that their losses stemmed from the states' use of Medicaid default assignment procedures, as noted above. Health center patients involuntarily as-signed to other providers often return to the health center to receive care, citing difficulties accessing care through their assigned provider. Any care provided to these patients is typically uncompensated.

Simultaneous with the decline in Medicaid patients and revenues has been an explosion in the number of uninsured patients. As managed care plans enroll ever greater numbers of publicly and privately insured Americans, they can successfully demand and secure deep pricing dis-counts from subcontracting providers. As a result, those providers are markedly less able to shift their uncompensated care costs to other revenue sources, leaving them to shift their uninsured patients to health centers and other local safety-net providers. Fully 95 percent of the health centers responding to the NACHC survey indicated that their numbers of uninsured patients have increased over the past three years. These new uninsured patients accounted for slightly more than half of all new health center patients reported over this time period. Translat-ing these reported increases into numbers, health centers have added nearly one million uninsured people to their patient rolls over the past three years. Much of this growth occurred in southern and midwestern states, where either the growth in the number of uninsured people or the declining rates of employer-sponsored insurance coverage have been most significant. However, above-average growth rates were also re-ported by centers in Tennessee, Oregon, and Washington—three states that had initially reduced the numbers of uninsured people through statewide health reforms, only to see them edging back up recently toward their previous levels. In fact, more than half of all new unin-sured patients were reported by health centers in the 20 states with the highest levels of managed care activity, and the average increase in these centers' uninsured population was greater than the average for all health centers. Although the number of new uninsured patients has been significant in communities that have experienced the loss of other safety-net providers, growth in the number of uninsured health center patients has been so widespread that it clearly underscores the declining ability of providers in nearly all communities to continue serving the uninsured.

Another important factor in the recent overall growth of health center patient populations is found in their response to the AIDS epi-demic. Nearly 70 percent of all health centers, and 82 percent of all urban centers, reported that they are serving people with HIV or AIDS. This population is disproportionately uninsured for needed services, further exacerbating the fiscal pressures on health centers.

Although state and local funding of health centers has shown substantial growth over the years, it has not been adequate to replace the declining federal revenues. In 1995, state, local, and private sources accounted for nearly $400 million, or 16 percent, of all health center revenues, compared with only $150 million (8 percent) a decade ago (National Association of Community Health Centers 1996a; U.S. Bureau of Primary Health Care 1996a). A recent survey of state health agencies found that 21 states provided in excess of $150 million nationally in 1995 for the development and operation of health centers and similar primary care providers. Most of the state programs are patterned after the federal health center model to a substantial degree (Rosenbaum, Hawkins, and Rosenbaum, forthcoming). Sixty-one percent of centers reporting that they were serving increased numbers of uninsured people cited new or increased funding from state, local, or private sources as the main reason for service expansions. At the same time, however, 40 percent of all centers reporting declines in their patient populations pointed to cuts in state, local, and private funding as a primary cause.

Conclusion

The experience of health centers underscores the critical importance of (and the direct relationship between) the operating subsidies they receive and their ability to care for low-income and underserved populations. For the first 20 years of their existence, the health centers remained a small but important step in addressing the basic healthcare needs of the uninsured and underserved in the United States. Over the past decade, they have experienced exponential growth, fueled principally by huge increases in Medicaid funding. Health centers now represent a substantial commitment of public funds and are a major source of care for the poor. Recent events, most notably the actual or threatened loss of Medicaid coverage and the effects of a competitive healthcare environment generally on the availability of either free or discounted healthcare, suggest that the need for health centers can only be expected to increase in the coming years.

Unfortunately, those very same events pose the greatest threat to the centers' future (and that of other safety-net providers, as well). The same Medicaid program that fueled their recent growth appears to be in decline, both in the number of people it covers and in its payment levels. Across the country, health centers are confronted with a simultaneous "one–two" punch of declining overall revenues and increasing numbers of uninsured people seeking their care. Because health centers cannot survive financially in poor communities—much less remain true to their mission—without adequate revenues to serve both their insured and uninsured patients, they face a threat of decline in most localities, and perhaps outright collapse in a number of places. Because of who they are and what they do, health centers have had remarkable staying power over the years. But this challenge is daunting, and unlike earlier times, the heights from which the fall could begin are much greater.

If health centers are to survive, they need operating subsidies tied to the size of their uninsured populations and to the typically nonreimbursable services they must furnish to all patients. For the first two decades of their existence, health centers relied principally on discretionary federal grant support for these subsidies. But the declining value of these annual appropriations underscores their tenuousness; given the heightened pressures to contain and reduce overall federal spending, there is no indication that federal discretionary funding can do more than maintain its current level over the next several years. At that rate, these grant funds will permit centers to serve no more than a fraction of those who might need their care.

One approach to maintaining the revenue base of health centers would be to adopt a series of related and highly regulatory measures designed to insulate them from the effects of competition. For example, managed care plans could be required to contract with all health centers in their service area, to assign patients to them consistent with their service capacity, and to pay them a rate that covers their reasonable costs. Simply put, such proposals, no matter how meritorious, are not politically realistic; indeed, federal and state governments do not appear either willing or able to enforce the lesser requirements now in place. Moreover, such measures, even if enacted, would not address the underlying problem of declining Medicaid coverage itself, nor would they address the fact that many health center patients experience limited, sporadic periods of Medicaid coverage and are otherwise uninsured. In addition, it is not a good idea, in the long run, to isolate health centers from the effects of change in the healthcare system. The move toward managed care is complicated, particularly for safety-net providers, but the transformation does promise greater efficiencies and more integrated services over time.

Another approach, and one that appears more viable, would be to replace both the current Medicaid and the Medicare FQHC payment requirements with a directed spending program that provides underwriting support directly to health centers in relation to their overall uncompensated care costs. In the absence of a new insurance system for the poor, this payment system (which is similar to the payment reforms under discussion with regard to graduate medical education under Medicare) would supplement the revenues that health centers receive from managed care plans, other payors, patients, and other sources (including their federal grants), allowing a sum that is certain to be budgeted and spent annually to support the operations of federally qualified health centers. Such support could help stabilize health centers and allow them to participate more effectively in the new health system without being threatened by the twin burdens of more uninsured patients and excess uncovered, uncompensated-care costs.

The obstacles to enactment of such a program are principally monetary and structural, because health centers enjoy fairly widespread, bipartisan support in Congress. Should only federal funds be used to support such a program? Should the program be administered at the federal or state level? What rules should govern the disbursement of funds? Should the funds be sufficient to support care for additional numbers of uninsured patients and the establishment of new centers in currently underserved areas? If so, how would these funds interact with the current federal health center grants, which are intended to support similar purposes? These questions and others would need to be answered in fashioning such a new program, but the result would be the stabilization of a crucial source of primary healthcare for the poor in the face of great, and still growing, need—a goal that we believe is well worth pursuing.

Notes

1. Specifically, discussion focuses on trends affecting all health centers that are certified as federally qualified health centers under the Medicare and Medicaid statutes. These health centers include entities that receive federal grants under sections 329, 330, 340, and 340A of the Public Health Service Act (all four grant authorities were consolidated into a revised Section 330 of the Public Health Service Act under the Consolidated Health Centers Act of 1996, P.L. 104-299); certain other federally funded entities (i.e., urban Indian health clinics funded under Title V of the Indian Health Improvement Act as well as tribally operated clinics under the Indian Self Determination Act); and entities that meet all of the qualifications applicable to grantees under the community health centers program but that do not receive federal funds (e.g., community clinics supported with state and local grant revenues).
2. Examples of similar programs are clinics operated by local health agencies, federally funded family planning clinics, and community free clinics. For a

review of the relationship between managed care and federally supported family planning programs see Rosenbaum et al. (1995).

3. Even in the case of public hospitals, medical staffs maintain authority over medical practice and staffing matters, independent of other aspects of hospital operations. See, generally, Rosenblatt, Law, and Rosenbaum 1997).

4. P.L. 94-63. Legislative authority for the migrant health program actually dates back to 1962. In 1975 this early law was revised and enacted as companion legislation to the community health centers program.

5. P.L. 101-239, which amended several provisions of Title XIX of the Social Security Act (Medicaid); and P.L. 101-508, which amended provisions of Title XVIII of the Act (Medicare). Federally qualified health centers were defined to include all federally supported health centers, as well as urban Indian health clinics, and clinics operated by Indian tribal organizations and other entities that met the conditions of grant receipt applicable to health centers but that did not receive federal funding.

6. The term "FQHC services" means the following services when furnished by a federally qualified health center: physician services and services incident to physician services; the services of nurse practitioners and physician assistants and services incident to these services; services of clinical psychologists and social workers; and, in the case of Medicare, preventive health services (sections 1861(aa) and 1905(l) of the Social Security Act).

7. Several reviews over the years have cataloged and summarized the major findings of such studies and evaluations. See, for example, Zwick (1972), Geiger (1984), Rosenbaum (1987), Zuvekas (1990), and Darnell and Rosenbaum (1992).

8. These more recent evaluations reaffirm similar findings contained in earlier studies. See, for example, Morehead (1970); Morehead, Donaldson, and Seravalli (1971); Hershey and Moore (1975); Wingate et al. (1976); Sussman et al. (1979); and Davis, Gold, and Makuc (1981).

9. Here, too, the recent studies confirm the findings of earlier reports. See, for example, Alpert et al. (1968); Bellin, Geiger, and Gibson (1969); Chabot (1971); Hochheiser, Woodward, and Charney (1971); Bellin and Geiger (1972); Moore, Bernstein, and Bonnano (1972); Gordis (1973); Klein et al. (1973); Moore and Bonnano (1974); Gold and Rosenberg (1974); Davis and Schoen (1977); Cowan et al. (1978); Columbo et al. (1979); and Biscoe et al. (1980).

10. The findings of these studies are also consistent with those found in earlier reports. See, for example, Sparer and Anderson (1972); Okada and Wan (1980); Duggar, Balicki, and Zuvekas (1981); and Fleming and Andersen (1984).

11. States also have the option to roll back their 1996 AFDC income eligibility standards to levels that were in effect on May 1, 1988, for purposes of determining Medicaid eligibility.

12. The waivers of these statutory provisions are listed specifically in letters from the Health Care Financing Administration that grant federal waivers to state Medicaid agencies.

13. See February 8, 1996, letter from the Health Care Financing Administration to State Medicaid agencies (National Association of Community Health Centers 1996b).
14. Data from an analysis of contracts between state Medicaid agencies and full-risk managed care plans indicate that contractors are encouraged but not required to allow members to select their own providers.

References

Alpert, J. J., M. C. Heagarty, L. Robertson, J. Kosa, and R. J. Haggerty. 1968. "Effective Use of Comprehensive Pediatric Care." *American Journal of Diseases of Children* 116: 529–33.

Bellin, S., and H. Geiger. 1972. "The Impact of a Neighborhood Health Center on Patients' Behavior and Attitudes Relating to Health Care: A Study of a Low Income Housing Project." *Medical Care* 10: 224–39.

Bellin, S., H. Geiger, and C. Gibson. 1969. "Impact of Ambulatory-Health-Care Services on the Demand for Hospital Beds." *New England Journal of Medicine* 280: 808–12.

Biscoe, M., D. Hochstrasser, G. Somes, D. Cowen, and G. Culley. 1980. "Follow-up Study of the Impact of Rural Preventive Care Outreach Program on Children's Health and Use of Medical Services." *American Journal of Public Health* 70 (2): 151–56.

Blendon, R. J., L. H. Aiken, H. E. Freeman, and C. R. Corey. 1989. "Access to Medical Care for Black and White Americans." *Journal of the American Medical Association* 261 (2): 278–81.

Braddock, D. 1994. *Using Medicaid Fee-For-Service Data to Develop Health Center Policy.* Seattle, WA: Washington Association of Community Health Centers and Group Health Cooperative of Puget Sound.

Center for Health Policy Studies/SysteMetrics. 1994. *Health Services Utilization and Costs to Medicaid of AFDC Recipients in New York and California Served and Not Served by Community Health Centers.* Washington, DC: U.S. Department of Health and Human Services.

Chabot, A. 1971. "Improved Infant Mortality Rates in a Population Served by a Comprehensive Neighborhood Health Program." *Pediatrics* 47: 989–94.

Columbo, T., D. Freeborn, J. Mullooly, and V. Burnham. 1979. "The Effect of Outreach Workers' Educational Efforts on Preschool Children's Use of Preventive Services." *American Journal of Public Health* 69 (5): 465–68.

Congressional Budget Office. 1996. Cost Estimates and Underlying Assumptions for H.R. 4174, The Personal Responsibility and Work Opportunity Act of 1996. Washington, DC (July), Congressional Budget Office.

Cowan, D., G. Culley, D. Hochstrasser, M. Biscoe, and G. Somes. 1978. "Impact of a Rural Preventive Care Outreach Program on Children's Health." *American Journal of Public Health* 68 (5): 471–76.

Darnell, J., and S. Rosenbaum. 1992. *Community and Migrant Health Centers: A Literature Review.* Washington, DC: Center for Health Policy Research, The George Washington University Medical Center.

Davis, K., and C. Schoen. 1977. *Health and the War on Poverty: A Ten-Year Appraisal.* Washington, DC: The Brookings Institution.

Davis, K., M. Gold, and D. Makuc. 1981. "Access to Health Care for the Poor: Does the Gap Remain?" *Annual Review of Public Health* 2: 159–82.

De Prez, R., B. Pennell, and M. Libby. 1987. "The Substitutability of Outpatient Primary Care in Rural Community Health Centers for Inpatient Hospital Care." *HSR: Health Services Research* 22: 207–33.

Donelan, K., R. J. Blendon, C. A. Hill, C. Hoffman, D. Rowland, M. Frankel, and D. Altman. 1996. "Whatever Happened to the Health Insurance Crisis in the United States? Voices from a National Survey." *Journal of the American Medical Association* 276 (16): 1346–50.

Duggar, B., B. Balicki, and A. Zuvekas. 1981. *Costs and Utilization Patterns for Comprehensive Health Center Users.* Washington, DC: U.S. Department of Health and Human Services.

Employee Benefit Research Institute. 1996. *Sources of Health Insurance and Characteristics of the Uninsured: An Analysis of the 1996 Current Population Survey.* EBRI Issue Brief No. 178. Washington, DC: The Institute.

Farley-Short, P., and J. Banthin. 1995. "New Estimates of the Underinsured Younger Than 65 Years." *Journal of the American Medical Association* 274 (16): 1302–5.

Fleming, G., and R. Andersen. 1984. "The Municipal Health Services Program: Improving Access to Primary Care without Increasing Expenditures." *Medical Care* 24 (7): 565–79.

Fossett, J., and J. Perloff. 1995. "The 'New' Health Reform and Access to Care: The Problem of the Inner City." Paper presented to the Kaiser Commission on the Future of Medicaid (15 December), Washington, DC.

Freeman, H., K. Kiecolt, and H. Allen. 1982. "Community Health Centers: An Initiative of Enduring Utility." *Milbank Memorial Fund Quarterly* 60 (2): 245–67.

Geiger, H. 1984. "Community Health Centers: Health Care as an Instrument of Social Change." In *Reforming Medicine,* edited by V. Sidel and R. Sidel. New York: Pantheon Books.

Gold, M., and R. Rosenberg. 1974. "Use of Emergency Room Services by the Population of a Neighborhood Health Center." *Health Services Reports* 89 (1): 65–70.

Gordis, L. 1973. "Effectiveness of Comprehensive Care Programs in Preventing Rheumatic Fever." *New England Journal of Medicine* 289 (7): 331–35.

Gorman, S., and H. Nelson. 1984. "Meeting the Data Needs of Neighborhood Health Centers." Paper delivered at the 102nd meeting of the American Public Health Association.

Grossman, M., and F. Goldman. 1982. *An Economic Analysis of Community Health Centers.* Washington, DC: National Bureau of Economic Research.

Grumbach, K., S. Siefer, K. Vranizan, D. Keane, D. Osmond, D. Soffel, K. Huang, and A. B. Bindman. 1995. "Primary Care Resources and Preventable Hospitalization in California." CPS Report, California Policy Seminar, Berkeley, CA.

Guyer, J., C. Mann, and D. Super. 1996. *The Timeline for Implementing the New Welfare Law.* Washington, DC: Center on Budget and Policy Priorities.

Hawkins, D., and S. Rosenbaum. 1993. *Lives in the Balance: A National, State, and County Profile of America's Medically Underserved.* Washington, DC: National Association of Community Health Centers.

Hershey, J., and J. Moore. 1975. "The Use of an Information System for Community Health Services Planning and Management." *Medical Care* 13: 114–19.

Hochheiser, L., K. Woodward, and E. Charney. 1971. "Effect of Neighborhood Health Center on the Use of Pediatric Emergency Departments in Rochester, New York." *New England Journal of Medicine* 285 (3): 148–52.

JRB Associates. 1981. *Final Report for Community Health Center Cost Effectiveness Evaluation.* Washington, DC: U.S. Department of Health and Human Services.

Kaiser Commission on the Future of Medicaid. 1996. *Medicaid and Managed Care.* Washington, DC: The Commission.

Kindig, D. 1994. "What Is Rural Underservice?" Paper presented to the Kaiser Commission on the Future of Medicaid (17 November) Washington, DC.

Kindig, D. A., and G. Yan. 1993. "Physician Supply in Rural Areas with Large Minority Populations." *Health Affairs* 12 (2): 177–84.

Klein, M., K. Roghmann, K. Woodward, and E. Charney. 1973. "The Impact of the Rochester Neighborhood Health Center on Hospitalization of Children." *Pediatrics* 51: 833–39.

Kohrs, F., and A. Mainous. 1995. "The Relationship of Health Professional Shortage Areas to Health Status." *Archives of Family Medicine* 4: 681–85.

The Lewin Group, Inc. 1996. *Recent Trends in Employer Health Insurance Coverage and Benefits.* Washington, DC: The Lewin Group, Inc.

Lipson, D., and N. Naierman. 1996. "Effects of Health System Changes on Safety-Net Providers." *Health Affairs* 15 (2): 33–48.

Moore, G., R. Bernstein, and R. Bonnano. 1972. "Effect of a Neighborhood Health Center on Emergency Room Use." *Medical Care* 10 (3): 240–47.

Moore, G., and R. Bonnano. 1974. "Health Center Impact on Hospital Utilization." *Journal of the American Medical Association* 282 (2): 332–33.

Morehead, M. 1970. "Evaluating Quality of Medical Care in the Neighborhood Health Center Program of the Office of Economic Opportunity." *Medical Care* 8 (1): 118–31.

Morehead, M., R. Donaldson, and M. Seravalli. 1971. "Comparisons Between OEO Neighborhood Health Centers and Other Health Care Providers of the Ratings of the Quality of Health Care." *American Journal of Public Health* 61 (7): 1294–1306.

National Association of Community Health Centers. 1995. Letter to Ms. Debbie Chang, Director, Office of Legislation and Policy, U.S. Health Care Financing Administration, Washington, DC.

———. 1996a. *Access to Community Health Care: A National and State Data Book.* Washington, DC: The Association.

———. 1996b. *NACHC Managed Care Technical Assistance Issue Brief #24: FQHC and Medicaid Managed Care—Recent Policy Guidance.* Washington, DC: The Association.

Okada, L., and T. Wan. 1980. "Impact of Community Health Centers and Medicaid on the Use of Health Services." *Public Health Reports* 95 (4): 520–34.

Rosenbaum, S. 1987. *Community and Migrant Health Centers: Two Decades of Achievement.* Washington, DC: National Association of Community Health Centers.

———. 1992. "Medicaid Reforms Enacted During the 1980s." In *The Medicaid Financing Crisis,* edited by D. Rowland. Baltimore, MD: AAAS Press.

Rosenbaum, S., and A. Zuvekas. 1993. *An Analysis of Data for Health Centers and Medically Underserved Populations.* Washington, DC: Center for Health Policy Research, The George Washington University Medical Center.

Rosenbaum, S., R. Serrano, and E. Wehr. Forthcoming. "Negotiating the New Health System: An Analysis of Contracts Between Managed Care Organizations and Primary Health Care Group Practices." *Journal of the American Medical Association.*

Rosenbaum, S., and J. Darnell. 1996. *A Review of Comprehensive Medicaid Managed Care Demonstrations Under Section 1115 of the Social Security Act: Implications for Federal Policy.* Washington, DC: Kaiser Commission on the Future of Medicaid.

Rosenbaum, S., D. Hawkins, and E. Rosenbaum. Forthcoming. "State Funding of Comprehensive Primary Care Service Programs for Medically Underserved Populations." *American Journal of Public Health.*

Rosenbaum, S., P. Shin, A. Mauskopf, K. Fund, G. Stern, and A. Zuvekas. 1995. "Beyond the Freedom to Choose: Medicaid Managed Care, and the Freedom of Choice Requirement." *Western Journal of Medicine* 103 (Supplement): 33–38.

Rosenbaum, S. 1996. *An Analysis of the Medicaid and Health-Related Provisions of the Personal Responsibility and Work Opportunity Act of 1996 (P.L. 104-193).* Washington, DC: Center for Health Policy Research, The George Washington University Medical Center.

Rosenblatt, R., S. Law, and S. Rosenbaum. 1997. *Law and the American Health System.* St. Paul, MN: Foundation Press.

Schwartz, R., and P. Poppen. 1982. *Measuring the Impact of Community Health Centers on Pregnancy Outcomes.* Boston, MA: Abt Associates.

Sparer, G., and A. Anderson. 1972. "Cost of Services at Neighborhood Health Centers." *New England Journal of Medicine* 286: 1241–45.

Starfield, B., N. R. Powe, J. R. Weiner, M. Stuart, D. Steinwachs, S. H. Scholle, and A. Gerstenberger. 1994. "Costs vs. Quality in Different Types of Primary Care Settings." *Journal of the American Medical Association* 272 (24): 1903–8.

Stevens, R., and S. Stevens. 1975. *Welfare Medicine.* New York: Basic Books.

Stuart, M., and D. Steinwachs. 1993. "Patient-Mix Differences Among Ambulatory Providers and Their Effects on Utilization and Payments for Maryland Medicaid Users." *Medical Care* 31 (12): 1119–37.

Stuart, M., D. Steinwachs, B. Starfield, S. Orr, and A. Kerns. 1995. "Improving Medicaid Pediatric Care." *Journal of Public Health Management Practice* 1 (2): 31–38.

Sussman, E., H. Rosen, A. Siegel, J. Witherspoon, and H. Nesson. 1979. "Can Primary Care Deliver?" *Journal of Ambulatory Care Management* 2 (3): 29–39.

U.S. Bureau of Primary Health Care. 1996a. Data provided to U.S. House and Senate Appropriations Committees. U.S. Department of Health and Human Services, Washington, DC.

————. 1996b. Briefing materials on health centers for HHS Assistant Secretary for Planning and Evaluation (September). U.S. Department of Health and Human Services, Washington, DC.

U.S. Congressional Research Service. 1995. *Medicaid Source Book: Background Data and Analysis (A 1995 Update)*. House Commerce Committee. Washington, DC: U.S. Government Printing Office.

U.S. Senate Labor Committee. 1975. *Report to Accompany S. 66, the Health Services and Nurse Training Amendments of 1975*. Senate Report 94-29. Washington, DC: U.S. Government Printing Office.

Weiner, J., and J. Engel. 1991. *Improving Access to Health Services for Children and Pregnant Women*. Washington, DC: National Governors' Association.

Wennecker, M., and A. Epstein. 1989. "Racial Inequalities in the Use of Procedures for Patients with Ischemic Heart Disease in Massachusetts." *Journal of the American Medical Association* 261 (2): 2683–92.

Wingate, M. B., T. Silbert, M. McMillen, and J. Zeccardi. 1976. "Obstetric Care in a Family-Health Oriented Neighborhood Health Center." *Medical Care* 14 (4): 315–25.

Zuvekas, A. 1990. "Community and Migrant Health Centers: An Overview." *Journal of Ambulatory Care Management* 13 (4): 1–12.

Zwick, D. 1972. "Some Accomplishments and Findings of Neighborhood Health Centers." *Milbank Memorial Fund Quarterly* 50: 387–420.

7

The Future of Safety-Net Hospitals

Larry S. Gage

The past decade has seen a dramatic transformation of the role of the hospital in the nation's health system, with a profound impact on every important element of that system. From the way people purchase and pay for health coverage, to where and how care is provided, the metamorphosis has been swift and intense. New systems and networks spring to life overnight, mergers and acquisitions dramatically shrink the number of players, and traditional payment mechanisms turn upside down in a heartbeat. All the buzzwords are well-known by now—vertical and horizontal integration, consolidation, networks, decentralization, privatization, managed care, subacute care, alternate site delivery, rightsizing.

Although all hospitals are affected by these trends, safety-net hospitals and health systems have felt their impact disproportionately. The pressure for change is especially acute for those providers who rely most heavily on federal, state, and local government funding to pay for their wide range of primary, acute, and public health services. For such systems, marketplace pressures are intensified by a variety of other factors, including the growth in the uninsured, reductions in Medicaid funding and local support, greater competition for Medicaid patients, the explosion in managed care, the need to provide public health and communitywide services, inadequate governance, and often cumbersome political or bureaucratic obstacles.

As a result of these challenges, safety-net hospitals and systems face major threats to their future survival. The health of many millions of low-income patients and the viability of the health system for rich

National Association of Public Hospitals and Health Systems

The purpose of this chapter is to provide an overview of the current situation and future viability of America's safety-net health systems. This overview focuses, in particular, on hospital-based systems in the nation's metropolitan areas, because these are the institutions that primarily constitute the membership of the National Association of Public Hospitals and Health Systems (NAPH).

The NAPH was founded in 1981 by a handful of urban public hospitals. Today, NAPH's membership includes more than 100 metropolitan area safety-net hospitals and health systems. The association also works closely with many nonmember safety-net systems, and the findings, trends, and recommendations expressed in this chapter can thus be generalized to most systems that share common characteristics with NAPH members. Those characteristics include a mandate to treat anyone in need of care regardless of their ability to pay, and the provision of high volumes of inpatient, outpatient, and primary care to the poor and uninsured. In addition, such systems often play an essential role in the provision of public health services and also provide many specialty services to their entire communities, such as trauma, burn, and neonatal intensive care, that are too costly for other hospitals to provide. Finally, such systems also typically serve as major teaching hospitals for both undergraduate and graduate medical education, as well as the training of nursing and ancillary medical personnel.

and poor alike in many metropolitan communities are likely to be in danger if these threats are not adequately addressed and if policymakers do not respond with adequate funding and innovative programmatic solutions.

At the Princeton conference in June 1996 that led to this volume, there was considerable concern and support expressed for the survival of safety-net providers. Even economist Alain Enthoven—an acknowledged champion of health reform based on competition rather than institutional support—allowed that "we will always need County systems for those on the margins."

Enthoven, like others, appears to define the safety net rather narrowly, as if it were composed entirely of aging public "charity" hospitals cut from the same (antique) mold. Although such hospitals clearly do exist today, they constitute a diminishing minority of safety-net providers. And while there are numerous threats to the continued stability of all safety-net providers, their numbers increasingly include many successful, dynamic health systems that provide high-quality care. These hospitals and systems have adopted a wide range of innovative approaches to meeting the needs of the vulnerable patients and urban communities they serve.

This chapter focuses on improving the common understanding of the quality and diversity of the nation's safety-net hospitals and health systems, while also describing the threats and challenges they face. These threats include the growth in the number of uninsured, a heavy reliance on shrinking government funding sources, the increased competition for Medicaid patients, the explosion in managed care, and the impact of new legislation (such as the recent caps on Medicaid disproportionate-share payments and the 1996 welfare and immigration reform laws).

In describing the current situation of safety-net systems, new 1995 data collected by the NAPH in its annual Hospital Characteristics Survey is used, augmented by data from the 1994 American Hospital Association's annual survey and other sources.

This chapter also provides an overview of the sources of funding for safety-net hospitals and systems, with particular attention to those funding sources that support services and programs for vulnerable populations and communitywide public health services. I include an assessment of trends in federal, state, and local support over the past several years, as well as a brief analysis of the most important current federal funding source for the uncompensated care provided by safety-net hospitals: the Medicare and Medicaid disproportionate-share hospital (DSH) payments.

Characteristics of Safety-Net Health Systems

The United States has long relied on an institutional safety net to fill in the gaps in the nation's health system. Despite legitimate concerns about equality of access for both insured and uninsured patients, America's institutional health safety net has been accomplishing the task of meeting at least the basic needs of the uninsured and underinsured in many areas. In fact, it can be argued that this success is the main reason that American politicians have had the luxury of endlessly (and fruitlessly) debating, rather than enacting, universal coverage for the past 50 years.

Prior to the enactment of the Medicare and Medicaid programs, America's health "safety net" consisted primarily of public hospitals that represented virtually the only treatment alternatives available to most low-income patients. Many functioned primarily (or even solely) as *charity hospitals* in the nation's urban areas—in effect, the successors to the old almshouses for the poor. Their reputation with the public at large during that period was—to be charitable—low.

Indeed, the history of hospitals in the United States generally, prior to the past 75 years, is almost exclusively a history of such charity hospitals. Health policy analyst Emily Friedman has described this history eloquently. Until early in this century, with the advent of immunizations and antibiotics, hospitals in general were extremely dangerous places to be, even for healthy people. Apart from a few pioneering institutions such as Bellevue, Philadelphia General, and Massachusetts General hospitals, which treated rich and poor alike, only those patients who could not afford to be sick at home found their way to the public sanitaria (Friedman 1987).

Following World War II, hospitals began to take on a far greater importance to the health of the American population. Through the Hill-Burton Act, and augmented by local fundraising, bond campaigns, and the entreprenuerialism of local physicians, community hospitals grew up all over the United States. Still, the poor gained little access to many of these new facilities, and the major urban public hospitals continued to represent an important source of medical care for vulnerable patients.

Many thought that the enactment of the Medicare and Medicaid programs would eliminate the need for public charity hospitals. But that just didn't happen. From the outset, the Medicaid program never covered all of the population living in poverty, and after a few years of early growth, Medicaid coverage declined dramatically. From a 1976 high-water mark of 65 percent of all individuals living in poverty or near poverty, Medicaid covered fewer than 45 percent by the early 1980s. And while some expansion occurred in the late 1980s among certain populations (such as children and pregnant women), barely more than half of the poor remain covered today.

Although it provides coverage to most Americans over age 65, Medicare, too, has covered less and less of the total cost of care for the elderly in recent years, shrinking to well below half in the 1990s. The Health Care Financing Administration (HCFA) estimates today that the average elderly person in America spends 18 percent of after-tax income on healthcare, up from 10 percent in 1972, as opposed to just 5 percent for the nonelderly. This can be particularly devastating for the low-income elderly, who may spend half or more of their income on healthcare if they are ineligible for Medicaid (Health Care Financing Administration 1996).

In the meantime, in addition to the continued need to serve the Medicaid and non-Medicaid poor over the past 30 years, urban public hospitals and health systems have also contributed significantly in other areas, including medical education, the provision of high-cost tertiary medical specialties, outpatient care, and important public health services that are of benefit to their entire communities.

In the mid-1970s, the Kellogg Foundation, together with the American Hospital Association (AHA), financed the establishment of a Commission on Public General Hospitals, for the purpose of "examining the present healthcare delivery roles of public general hospitals, and to identify future roles, if any, for these hospitals" (Kellogg Commission on Public General Hospitals 1978). The 1978 report of this commission was probably the first step toward the formal national recognition by federal decision makers of the existence of, and the need to support, the DSH hospital safety net as we know it today.

The Kellogg Commission divided public hospitals into four groups: urban public general hospitals, or those located in our nation's 100 largest cities; public general hospitals in standard metropolitan statistical areas (SMSAs) outside the 100 largest cities; rural hospitals; and state university hospitals. The commission's final report targeted particular attention on the large urban public general hospitals, 90 of which were identified, and hospitals owned by public universities, which then numbered 45. Medium-sized public hospitals in smaller SMSAs (357) were found to be similar in many ways to private hospitals in the same setting. The remainder of our nation's public hospitals were small rural facilities that often fulfilled a safety-net role in their regions or communities. In all, public hospitals accounted for more than one-fourth of all the hospitals in America in the mid-1970s.

Safety-net health systems continue to differ widely across our nation today. Yet, there are many other types of organizations that make up the safety net. In the public sector, in addition to traditional city or county hospitals and health systems, the safety net includes freestanding government entities such as authorities, districts, and public benefit corporations; state hospitals (and especially state university health systems); public health departments and clinics; federally qualified community, migrant, and rural health centers (FQHCs); and a fairly wide range of other federal facilities, such as veterans' hospitals and Indian health facilities.

The safety net has also historically included private institutions that have been willing (or sometimes required by law, their enabling charter, or their geographic location) to play this role.

Because the situation of other provider groups, such as FQHCs, is addressed elsewhere in this volume, the remainder of this chapter focuses on hospital-based safety-net systems. There have been several recent efforts to quantify the number of hospital-based safety-net systems in America. In 1996, the Georgetown Institute for Health Care Research and Policy estimated that there are 369 "urban safety-net hospitals" in America, using the Medicaid statutory definition of Medicaid volume greater than 1 standard deviation above the mean (Gaskin 1996). Of those, 33 percent are public, 57 percent private nonprofit, and 10 percent investor owned. Alternatively, The Lewin Group has estimated that there are 696 hospitals nationally that meet the optional Medicaid statutory definition of a greater than 25 percent "low-income utilization rate" (or the combination of Medicaid revenues and direct local subsidies as a proportion of total net revenues) (Sheils and Alecxih 1996). The fact is that the total is probably between these two numbers, and, in any case, fewer than 10 percent of all hospitals in America.

Safety-Net Hospitals Provide a Large Volume of Inpatient and Outpatient Care

It is possible to begin to quantify the mission and services of safety-net health systems, based on data provided by a significant proportion of NAPH members in an annual hospital characteristics survey. Seventy hospitals responded to NAPH's 1995 survey, and most of the statistics cited for 1995 are drawn from the entire sample (see Table 7.1). Occasionally, fewer hospitals are used because of incomplete data from particular respondents. Comparative data over time can also be presented in a number of these areas, but only for those hospitals responding in all of the years selected. Some comparative data are drawn from the 1994 AHA survey, which we were able to obtain for 90 urban safety-net hospitals. This sample, while not a purely random one, includes the major urban safety-net hospitals and health systems in a substantial majority of the nation's 50 largest SMSAs, and the data is thus offered as illustrative of trends and characteristics of urban safety-net systems in general.

Perhaps the most dramatic characteristic of hospital-based safety-net systems is simply the tremendous volume of *both* inpatient and

Safety-Net Hospitals Serve a Wide Range of Vulnerable Populations

Just as they provide a great variety of services, safety-net health systems are by no means monolithic in the patient populations they serve. In considering solutions to the problems faced by such systems, it is important to understand the broad range of vulnerable populations who rely on safety-net hospitals. Although many of the characteristics of the uninsured and underinsured are described elsewhere in this volume, it may be helpful to simply provide a partial list of many of the different categories of vulnerable patients who may often be found in just a single safety-net hospital:

- Uninsured/Underinsured
  - working poor with no employer-provided coverage
  - non-Medicaid unemployed poor (including single nonpregnant adults, childless couples, poor families above certain income levels)
  - uninsurables (people with high-cost illnesses who are denied coverage)
  - children who are not included in parents' coverage
  - young single middle- (and upper-) class adults (they become ineligible for parents' policy and do not have employer-provided coverage)
  - employed people who choose not to purchase employer-sponsored coverage
- Legal and undocumented immigrants
- Minorities
- Homeless
- Chronically ill and disabled (even those who are insured, as they often exceed policy limits)
- High-risk mothers and infants
- Victims of violence
- Mentally ill
- Substance abusers
- Persons with communicable diseases (including HIV and tuberculosis)
- Boarder babies
- Migrant farm workers
- Prisoners
- Persons with limited or no English-speaking abilities
- Noncompliant managed care enrollees (individuals who seek care outside of the managed care organization provider network, often due to the inaccessibility of network providers)

Table 7.1   Hospitals Responding to 1995 NAPH Hospital
Characteristics Survey

Hospital	City	State	Zip
Alameda County Medical Center	Oakland	CA	94602
Boston City Hospital	Boston	MA	02118
Cambridge Hospital	Cambridge	MA	02139
Cook County Hospital	Chicago	IL	60612
Cooper Green Hospital	Birmingham	AL	35233
Denver Health Medical Center	Denver	CO	80204
Erie County Medical Center	Buffalo	NY	14215
Grady Health System	Atlanta	GA	30335
Harborview Medical Center	Seattle	WA	98104
Harris County Hospital District	Houston	TX	77054
Hennepin County Medical Center	Minneapolis	MN	55415
Hermann Hospital	Houston	TX	77030
Hurley Medical Center	Flint	MI	48503
Jackson Memorial Hospital	Miami	FL	33136
Kern Medical Center	Bakersfield	CA	93305
LAC–Harbor/UCLA Medical Center	Torrance	CA	90509
LAC–High Desert Hospital	Lancaster	CA	93536
LAC–King/Drew Medical Center	LosAngeles	CA	90059
LAC–LAC/USC Medical Center	LosAngeles	CA	90033
LAC–Olive View Medical Center	Sylmar	CA	91342
LHCA–E.A. Conway Medical Center	Monroe	LA	71210
LHCA–Huey P. Long Medical Center	Pineville	LA	71361
LHCA–Medical Ctr of Louisiana at New Orleans	New Orleans	LA	70112
LHCA–W.O. Moss Regional Medical Center	Lake Charles	LA	70605
Maricopa Medical Center	Phoenix	AZ	85010
Medical Center of Central Georgia	Macon	GA	31201
Memorial Regional Hospital	Hollywood	FL	33021
Merrithew Memorial Hospital and Health Center	Marinez	CA	94553
Metro Nashville General Hospital	Nashville	TN	37210
MetroHealth Medical Center	Cleveland	OH	44109
Nassau County Medical Center	East Meadow	NY	11554
Natividad Medical Center	Salinas	CA	93912
NBHD–Broward General Medical Center	Ft. Lauderdale	FL	33316
NBHD–Coral Springs Medical Center	Coral Springs	FL	33065
NBHD–Imperial Point Medical Center	Ft. Lauderdale	FL	33308
NBHD–North Broward Medical Center	Pompano Beach	FL	33064
North Oakland Medical Center	Pontiac	MI	48341
Nueces County Hospital District	Corpus Christi	TX	78405

Continued

Table 7.1   Continued

Hospital	City	State	Zip
NYCHHC–Bellevue Hospital Center	New York	NY	10016
NYCHHC–Coney Island Hospital	Brooklyn	NY	11235
NYCHHC–Elmhurst Hospital Center	New York City	NY	11373
NYCHHC–Harlem Hospital Center	New York	NY	10037
NYCHHC–Jacobi Medical Center	Bronx	NY	10461
NYCHHC–Kings County Hospital Center	Brooklyn	NY	11203
NYCHHC–Lincoln Medical & Mental Hlth Ctr	Bronx	NY	10451
NYCHHC–Metropolitan Hospital Center	New York	NY	10029
NYCHHC–North Central Bronx Hospital	Bronx	NY	10467
NYCHHC–Queens Hospital Center	Jamaica	NY	11432
NYCHHC–Woodhull Medical & Mental Hlth Ctr	Brooklyn	NY	11206
Parkland Health and Hospital System	Dallas	TX	75235
Regional Medical Center at Memphis	Memphis	TN	38103
Riverside General Hospital	Riverside	CA	92503
San Bernardino County Medical Center	San Bernardino	CA	92415
San Francisco General Hospital	San Francsico	CA	94110
San Joaquin General Hospital	French Camp	CA	95231
San Luis Obispo General Hospital	San Luis Obispo	CA	93401
Santa Clara Valley Medical Center	San Jose	CA	95128
St. Mary's Hospital (East St.Louis IL)	East St. Louis	IL	62201
St. Paul–Ramsey Medical Center	St. Paul	MN	55101
Tampa General Healthcare	Tampa	FL	33601
Thomason General Hospital	El Paso	TX	79905
Truman Medical Center West	Kansas City	MO	64108
UMDNJ–University Hospital	Newark	NJ	07107
University Hospital of Brooklyn	Brooklyn	NY	11203
University Medical Center of Southern Nevada	Las Vegas	NV	89102
University of Chicago Hospitals	Chicago	IL	60637
University of Texas Health Center at Tyler	Tyler	TX	75710
University of Texas Medical Branch Hospital	Galveston	TX	77555
Valley Medical Center of Fresno	Fresno	CA	93702
Wishard Memorial Hospital	Indianapolis	IN	46202

outpatient services they provide. Safety-net health systems tend to be centered around large teaching hospitals. According to the 1994 AHA survey, 90 urban safety-net hospitals surveyed reported total staffed beds of 39,741, for an average of 442 each. These hospitals reported total admissions of 1,437,932, for a per-hospital average of 15,977, and total inpatient days of 10,912,944, for an average of 121,255 each.

The National Public Health and Hospital Institute's (NPHHI) 1995 analysis of data reported by hospitals in smaller cities reveals that safety-net hospitals provide higher volumes of service than their hospital-industry counterparts. (The 100 largest cities are ranked according to population and defined as central cities, not SMSAs. This analysis was conducted using data from the 1994 AHA annual survey.) Compared with the average hospital in the 100 largest cities, safety-net hospitals reported 30 percent more admissions, 39 percent more inpatient days, and an average occupancy rate (75 percent) that was 11 percentage points higher.

Although safety-net systems provide higher volumes of inpatient services than their private-sector counterparts, the volume of these services has decreased in recent years, reflecting industry trends. Since 1988, the number of discharges per hospital from all safety-net hospitals in the 100 largest cities dropped 8.1 percent, from 22,374 to just over 20,698 per hospital. At the same time, the average number of inpatient days decreased by a much more dramatic 18.5 percent, from 173,602 per hospital to 146,548 per hospital, reflecting decreased lengths of stay over time.

In addition to general inpatient care, safety-net hospitals provide a high level of obstetric and gynecological care. Seventy-six such hospitals delivered an average of 3,194 babies in 1994, more than twice the number reported at the average hospital in the 100 largest cities. Since 1991, however, the number of births at such hospitals has decreased 23 percent. This decrease reflects the tremendous competition among providers for Medicaid obstetrics patients over the past several years. In 1993, public general hospitals in the 100 largest cities represented 9 percent of hospitals but also provided more than 18 percent of neonatal intensive care days, 21 percent of pediatric intensive care days, 27 percent of burn care days, and 18 percent of emergency visits (Andrulis et al. 1995).

Although some observers think of safety-net hospitals primarily as inpatient facilities, in fact, safety-net hospitals have always served as family doctors for large numbers of low-income or uninsured patients. Hospitals thus also provide huge (and growing) volumes of emergency, outpatient, and primary care. In 1995, just 67 hospital-based safety-net health systems reported a total of 22,331,800 outpatient and emergency department visits, for an average of 331,818 per hospital (as compared, e.g., with the 7 million visits reported by all 2,000 FQHCs in 1995).

Although the volume of care provided in the inpatient setting has decreased, the volume of emergency and outpatient care has increased dramatically. Since 1988, the average number of outpatient visits provided at 24 safety-net systems increased 17.6 percent (see Figure 7.1).

It is often maintained that outpatient care in hospital-based systems is too costly and too often provided in inappropriate settings, such as the emergency department (ED). This is not true. Fewer than 20 percent of the 22 million reported ambulatory visits were in the ED. The vast majority (more than 80 percent) of these visits were provided in appropriate, cost-effective outpatient clinic and primary care settings. A 1991 survey conducted by the NPHHI found that 37 percent of the ED utilization in safety-net hospitals was considered by respondents to be inappropriate—a proportion that has likely been reduced since that study was undertaken. However, even if that proportion were the same in 1995, it would represent only 7 percent of all visits—still too high, perhaps, but not a particularly alarming percentage (Andrulis et al. 1991).

Figure 7.1 Outpatient Visits per Hospital for a Matched Set of NAPH Members, 1988–95

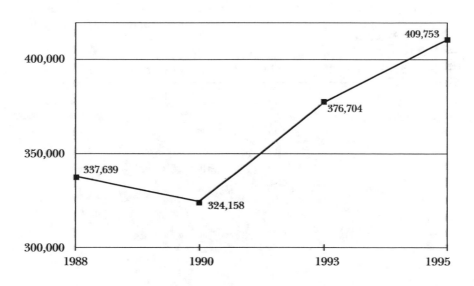

Source: 1988–95 NAPH Hospital Characteristics Survey Data
Number of Hospitals in Matched Set = 24

Safety-Net Hospitals Provide Disproportionate Levels of Medicaid, Medicare, and Uncompensated Care

Another defining characteristic of safety-net health systems is the huge proportion of care provided to Medicaid, Medicare, and uninsured patients. Payor mix, using gross revenues, is a good measure of the volume of patients because each unit of service is valued the same regardless of the payor. (Net revenue payor mix, on the other hand, measures how much payors actually reimburse hospitals for services.) Seventy percent of inpatient care provided in 70 safety-net hospitals studied was for Medicaid and self-pay individuals (typically, self-pay patients in safety-net hospitals are medically indigent individuals who cannot afford to pay for services), a proportion that jumps to 90 percent when Medicare patients are included (see Figure 7.2). For outpatient and emergency care, the proportion of Medicaid and self-pay visits was 77 percent (see Figure 7.3).

As safety-net providers, urban safety-net hospitals have historically provided large amounts of uncompensated care in their communities. Moreover, the level of uncompensated care (defined by AHA as bad debt and charity care, but excluding so-called "contractual allowances") provided by such hospitals has increased over time. Sixty-seven safety-net hospitals reported in 1995 incurring $5.8 billion in deductions from revenue for bad debt and charity care, for an average of just over $86

Figure 7.2 Inpatient Days for NAPH Members by Payor Source

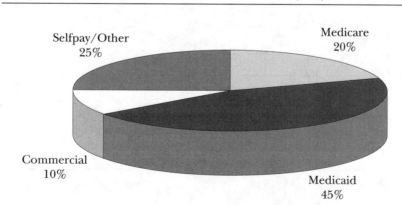

Selfpay/Other
25%

Medicare
20%

Commercial
10%

Medicaid
45%

Source: 1995 NAPH Hospital Characteristics Survey

Figure 7.3 Outpatient Visits for NAPH Members by Payor Source

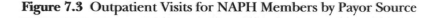

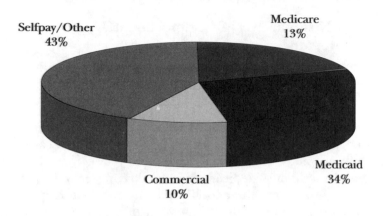

Source: 1995 NAPH Hospital Characteristics Survey

million per hospital. Bad debt and charity care charges represented 25 percent of total gross charges at these hospitals.

According to the AHA, $28.1 billion in bad debt and charity care was provided nationwide in 1994. The AHA data show that safety-net hospitals, representing fewer than 2 percent of all hospitals in the United States, provided more than 20 percent of the bad debt and charity care nationally in 1994. Moreover, the proportion of uncompensated care provided by these hospitals has increased since 1990. As a percent of total gross charges, bad debt and charity care charges increased from 26.0 percent in 1990 to 27.7 percent in 1995 for 33 hospitals for which data were available over that period.

Market trends indicate that uncompensated care is increasingly being concentrated among a smaller number of providers. The AHA data on public general hospitals in the 100 largest cities between 1980 and 1993 indicate that the category of self-pay patients increased from 16.8 percent of gross charges to 22.2 percent of gross charges, or an increase of more than 30 percent (Andrulis et al. 1995). Among private general hospitals during the same period, self-pay patients decreased from 7.4 percent of gross charges to 5.5 percent, a 26 percent decrease. Self-pay, as defined in the AHA survey, does not include Blue Cross or commercial payors or other governmental or nongovernmental sources of revenue. During the same period, the share of Medicaid patients among private general hospitals increased 15 percent, reflecting increasing competition for any patient with a payor source.

Safety-Net Hospitals Rely Disproportionately on Medicare, Medicaid, and Local Subsidies to Cross-Subsidize Uncompensated Care

A comparison of payor mix for gross and net revenues reveals that the huge amounts of uncompensated care provided by urban safety-net hospitals are subsidized by Medicare, Medicaid, and direct subsidies from state and local governments, unlike uncompensated care of most community hospitals, where it may be subsidized by commercial payors. Although Medicaid and Medicare combined represented 55 percent of gross revenues, they accounted for 61 percent of net revenues. Although self-pay patients accounted for 43 percent of outpatient visits and 28 percent of inpatient days, the combined direct local subsidies and other revenues for this population amounted to only 22 percent of collections (see Figure 7.4).

In effect, state and local subsidies today cover just over half the cost of uncompensated care in safety-net hospitals. To make up the difference, such systems finance uncompensated care primarily through Medicaid DSH payments (40 percent) and Medicare DSH payments (9 percent) (see Figure 7.5).

Figure 7.4 Net Patient Revenues for NAPH Members

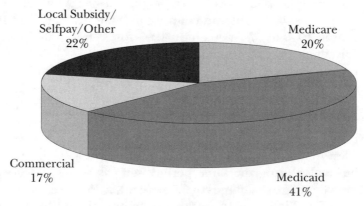

Source: 1995 NAPH Hospital Characteristics Survey

Figure 7.5 Sources of Financing of Uncompensated Care for NAPH
Members, 1995

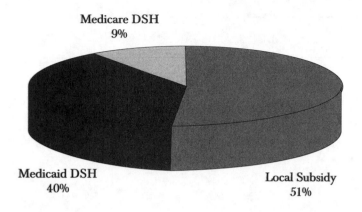

Medicare DSH
9%

Medicaid DSH
40%

Local Subsidy
51%

Source: 1995 NAPH Hospital Characteristics Survey
  Local Subsidy = $1.87 billion; Medicaid DSH = $1.44 billion; Medicare DSH = $0.32
billion

Although local subsidies continue to represent the largest proportion of funding for uncompensated care, such subsidies have been
declining for several years, while the proportion of Medicaid revenues, in
particular, has risen (see Figures 7.6 and 7.7). This rise is based largely
on the increase in DSH payments. But Medicare and Medicaid DSH
payments have also come under severe pressure in recent years.

The Medicaid DSH program was originally established in 1981 as
a means of assisting hospitals providing large volumes of care to low-
income and Medicaid patients. Throughout the early- and mid-1980s
the program was relatively small, but in the late 1980s and early 1990s,
DSH payments grew exponentially due primarily to creative (and to
some extent, abusive) financing mechanisms used by states to draw down
large federal matching payments. As of FY 1995, DSH payments totaled
$19 billion, of which $11 billion was federal and $8 billion was the states'
share. In 1991, and again in 1993, Congress closed some of the loopholes
that fueled this extraordinary growth, and capped future growth in the
DSH program. Despite the abuses in this program, it has, nevertheless,
provided crucial funding for hospitals that truly serve a disproportionate
share of low-income patients. However, DSH spending in both the Medicaid and Medicare funding has been targeted for further reductions in
coming years, both to reduce the deficit generally and to pay for other
programs or services in a "budget neutral" environment.

Figure 7.6 Local Subsidy and Selfpay/Other Revenues as a Percent of
Total Revenues for a Matched Set of NAPH Members,
1988–95

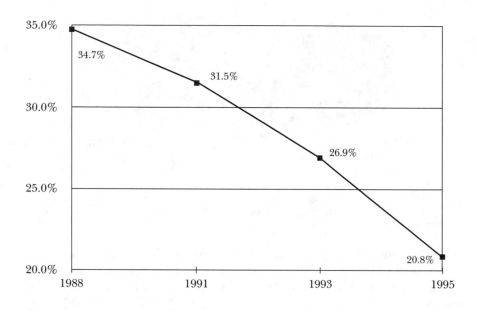

Source: 1988–95 NAPH Hospital Characteristics Surveys
Number of Hospitals in Matched Set = 30

Other current sources of funding for safety-net health systems
include Medicare medical education, grants to federally funded clinics
(Public Health Service Act granted under sections 330, 340, 326, etc.),
Medicaid and Medicare FQHC Reasonable Cost Reimbursement, state
general relief medical programs (i.e., state programs to provide non-
Medicaid coverage for the poor and uninsured), research funding (i.e.,
free care for research subjects), and other categorical federal funding
(e.g., the Ryan White Act). However, it is unlikely that these funding
sources will be adequate to make up for past and future reductions in
local subsidies and DSH funding. It is therefore essential to look for
other sources to help fund indigent care, as well as to seek competitive
or marketplace solutions to broaden the payor mix and base of support
for safety-net hospitals.

Figure 7.7 Medicaid Revenues as Percent of Total Net Patient
Revenues, 1988–95

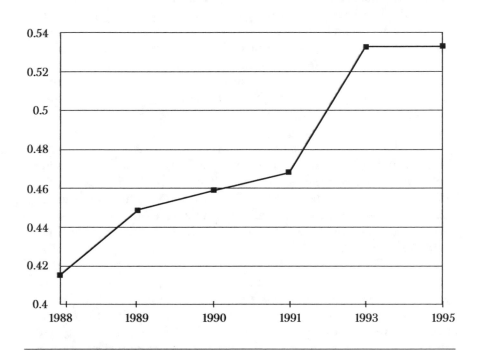

Source: NAPH Hospital Characteristics Survey

The Impact of Managed Care

The healthcare marketplace brings an entire series of other perils to bear
on other safety-net systems. In addition to constraints on their traditional
sources of funding, such systems today face significant pressures as a
result of the restructuring of the delivery and financing of care for the
patient populations traditionally served by such systems. This restructuring is primarily centered around the explosive growth in managed
care, both as a financing mechanism (through capitation) and as a way
to control costs and reform the delivery systems.

Although managed care has played a role in the delivery of healthcare in this country for decades, only in recent years has it been a
significant system for delivering care to low-income populations (Gage

and von Oehsen 1995). The explosion of Medicaid managed care has been a powerful one: Between 1992 and 1995 Medicaid managed care enrollment more than tripled to 11.6 million people, or nearly one-third of the Medicaid population. In 1995 alone, two-thirds of the states applied for Medicaid managed care waivers or expanded existing waivers to encompass broader populations. Yet, in the rush to expand managed care to ever greater portions of the Medicaid and low-income populations, relatively little effort has been made to protect the unique characteristics of the current healthcare delivery system for the poor. The trend has been to implement managed care first and iron out the kinks later.

The basic outline of state-based Medicaid managed care programs has been similar from state to state, but the details of the programs have varied widely across states. Some states have been more sensitive than others to the unique needs of Medicaid's vulnerable patient population and the safety-net providers. Some providers have been more assertive than others in shaping state or local managed care programs to meet these needs.

Whether Congress enacts sweeping Medicaid reform in the future, the trend among states to turn to managed care to gain control over Medicaid costs will only intensify. States will continue to seek and obtain flexibility in designing Medicaid managed care programs through the current waiver process. Moreover, federal reforms are inevitable. They will involve, at a minimum, a retooling of the Medicaid program to eliminate the need for waivers for most managed care activities.

The impact on safety-net providers can be devastating. The advent of TennCare, for example, nearly destroyed the Regional Medical Center at Memphis—a safety-net system for low-income patients from a three-state region—and severely damaged the Meharry Medical College and a range of other providers (Blumenthal and Meyer 1996).

Texas State Comptroller John Sharp has estimated that the Harris County Hospital District (HCHD) could lose between $72.3 million and $196.2 million in Medicaid funds over the next several years under a Texas managed care proposal. One result is that large urban public health systems such as HCHD is assured participation under the plan as an "historical" provider of care to Medicaid patients—but only for five years, and it is not at all clear what special advantages this status will convey (Sorelle 1995). The HCHD is also planning to enroll its own employees in its managed care plan, bringing revenues to the District and saving up to $10 million in health costs in the bargain.

Medicare is viewed by many observers as the next great frontier for managed care growth and expansion. The number of enrolled lives covered by risk-based plans has more than tripled in just six years from 1.2 million in 1990 to 3.9 million in 1996 (Health Care Financing Administration 1996). In 1995, more than 9 percent of total Medicare beneficiaries were enrolled in managed care plans (Fubini and Anonelli 1996), with some observers estimating that as many as 25 percent will enroll in such plans by the end of 1997. As of April 1996, approximately 45 percent of health maintenance organizations either had Medicare risk contracts or had applied for one, with a full 70 percent expecting to have risk contracts by 1997 (Zarabozo, Taylor, and Hicks 1996). This trend is sure to intensify in the coming years. By the year 2020, 17.5 percent of the population of the United States will be over age 65, as compared with just 12.7 percent in 1994 (Administration on Aging 1995). Despite some current apprehension, it is likely that more and more of the elderly will find managed care acceptable over the next several years, and that more and more employers will seek to shift their retirees into health plans with Medicare risk contracts.

Options for Protecting Safety-Net Health Systems

Although the general stability of Medicaid financing appears to be assured at this writing, due to the much slower rate of growth now projected for the next several years, it appears unlikely that major reforms or coverage expansions will be enacted at any time in the foreseeable future. While there appears to be some support for coverage expansions for children or the newly unemployed, any such initiatives are likely to be modest in scope, more like the incremental reforms of the 1996 Kennedy-Kasscbaum legislation than any of the Democratic *or* Republican proposals of 1993–94. At the same time, as is described eloquently elsewhere in this volume, the numbers of uninsured are actually increasing at a fairly alarming rate. These increases are caused, in part, by the actions of employers, the types of new jobs being created in the economy, and are the intended and unintended consequences of welfare and immigration reform laws passed in 1996. As a result, it is more essential than ever that policymakers consider measures to preserve and protect safety-net health systems that serve vulnerable patient populations—and that such systems also take steps of their own to improve their viability and competitiveness in their local health markets.

In support of a number of the proposals set forth elsewhere in this volume for expanding coverage, improved funding for FQHCs, etc., in the remainder of this chapter I focus on three areas that are directly applicable to safety-net health systems.

The Need to Reform DSH

Medicaid DSH is a sizable, stand-alone pool of federal funds that is not tied to specific services. Therefore, it is "the most vulnerable part of the Medicaid program," as HCFA Deputy Administrator Sally Richardson said in a speech to the NAPH at its conference in November 1996. If we assume that DSH reductions may be inevitable, the key question is how best to target those funds that remain. It has long been clear that only a portion of current Medicaid DSH spending flows to facilities that the DSH program was originally intended to support—hospitals providing significantly disproportionate amounts of care to low-income and uninsured patients. The remainder of the $19 billion in DSH funding—the level to which the program had grown by 1994—has been used by states for other purposes. In some cases, it has been paid out to a wide range of hospitals other than those originally intended to benefit from this program. Some states, for example, have used DSH funds to settle Boren Amendment lawsuits or to support entire categories of hospitals, such as rural facilities or state mental hospitals. Although savings can thus clearly be achieved in this program, a DSH targeting approach is also needed that will return the remainder of the program to its original purpose.

For all of the reasons set forth in this chapter, it is more important now than ever that the DSH program meet the original need for which it was created: assisting high-volume providers of care to the poor. Nevertheless, this need can be met with less than the full $19 billion currently allocated to DSHs. It is thus proposed to establish a "core" DSH program that would target a portion of current DSH funds to high-volume providers of care to the poor. By targeting a smaller pool of funds to those hospitals and health systems with the greatest need, the program can be returned to its original purpose of supporting an institutional healthcare safety net for the poor. Remaining savings in the program could be used for a variety of purposes.

It is important, as others have suggested (Davis 1996), that any DSH savings achieved be used to fund other services or coverage expansions. However, it is also essential that those DSH funds currently flowing to the highest volume safety-net providers be continued, even if some modest incremental expansions are achieved to support the vast need for uncompensated care and communitywide safety-net services that are certain to remain. Even if reductions are not proposed, the DSH statute is in need of modernization. The American healthcare system has undergone major change in the years since the original enactment of the program, and the statute no longer conforms to marketplace realities in a number of respects. For example, the DSH statute is focused primarily on inpatient hospital care, yet the marketplace incentives now dictate a shift toward more outpatient and primary care. Similarly, when the statute was enacted, most providers were uninterested in serving the Medicaid population, given the low reimbursement rates. Yet today, with Medicaid managed care and other forces in effect, competition for Medicaid patients is quite keen, whereas competition for the uninsured and other vulnerable populations remains nonexistent. In the long run, assuming Congress continues to be incapable of enacting any form of universal coverage, it may be best to convert a significant part of the Medicaid DSH program to some form of national indigent care trust fund, which could then be financed by a variety of sources.

The Need for Managed Care Safeguards

As states exercise their enhanced flexibility to expand their managed care programs, it is essential that safeguards be adopted to protect safety-net providers. In the frenzy to control Medicaid costs, states will continue to design managed care programs with single-minded devotion to their bottom line. At the same time, as revenues are squeezed across the industry, more providers and health plans than ever before are gearing up to compete for the Medicaid patient.

Safety-net providers traditionally have been the backbone of most Medicaid systems, and they will continue to play this role for the uninsured and the other vulnerable populations. There are a number of key issues to be addressed to protect such providers in the further development of Medicaid managed care. These issues include:

- tailoring licensure and other regulatory requirements to meet the needs of safety-net health systems that wish to develop their own managed care plans, either as provider-sponsored organizations, Medicaid-only plans, public plans, non-risk-bearing plans, or otherwise;
- adopting auto assignment procedures for individuals who do not select a plan—procedures that take into account the providers that traditionally serve such individuals;

- ensuring that all provider networks are accessible to plan enrollees and requiring all plans to contract with providers that traditionally serve low-income patients;
- imposing marketing protections essential to avoid improper enrollment of participants and skewed enrollment patterns;
- adopting managed care organization reimbursement guidelines that are sensitive to the needs of safety-net plans, including actuarially sound capitation rates, risk adjustments for plans enrolling high-risk populations, programs for high-cost populations, and enhanced rates for safety-net plans; and
- requiring plans to pay adequate provider reimbursement rates, including requiring that DSH and medical education payments continue to be made apart from plan premiums, and/or developing supplemental provider payments for those providers that continue to serve large numbers of ineligible, uninsured patients.

The Need for a Level Playing Field for Safety-Net Health Systems

With traditional sources of public revenues evaporating, and with new competitors for many of the traditional safety-net patients, these systems will have to rely on aggressive reforms of their own to keep pace and continue to finance their safety-net mission. The emergence of managed care as the predominant delivery model in the healthcare marketplace will require safety-net providers to develop strategies to compete in all segments of this environment.

Even if current funding sources can be protected and appropriate restraints placed on the growth of managed care, safety-net hospitals and health systems must recognize that they are part of an industry in which all hospitals are fighting for survival. Many will lose. If safety-net providers are to be among the winners, they must also begin to take matters into their own hands, take steps to level the playing field, and become better able to compete for all patients, not just the poor.

Success or survival in today's market will hinge on cost containment, patient satisfaction, demonstrated quality, and the ability to offer payors a fully integrated health system or one or more of its critical components. To respond to the challenges of capitation and greater patient choice, today's safety-net hospital must be able to demonstrate mastery—or at least substantial progress—in all of these areas. There are a number of different ways for safety-net hospitals to accomplish this, such as through mergers and partnerships with other systems or the development of their own integrated delivery systems. Fortunately, although it is not widely appreciated, many safety-net providers have already implemented such reforms. These systems are already positioning themselves not only to protect and preserve their ability to serve the uninsured and disenfranchised, but also to compete at the highest levels of quality and patient satisfaction with the rest of the industry.

One myth that continues to affect safety-net hospitals is the public perception that they are of lower quality than the rest of the industry—that theirs is inevitably going to be the second tier in a two-tier system. In fact, nothing could be farther from the truth. To be sure, there are financially troubled safety-net hospitals, including some with older physical plants that make them less attractive to the public at large. But this is also true today of many non-safety-net hospitals, at least in urban areas. At the same time, there are also many outstanding, award-winning safety-net hospitals that can and do compete with the best—or could, if public perception matched reality. The reality is that many safety-net hospitals have attained the highest levels of accreditation, clinical care, and patient satisfaction, even while filling their unique mission. By way of example, safety-net hospitals are disproportionately represented in a number of well-recognized categories of "excellence," such as among winners of the AHA's prestigious Foster McGaw awards, as well as in lists of "America's Best Hospitals," published annually by *Modern Healthcare* and *U.S. News and World Report.*

Many *public* safety-net hospitals have taken steps in recent years to restructure their governance and management to enable them to compete more effectively. In fact, there are as wide a variety of legal structures among urban safety-net systems in America today as in the hospital industry in general. Along with historically private institutions, in the past several years, a surprising number of public hospitals have restructured their governance and legal organization to become quasi-independent authorities or nonprofit corporations. Many have entered into mergers or affiliations with private institutions, and this trend seems to be accelerating. A recent survey of NAPH members indicated that fewer than a third remain under the direct ownership and operation of a city or county. The rest range over a wide spectrum of quasi-governmental or private structures and relationships.

Although it is by no means a panacea, reorganization can be an important tool to public hospitals and health systems. Reorganization can take many forms—from the straightforward restructuring of a city or county agency into a freestanding governmental entity (such as an authority, district, or public benefit corporation), to its conversion to a new nonprofit corporation, or to the privatization through sale or merger with an existing private nonprofit or for-profit organization.

Public hospital reorganizations are undertaken for a variety of reasons, with the reason often dictating the structure selected. Reasons range from the negative (taxpayer opposition to continued subsidies or fear of future increases in those subsidies) to the positive (a desire to improve the efficiency and competitiveness of a safety-net system—in effect to meet and beat the private sector on their own turf).

The goals of reorganization are usually multifaceted and include at least some of the following (Camper et al. 1996):

- enhance competitiveness;
- reduce or stabilize dependence on tax dollars;
- maintain public/safety-net mission;
- enhance access to capital;
- enhance professionalism and managerial autonomy;
- depoliticize operations;
- maintain public accountability;
- retain public funding;
- reduce financial risk to local government;
- reduce bureaucracy;
- streamline purchasing;
- improve personnel system;
- maintain medical education program; and
- improve patient care.

Another potent tool to level the playing field is a partnership, affiliation, or merger with other public or private organizations. Such efforts are not always without controversy and typically involve broad consensus building.

The merger of Boston City Hospital (BCH) and Boston University Medical Center (BUMC), for example, was implemented on July 1, 1996, and grew out of the 1994 report of a mayoral commission. The commission was charged with identifying the needs of the population served by BCH and developing recommendations to meet those needs in light of ongoing changes in the healthcare marketplace. The commission included representatives from the Department of Health and Hospitals, other city departments, BUMC, labor, community health centers, private teaching hospitals, and community organizations. The commission's credibility and broad representation facilitated the legislative, regulatory, financial, and operational changes needed to achieve both the reorganization of BCH into a freestanding governmental entity and the merger of that entity with BUMC.

Numerous other examples of successful safety-net restructuring or partnerships could be cited, including the Denver Health & Hospital Authority; the Cambridge Hospital; the University of Cincinnati; Brackenridge Hospital in Austin, Texas; Milwaukee County; John Doyne Hospital; the Detroit Medical Center; the St. Paul–Ramsey Medical Center; Memorial Medical Center of Savannah; the North and South Broward Hospital Districts; the Hawaii Health Systems Corporation; and the State University Medical centers of Maryland, Florida, Colorado, and West Virginia—among others.

Conclusion

The healthcare industry is undergoing a metamorphosis. The shift to managed care and other changes in delivery of care, new technology, and federal and state reimbursement pressures have placed public and other safety-net hospitals under increasing duress. Recent moves in Congress have exacerbated these pressures. Whatever direction the debate takes in the second Clinton administration, it is clear that safety-net health systems can no longer count on the federal government to maintain funding at even its previous level. The problem of preserving an institutional safety net is not merely for "those on the margins." Nor will the need for safety-net institutions magically evaporate if, as President Clinton and others suggest, Congress can begin enacting incremental expansions of coverage for certain targeted populations during his second term. In fact, there may be a considerable danger if either, in the name of cost containment and budget balancing, or of incremental coverage expansions, further erosion is permitted in the already fragile base of federal, state, and local/public and private funding sources for this institutional safety net. But the reality is that safety-net hospitals, as all hospitals, will continue to be squeezed by their payors. In addition to protecting and preserving their essential governmental funding sources, ways must also be found to broaden their base of support, empower them to establish integrated delivery systems and improve their quality and competitiveness—and otherwise level the playing field—in the overall health industry.

Acknowledgments

I am indebted to NAPH analyst Jennifer Tolbert and chief financial officer Lynne Fagnani for their outstanding work in gathering and analyzing the data included in this chapter.

References

Administration on Aging. 1995. *A Profile of Older Americans: 1995*. Washington, DC: U.S. Department of Health and Human Services.

Andrulis, D., A. Kellerman, E. Hintz, B. Hackman, and V. Beers-Weslowski. 1991. *Emergency Departments and Crowding in United States Teaching Hospitals*. Washington, DC: National Public Health & Hospitals Institute.

Andrulis, D., K. Ginsberg, V. Martin, and Y. Shaw-Taylor. 1995. *Urban Social Health, a Chartbook Profiling the Nation's Largest Cities*. Washington, DC: National Public Health & Hospitals Institute.

Blumenthal, D., and G. Meyer. 1996. "The Initial Effects of TennCare on Academic Health Centers." The Commonwealth Fund Task Force on Academic Health Centers. *Journal of the American Medical Association* 276 (9): 672–76.

Camper, A., L. Gage, B. Eyman, J. Myers, B. Carrier, and A. Lewis. 1996. *The Safety Net in Transition. Monograph II: Reforming the Legal Structure and Governance of Safety Net Health Systems*. Washington, DC: National Association of Public Hospitals.

Davis, K. 1996. "Incremental Coverage of the Uninsured." *Journal of the American Medical Association* 276 (10): 831–32.

Friedman, E. 1987. Public Hospital Series: "Public Hospitals: Doing What Everyone Wants Done, but Few Others Wish to Do"; "Demise of Philadelphia General, An Instructive Case: Other Cities Treat Public Hospitals' Ills Differently"; "Public Hospitals Often Face Unmet Capital Needs, Underfunding, Uncompensated Patient Care Costs"; "Problems Plaguing Public Hospitals: Uninsured Patient Transfers, Tight Funds, Mismanagement and Misperception." *Journal of the American Medical Association* 257 (11–14).

Fubini, S., and V. Anonelli. 1996. "Medicare HMOs—The Last Frontier." *Healthcare Trends Report* 10 (3): 1.

Gage, L. S., and W. H. E. von Oehsen. 1995. *Managed Care Manual: Medicaid and State Health Reform*. New York: Clark Boardman Callaghan.

Gaskins, D. 1996. "The Impact of Managed Care and Public Safety Policy Changes on Urban Safety Net Hospitals." Unpublished proposal, Institute for Health Care Research and Policy, Georgetown University Medical Center, Washington, DC.

Health Care Financing Administration. 1996. *Profiles of Medicare*. Washington, DC: U.S. Department of Health and Human Services.

Kellogg Foundation Commission on Public General Hospitals. 1978. *Hospital Research and Education Trust*. Kellogg Foundation.

Sheils, J., and L. Alecxih. 1995. *Recent Trends in Employer Health Insurance Coverage and Benefits.* Washington, DC: The Lewin Group, Inc.

Sorelle, R. 1995. "Hospital District Chief Views Medicaid Shift as Opportunity." *Houston Chronicle.* (30 July): 26.

Zarabozo, C., J. Taylor, and J. Hicks. 1996. "DataView: Medicare Managed Care: Numbers and Trends." *Health Care Financing Review* 17 (3): 243.

8

The Role of Academic Health Centers and Teaching Hospitals in Providing Care for the Poor

James Reuter
Darrell J. Gaskin

Academic health centers are cornerstones of the American healthcare delivery system. They have a unique combination of missions that includes care to the poor and medically indigent, medical education and training, basic and applied research on new medical practices and technologies, and the provision of state-of-the-art and technologically advanced healthcare services. Their mission of caring for the poor is a result of their history and tradition, their location in the center of our largest cities, and the fact that many are public institutions.

The origins of these missions go back to prerevolutionary times, when the first teaching and research hospitals were being established. In 1769, Dr. Samuel Bard gave a commencement speech to the first graduating class of King Colleges medical school in New York City. While urging the establishment of a hospital, Dr. Bard laid out what he believed the basic missions of this new institution should include: patient care, research, and teaching. In regard to patient care, Dr. Bard said, "Let those who are at once the Victims, both of Poverty and Disease, claim your particular Attention" (Larrabee 1971). This statement contributed to the founding of the institution now commonly known as New York Hospital, the second oldest hospital in the United States.

Dr. Bard's statement on the need to provide care to the poor was as much a reflection of the role of the hospital in eighteenth and

This work was supported by a grant from the Commonwealth Fund.

nineteenth century America as anything else. Middle- and upper-class patients were treated in their homes. Only the poor were left to seek care from hospitals. Yet, despite all the changes that have occurred during the intervening 230 years, Dr. Bard's vision remains valid as an expression of the missions of academic health centers today.

Although the missions have remained the same, the methods of financing have changed dramatically. As do most other providers, academic health center hospitals and other teaching hospitals finance much of their indigent care through an ill-defined system of internal transfers and subsidies from revenues earned providing care to paying patients. Publicly owned academic health centers and teaching hospitals also draw on state and local government subsidies, known as tax appropriations, that provide earmarked funds for specific programs as well as general operating support.

Unlike hospitals that are not engaged in teaching or research, academic health center hospitals also use patient care and tax revenues to subsidize their teaching and research missions. They provide direct subsidies to their affiliated medical schools and schools of allied health professions, to the training of interns and residents, to the costs of some clinical research, and to the high cost of keeping specialized, advanced technology services available. It is this unique balancing of multiple missions, and the competition among them for limited resources, that distinguishes the demands placed on the internal subsidies in academic health centers from the systems of internal subsidies in other hospitals, generally public institutions, that focus on providing care to the poor.

This chapter has three objectives. First, academic health centers are defined and their role in providing care to the poor and medically indigent in their communities is described. Second, the impact of the changing medical market on academic health centers and their missions is explored, including the impact on the provision of uncompensated care. Finally, the challenges for the future of academic health centers and their missions of providing care for the poor, teaching, and research are discussed.

Academic Health Centers and Care to the Poor

An academic health center (AHC) is defined as an entity that includes, at minimum, a medical school and one or more hospitals. Academic health centers often also include schools for training nurses, dentists, and other health personnel. Not all medical schools are part of an AHC. Some of the newer medical schools, established during the 1970s, rely on relatively loose affiliations with independent, local hospitals. Some AHCs include two or more hospitals. Depending on the exact definition used, there are currently between 115 and 130 hospitals that are closely integrated with medical schools and that are generally recognized as being part of an AHC.[1]

Nearly all AHC hospitals are located in urban areas, often in the central core of the largest U.S. cities. Only two AHC hospitals, those affiliated with the University of West Virginia and Dartmouth College, are not located within a metropolitan statistical area (MSA). Compared with other types of hospitals, a high proportion (44 percent) of AHC hospitals are publicly owned. However, unlike other public hospitals that are sponsored predominantly by county or municipal governments, two-thirds of the public AHC hospitals are sponsored by state governments. Academic health center hospitals are large institutions. Based on data from the American Hospital Association (AHA), they average just under 600 beds. In 1994 they had total net patient care revenues of approximately $35 billion, or an average of more than $275 million per hospital.

By virtually any measure used, AHCs and other major teaching hospitals are a major source of care for the poor and uninsured in their communities. To explore the role of the AHCs and teaching hospitals in the provision of care to the poor and uninsured in their communities, the amount of Medicaid and uncompensated care provided in the 76 MSAs served by at least one AHC hospital were analyzed. The universe of hospitals used for this analysis are the 1,708 hospitals located in 76 MSAs that include at least one AHC hospital. These hospitals are divided into three groups: AHC hospitals; other major teaching hospitals, defined here as hospitals that are not AHCs but are members of the Council of Teaching Hospitals (COTH); and all other hospitals.

Table 8.1 shows the level of uncompensated care and care to the poor by hospital type and ownership for the 1,708 hospitals located in one of the 76 MSAs with at least one AHC. Uncompensated care represents more than twice the proportion of gross patient revenues in AHC hospitals than in either of the other two categories of hospitals within these MSAs.

The high proportion of uncompensated care provided in AHC hospitals is due largely to the fact that public institutions are overrepresented substantially in the group of AHC hospitals. As mentioned above, 44 percent of these urban AHC hospitals are public. Public hospitals account for only 6.6 of the other COTH hospitals and 10.2 percent of all other hospitals in these MSAs. As shown in Table 8.1, the public major teaching hospitals (AHCs and other COTH member hospitals) have

Table 8.1   Medicaid and Uncompensated Care by Type of
Hospital and Ownership in MSAs with Academic
Health Centers, 1994

Type of Hospital	AHC (n = 125)	Other COTH (n = 151)	Other (n = 1,432)
Public			
Uncompensated care (percentage of gross patient revenues)	20.2	19.3	10.7
Medicaid (percentage of net patient revenues)	34.0	38.5	26.2
Private			
Uncompensated care (percentage of gross patient revenues)	5.8	4.4	4.5
Medicaid (percentage of net patient revenues)	13.7	16.2	10.4
Total			
Uncompensated care (percentage of gross patient revenues)	11.7	5.6	5.0
Medicaid (percentage of net patient revenues)	22.0	18.1	11.6

Source: Georgetown University calculations based on AHA tabulations of the AHA
Annual Survey of Hospitals, 1994.

the highest levels of both uncompensated care and care to Medicaid
patients. Private hospitals of all types provide much less care for Medicaid and uninsured patients. Within the groups of public and private
hospitals, hospitals that are part of an AHC have the highest levels of
uncompensated care.

However, the level of uncompensated care provided within each
hospital understates the importance of AHCs in providing such care in
their communities. Table 8.2 displays the shares of total uncompensated
care, Medicaid, hospitals, and beds provided within the 76 MSAs served
by an AHC by hospital type and ownership.

As shown in Table 8.2, although AHC hospitals account for only 16
percent of the total beds in these MSAs, they account for 37 percent of the
total amount of uncompensated care and 31 percent of total payments
to hospitals by Medicaid. Although approximately two-thirds of this care
is concentrated within the 54 public AHC hospitals, the private AHC
hospitals also contribute disproportionately to the total amounts of such
care provided in these communities.

Table 8.2 Shares of Care to the Poor Provided in MSAs with AHCs by Type of Hospital and Ownership, 1994 (in percent)

Type of Hospital	AHC (n = 125)	Other COTH (n = 151)	Other (n = 1,432)
Public			
Share of uncompensated care	26.2	4.3	7.4
Share of Medicaid	19.8	4.3	18.2
Share of hospitals	3.3	0.5	8.6
Share of beds	7.2	1.5	5.5
Private			
Share of uncompensated care	10.8	11.6	39.7
Share of Medicaid	11.5	18.7	37.7
Share of hospitals	3.7	7.4	76.4
Share of beds	8.2	14.0	63.1
Total			
Share of uncompensated care	37.0	15.9	47.0
Share of Medicaid	31.2	22.8	45.9
Share of hospitals	7.0	8.0	85.0
Share of beds	16.0	15.5	68.5

Source: Georgetown University calculations based on AHA tabulations of the AHA Annual Survey of Hospitals, 1994.

Academic Health Centers and the New Medical Market

As are all other providers, AHCs are being confronted by the need to compete successfully in the new market for medical services. Absent the creation of new sources of revenue or reductions in costs, their ability to cross-subsidize their existing missions, including their mission of providing care to the poor, depends on how well they are able to maintain their revenue streams by attracting paying patients. Increasingly, this means attracting the enrollees of the various types of managed care plans: traditional health maintenance organizations (HMOs), preferred provider organizations (PPOs), and other types of network plans. In 1995, 62 percent of the population in MSAs where AHC hospitals are located were enrolled in a HMO or other type of managed care plan.[2] Only three AHCs are in MSAs with less than 50 percent managed care penetration, whereas 18 are in MSAs with over 70 percent managed care penetration.

There are a variety of factors that place AHC hospitals at a disadvantage in the market for managed care patients. They are often located in the central core of cities, away from the more affluent suburbs where higher proportions of the population are insured. Their organizational structures and management processes can be more cumbersome. The hospital, the school of medicine, and the faculty practice plan may be under different ownership. Each may have its own administrative structure. But by far the most important factor is the cost of care in AHC hospitals. Competing health plans, acting rationally in their own economic self-interest, contract with providers who can render services at the lowest possible costs, consistent with providing care of a reasonable quality. AHC hospitals are usually the most expensive sources of care in a community and simply do not compete well on the basis of price.

There have been a variety of attempts to measure the impact of graduate medical education on the cost of care in teaching hospitals. The most well known is Medicare's indirect medical education (IME) adjustment. The IME adjustment factor was intended originally to reflect the additional costs borne by teaching hospitals due to their participation in graduate medical education, net of the effects of the higher complexity of patients treated and the wage structure in their localities. These indirect costs of graduate medical education are usually attributed to higher numbers of tests ordered by interns and residents, other inefficiencies caused by these trainees' lack of experience, a higher severity of illness for patients in teaching hospitals (beyond that reflected in the diagnosis-related group classification system), and the need for the hospital to stay at the forefront of technology and research. In AHC hospitals, the indirect costs of teaching also may include the inefficiencies created by the presence of undergraduate medical students.

According to the most recent estimates (Prospective Payment Assessment Commission 1996), the indirect costs of teaching increase a hospital's Medicare cost per case by approximately 4.5 percent for each 10 percent increase in the ratio of the number of interns and residents to beds (IRB). AHC hospitals have the highest IRB, averaging nearly six residents for every ten beds. With the formula estimated by the Prospective Payment Assessment Commission (ProPAC), the indirect costs of graduate medical education add approximately 23.5 percent to the costs of each case treated in an AHC hospital. The estimated direct costs of graduate medical education add 5.1 percent to AHC hospitals' operating expenses.[3] Thus, net of wages and measured case mix, AHC hospitals are approximately 29 percent more expensive than the non-teaching hospitals in their communities. Other teaching hospitals, with a lower IRB, generally are less expensive than AHCs.

It is important to note that, although the most recent estimate places the difference in costs at 4.5 percent for each 10 percent increase in the IRB, Medicare has been paying an adjustment equal to 7.7 percent for each 10 percent increase in the IRB. This level of the adjustment was arrived at through a political compromise that was justified, in part, by the idea that major teaching hospitals also provide significant amounts of uncompensated care that is not subsidized directly by Medicare. Although there have been a variety of proposals to reduce the IME adjustment, these have not been successful. As a result, the IME adjustment has provided an important cushion during the period of rapid change in the market for privately insured patients.

Perhaps because of their competitive disadvantages, AHC hospitals have not been successful in attracting or retaining their shares of managed care patients. Reuter and colleagues examined hospital discharge data for patients under age 65 to determine where HMO patients are being treated (Reuter et al., forthcoming). The study included data from eight MSAs, each with at least one AHC hospital and with high levels of HMO penetration in 1991, ranging from 19.8 percent to 50.8 percent. The analysis computed a "relative risk" of HMO patients being treated in a particular type of hospital, compared with the proportion of privately insured patients being treated in hospitals of the same type. That is, a relative risk of 1.0 for a particular type of hospital would indicate that hospitals of that type were attracting the same share of non-HMO patients as HMO patients. A relative risk of less than 1.0 would indicate that a type of hospital had a smaller share of the HMO market than its share of the privately insured market.

Figure 8.1 shows the relative risks of HMO patients using different types of hospitals as compared with other privately insured patients in 1988 and 1991. AHCs are clearly failing to attract HMO patients in the same proportions as other privately insured patients. Although the categories of other COTH and other large hospitals are seeing increasing shares of HMO patients, the relative risk of HMO patients being treated in AHC hospitals was 85 percent of their share of other privately insured patients in 1988, falling to only 62 percent in 1991. In other words, AHC hospitals are treating a relatively small share of HMO patients. And as HMO and managed care enrollment continues to grow, AHC hospitals may lose a significant proportion of their privately insured patients. This would have a significant impact on their ability to continue to cross-subsidize their missions, including care to the poor, out of clinical revenues.

Figure 8.1 Relative Risk of HMO Patients' Use of Teaching Hospitals
Compared with Other Privately Insured Patients, 1988 and
1991

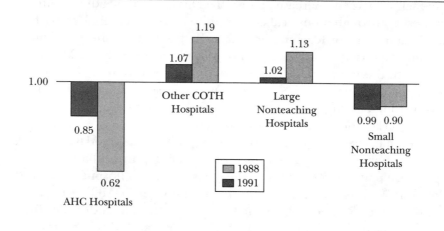

Source: Reuter et al., forthcoming.

There have been three factors that have allowed AHC hospitals to
maintain their revenues in spite of their failure to attract the growing
population of managed care patients. First, AHCs have benefited from
the political stalemate in Washington. There have been no Medicare
savings provisions enacted since 1993.

Second, many AHCs have been expanding their clinical enterprises. A few AHCs have purchased other hospitals, negotiated mergers, or joined networks. Others have established satellite clinics or purchased primary care practices. One measure of the growth in the clinical
enterprise of AHCs is the growth in the number of full-time clinical
faculty. According to the most recent data (Krakower, Ganem, and
Jolly 1996), the number of full-time clinical faculty increased by 11.8
percent between the 1992–93 and 1994–95 academic years. Over this
same period, the average faculty practice plan revenues generated per
faculty, in constant dollars, remained virtually constant at $133,000. In
effect, AHCs increased their clinical revenues by over $1 billion through
these expansions in faculty. Although most of these revenues were used
to support the operations related to the provision of these services, 13
percent was used to subsidize other activities of the medical schools and
their departments.

The third important contribution to AHCs' clinical revenues has been due to Medicaid disproportionate-share payments. Based on AHA data, while the number of Medicaid admissions in AHC hospitals remained virtually constant between 1989 and 1994, Medicaid revenues increased at an average annual rate of 20 percent. As a share of AHCs' net patient revenues, Medicaid increased from 14 percent in 1989 to 22 percent in 1994.

AHCs in competitive markets have also been working to control their costs. For example, AHC hospitals in high HMO penetration areas have limited their growth in staff. Between 1985 and 1993, personnel per 100 adjusted admission fell slightly, from 12.12 to 11.92, in AHC hospitals in high HMO penetrations. Academic health center hospitals in low HMO penetration areas increased their staff from 10.63 to 11.76 personnel per 100 adjusted admission.[4]

Reductions in the rate of growth in AHC hospital costs are related to the growth in managed care. Gaskin and Hadley (1996) used regression analysis to estimate a hospital technical cost function that related the costs of large urban hospitals to their patient volumes, input prices, and certain market factors, including HMO enrollment. Their analysis estimated the effect of HMO penetration on the rate of increase in hospital costs, controlling for other factors that may affect costs. These factors were patient volumes, hospital salaries, hospital capacity, patient mix, as well as fiscal pressure to contain costs. The results estimate the direct effect of HMO penetration on costs. The results, presented in Table 8.3, show that, net or all other factors, the increase of HMO enrollment reduced the rate of inflation in hospital costs between 1986 and 1993. Although the effect was greatest for nonteaching hospitals, an increase in HMO enrollment was associated with a drop in the annual rate of growth in costs in AHC hospitals. For AHC hospitals in areas with minimal HMO penetration (10 percent), the impact of

Table 8.3   Percentage Point Reduction in Hospital Cost Inflation Due to HMO Growth by Hospital Type, 1986–93

HMO Penetration Rate	10 Percent	25 Percent	40 Percent
Academic health centers	−0.59	−1.47	−2.35
Large other teaching hospitals	−0.53	−1.33	−2.11
Large nonteaching hospitals	−0.73	−1.82	−2.90

Source: Georgetown University analysis of data from the AHA Annual Survey of Hospitals, 1986–93.

HMO enrollment on costs was a reduction of 0.59 percentage points in the annual rate of inflation. For AHC hospitals in areas with substantial HMO penetration (40 percent), the rate of inflation in costs was reduced by 2.35 percentage points, from 8.80 to 6.45, the equivalent of a 26.7 percent reduction in the rate of inflation. These results were consistent for both public and private hospitals. A dummy variable for ownership was not significant in any of the equations estimated.

The overall effect of managed care penetration on the operating revenues and expenses of AHCs and other types of urban hospitals is shown in Table 8.4, which contrasts the experience in high and low HMO penetration areas.[5] Across all types of urban hospitals, higher HMO penetration was associated with slower growth in both revenues and expenses per adjusted admission. AHC hospitals and other teaching hospitals had higher growth in both revenues and expenses per adjusted admission than nonteaching hospitals. An important fact that emerges from these figures is that the gap in the relative costs of AHCs compared with other hospitals has grown larger. That is, the relative competitive position of AHCs became worse during this period.

The Impact of the Market on AHCs' Missions

Some of the efforts to reduce costs by AHC hospitals in competitive markets are coming at the expense of support for mission-related activities.

Table 8.4   Average Annual Change in Revenues and Expenses per Adjusted Admission by Teaching Status and HMO Penetration Area, 1985–93

Type of Hospital	HMO Penetration	Total Operating Revenues per Adjusted Admission %	Total Expenses per Adjusted Admission %
Academic health centers	High	9.24	8.34
	Low	11.15	9.96
Other teaching hospitals	High	9.31	8.28
	Low	9.84	9.11
Large nonteaching hospitals	High	7.15	6.96
	Low	10.53	9.68
Small hospitals	High	7.59	7.17
	Low	9.16	8.50

Source: Georgetown University calculations based on AHA tabulations of the AHA Annual Survey of Hospitals, 1985–93.

Between 1990 and 1993, expenses for graduate medical education in AHC hospitals in high HMO penetration areas grew at an average annual rate of only 6.6 percent, roughly half the rate of other operating expenses in these hospitals. In low HMO penetration areas, graduate medical education costs in AHC hospitals grew at an average annual rate of 10.7 percent.[6]

In spite of the evidence that AHC hospitals are including mission-related activities within the scope of their cost-reducing efforts, it does not appear that AHCs made any changes between 1989 and 1994 that significantly restricted access to care for the poor and uninsured. Table 8.5 shows the percent changes between 1989 and 1994 in uncompensated care as a proportion of gross charges and the share of uncompensated care provided in the community by hospital type and ownership for MSAs served by an AHC hospital.

Between 1989 and 1994, uncompensated care generally became more concentrated in public teaching hospitals. The share of uncompensated care provided by public AHC hospitals and other public major teaching hospitals each increased by more than one-third. The level of uncompensated care in other public hospitals increased by 12.4 percent. Private AHC hospitals appear to have maintained their level of effort; their amount of uncompensated care was unchanged. However, the data suggest that other private hospitals, including private teaching hospitals, are reducing their commitments to providing uncompensated care, leaving this burden to the public hospitals and private AHCs. Across all other private hospitals, uncompensated care decreased both as a percent of gross charges and as a percent of the total uncompensated care provided in the community.

Table 8.5   Percent Change in Amount and Shares of Uncompensated Care Provided in MSAs with AHCs by Type of Hospital and Ownership, 1989–94

Type of Hospital	AHC (n = 125)	Other COTH (n = 151)	Other (n = 1,432)
Public			
Level of uncompensated care	33.4	37.1	12.4
Share of uncompensated care in MSAs	30.2	29.3	−1.1
Private			
Level of uncompensated care	0.0	−11.1	−2.4
Share of uncompensated care in MSAs	−17.9	−20.2	−4.4

Source: Georgetown University calculations based on AHA tabulations of the AHA Annual Survey of Hospitals, 1989–94.

Looking to the Future

Thus far, AHC hospitals appear to be holding their own. Occupancy rates have remained high. They have, on average, been able to hold their costs below revenues. As a result, they do not appear to have taken any steps to set aside or dramatically deemphasize their long-standing mission of providing care to the poor and uninsured. However, this appearance of relative stability may be short lived.

Academic health centers are experiencing greater turmoil than these financial averages imply. One AHC hospital has been purchased by a for-profit corporation. The purchase of another is under active consideration. Several AHCs, including some of the nation's oldest, have merged, and additional mergers are under serious consideration.

Part of this turmoil is financial. Although AHCs may be doing well on average, some are doing very well, others are not. Fifteen AHC hospitals reported negative operating margins for the two most recent years for which data are available (1993 and 1994). Seven of those hospitals also had negative total margins in each of those two years.[7] Although most faculty practice plans reported increased revenues, the plans of 26 schools had decreasing revenues during the 1994–95 academic year (Krakower, Ganem, and Jolly 1996).

Academic health center administrators become even more concerned when looking toward the future. The IME adjustment under Medicare and the disproportionate-share payments under Medicaid have provided a significant cushion in recent years. These subsidies have enabled AHCs and teaching hospitals to maintain their commitments to their missions of indigent care, teaching, and research. However, both of these sources of revenues are under attack. Although new Medicare savings proposals have not been enacted since the Omnibus Budget Reconciliation Act of 1993, budget reconciliation will clearly be high on the agenda of the 105th Congress in 1997. Both the Clinton administration and Congress have previously proposed significant reductions in IME. The only question at the time of this writing is how low it will go when agreement on an overall bill is eventually reached. The status of Medicare's Hospital Insurance Trust Fund suggests that there also will be significant reductions in the payment updates.

Medicaid plans are moving rapidly to enroll beneficiaries in managed care arrangements. By 1995 nearly one-third of all Medicaid beneficiaries were in some type of managed care plan (Rowland and Hanson 1996). A case study of the initial experience under TennCare, the Medicaid managed care plan enacted in Tennessee in 1994, illustrates some of the potential issues that may face AHCs and other teaching hospitals as these types of reforms proliferate (Meyer and Blumenthal 1996). Initially, the supplemental funds for both charity and graduate medical education were suspended, although the graduate medical education payments were subsequently reinstated. Although the state of Tennessee expanded access, enrolling more than 400,000 new people in Medicaid, costs were controlled by the slashing of payment rates. In addition, the newly created managed care plans did not tend to use the available AHCs. One AHC in Tennessee reported an 80 percent drop in its Medicaid population.

Despite the fact that congressional proposals in 1995 to accelerate enrollment in Medicare managed care plans were not enacted, there are serious concerns about the long-range effects of growing enrollment in Medicare risk-contracting plans. Medicare enrollment in HMOs was 6.2 percent in 1994 and is projected to increase to 17 percent of beneficiaries by 2002 (Welch 1996).

In addition to the threats to AHCs' historical system of providing financial subsidies for their missions, AHCs are also having to cope with the more subtle effects of the growth of managed care on their teaching and research missions. The research mission may be affected in a variety of ways (Mechanic and Dobson 1996). First, clinical research requires access to patients. Managed care plans may either refuse to allow their patients to be research subjects or may create barriers to allowing their patients to participate in new projects. Second, third party payors have often (unknowingly) subsidized clinical research through payments for the routine care that is inextricably mixed with clinical research. As local markets become more competitive, plans are more likely to challenge these charges. Third, the research agendas of AHCs and managed care plans are different. Managed care plans are more interested in applied research, in answering questions about care for conditions that are common, expensive, or high risk. In contrast, academic researchers have focused more on basic research, with substantial focus on uncommon diseases and conditions.

Academic health centers' educational and training missions are also facing significant challenges related to the growth in managed care. The changes in medical technology and medical practice are moving care out of inpatient settings where medical education has traditionally been focused. Simultaneously, AHCs are being asked to reverse their decades-long trend toward greater specialization. An increase in the training of primary care physicians will place even greater emphasis on moving the focus of educational and training activities out of AHC hospitals and into community settings and on completing major revisions to medical schools' curricula.

The magnitude of the forces for change are such that some people are beginning to believe that AHCs will have to reinvent themselves, to take on some new form, if they are to serve the needs of the next century. This may or may not be true. But an obvious risk of any significant change is the possibility of leaving something behind that has real value, either to the organization itself or to society at large. Missions without supporting revenue streams, such as care to the poor and uninsured, would clearly fall into the category of "things that could be left behind."

So far there is no evidence that a process of revolutionary change has begun. Changes are preceding at an evolutionary pace. Nor is there evidence suggesting that the traditional mission of AHCs and teaching hospitals of providing care to the poor is being restricted and left behind. If anything, the opposite appears to be true. That is, while private nonteaching hospitals seem to be reducing their uncompensated care burdens, the public and teaching hospitals appear to be accepting an even larger role and commitment. But academic health centers are too important in the system of care to the poor for the potential long-range effects of these pressures to be ignored.

Notes

1. For this chapter, a list of 127 AHC hospitals developed at Georgetown University is used. This list is based, in part, on the membership lists of the Association of Academic Health Centers and the Association of American Medical Colleges. The list also includes other institutions that are generally recognized as part of the AHCs but that are not members of these two associations.
2. Inforum/The MEDSTAT Group, unpublished data from the Inforum 1995 PULSE Health Care Research Survey, the 1995 PULSE Managed Care Summary.
3. Association of Academic Medical Colleges, unpublished data from the 1994 Survey of the Council of Teaching Hospitals.
4. American Hospital Association, based on tabulations from the AHA Annual Survey of Hospitals, 1985 and 1993.
5. In this analysis, low HMO penetration areas were defined as having less than 10 percent HMO enrollment. High HMO penetration areas were defined as having greater than 15 percent penetration or having experienced at least a 10 percentage point increase in HMO penetration.
6. Association of Academic Medical Colleges, unpublished data from the 1990 and 1993 surveys of the Council of Teaching Hospitals.

7. Association of American Medical Colleges, unpublished data from the 1993 and 1994 surveys of the Council of Teaching Hospitals.

References

Gaskin, D., and J. Hadley. 1996. "The Impact of HMO Penetration on the Rate of Hospital Cost Inflation, 1984–1993." IWP #95-004. Institute for Health Care Research and Policy, Georgetown University, Washington, DC.

Krakower, J. Y., J. L. Ganem, and P. Jolly. 1996. "Review of U.S. Medical School Finances, 1994–1995." *Journal of the American Medical Association* 276 (4): 720–24.

Larrabee, E. 1971. *The Benevolent and Necessary Institutiion.* Garden City, NY: Doubleday & Company.

Mechanic, R. E., and A. Dobson. 1996. "The Impact of Managed Care on Clinical Research: A Preliminary Investigation." *Health Affairs* 15 (3): 72–89

Meyer, G., and D. Blumenthal. 1996. *The Initial Effects of TennCare on Academic Health Centers.* Task Force on Academic Health Centers. New York: The Commonwealth Fund.

Prospective Payment Assessment Commission. 1996. "Report and Recommendations to the Congress." Washington, DC: The Commission.

Reuter, J., D. Gaskin, J. Hadley, and D. Propp. Forthcoming. "HMOs Use of Academic Health Centers." IWP #96-103. Institute for Health Care Research and Policy, Georgetown University, Washington, DC.

Rowland, D., and K. Hanson. 1996. "Medicaid: Moving to Managed Care." *Health Affairs* 15 (3): 150–52.

Welch, W. P. 1996. "Growth in HMO Share of the Medicare Market, 1989–1994." *Health Affairs* 15 (3): 210–14.

9

The Hidden U.S. Healthcare Safety Net: Will It Survive?

Stuart H. Altman
Stuart Guterman

Much has been written about the growing number of uninsured in the United States and possible approaches for addressing this problem in the context of universal health coverage. There is also an increasing array of research studies that have documented the negative impact that being uninsured has on health status and the type of care received.[1] What is less well known is the amount of healthcare that is made available to those without insurance and those with very limited coverage. Much of this care is provided through the traditional "safety-net" healthcare delivery system, mostly funded or operated by various levels of government. What is happening to these traditional safety-net providers is discussed in other chapters in this volume.

An important adjunct to these publicly funded organizations in the safety-net chain is the care provided by the thousands of private community hospitals. Whether through the emergency room, other outpatient settings, or inpatient department, these hospitals accounted for $10.3 billion of the $13.5 billion in total uncompensated care losses in 1994 (see Table 9.1). This chapter focuses on the sources of funding for this safety-net care, the distribution of the burden of such care across types of hospitals, and, more important, whether this care will be available in the future at levels commensurate with the needs of the affected populations.

Financing the American Hospital

American hospitals received almost $290 billion in revenues in 1994.[2] Most of these funds were obtained from four sources: private patient

Table 9.1   Coverage of Uncompensated Care Costs by Government
Subsidies, 1980–94

	1980	*1986*	*1992*	*1994*
	In billions ($)			
Uncompensated care costs	3.9	8.9	14.9	16.8
Government subsidies	1.1	2.0	2.8	3.2
Uncompensated care losses	2.8	6.9	12.1	13.5
	In percent:			
Government subsidies as a proportion of uncompensated care costs	27.7%	22.3%	18.9%	19.3%

Source: Prospective Payment Assessment Commission analysis of data from the American Hospital Association Annual Survey of Hospitals.

care, Medicare, Medicaid, and other government payors. In addition, hospitals received other monies from private nonpatient care sources, including donations and auxiliary business activities. The relative importance of the four revenue sources varies greatly depending on the type of institution. For example, public institutions receive a far higher proportion of their funds from Medicaid and less from Medicare. At the other extreme, private nonteaching hospitals are much more dependent on privately insured patients, with private teaching hospitals falling somewhere in between. Important differences also exist as to whether each patient source pays fully for the care it uses, generates a surplus, or results in a shortage. These relationships are critical for how hospitals fund the free care they provide to those who cannot pay (Prospective Payment Assessment Commission 1995).

In response to a growing concern about people who lack health insurance or have limited coverage, government programs to support access to care have expanded substantially. In 1980, private pay patients accounted for 45.9 percent of total hospital patient care costs; by 1994, this proportion had declined to 36.8 percent.[3]

At the same time, the share of total hospital patient care costs accounted for by patients covered by government programs (predominately Medicaid and Medicare) rose from 48.5 to 56.9 percent.

For the most part, these government access programs were designed to compensate hospitals for the cost of care for low-income nonworking families, the elderly, and the disabled. This still left millions of limited-income Americans with little or no explicit financial protection against the high cost of healthcare expenses. In 1994, more than 39.7 million people, or 15.2 percent of the population, were uninsured at a given point in time (Prospective Payment Assessment Commission 1996, 45). This share was up from 12.9 percent in 1987 and 13.9 percent in 1990. Where do these people turn when they are in need of healthcare services? The answer is often the closest hospital.

Despite the fact that hospital care comprises a smaller share of personal healthcare spending than it did two decades ago, hospitals are still the most important single group of providers in the American healthcare system. In 1995, almost 40 percent of personal healthcare was provided by hospitals, down from almost 50 percent in 1980, but still almost twice as much as any provider group (Levit et al. 1996). Moreover, a large proportion of the services of physicians are provided in the hospital, and hospitals own many postacute-care facilities as well. Thus, hospitals are crucial in providing access to care to all populations, particularly people who face access problems because of a lack of funds.

Hospitals always have provided care to patients who cannot pay.[4] In 1980, the cost of this uncompensated care amounted to $3.9 billion nationwide (Table 9.1). This was 5.6 percent of hospitals' total patient care expenses in that year. By 1986, that amount had grown to $8.9 billion, or 6.5 percent of total patient care costs. In that period, uncompensated care costs grew 14.7 percent per year—almost three times the rate of general inflation (Table 9.2).

In addition to public programs specifically intended to cover the healthcare costs of certain populations, state and local governments provide limited subsidies to hospitals to cover the costs of uncompensated care.[5] However, government subsidies have consistently failed (and in fact are not intended) to match providers' costs for uncompensated care. In 1980, state and local governments contributed $1.1 billion toward the

Table 9.2 Growth in Uncompensated Care Costs and Government Subsidies, 1980–94 (in Percent)

	1980–86	*1986–92*	*1992–94*
Uncompensated care costs	14.7	8.9	6.1
Government subsidies	10.6	6.0	7.1
Uncompensated care losses	16.1	9.7	5.8

Source: Prospective Payment Assessment Commission analysis of data from the American Hospital Association Annual Survey of Hospitals.

costs of uncompensated care, covering 27.7 percent of those costs (Table 9.1). This left hospitals with uncompensated care losses of $2.8 billion. As the cost of healthcare services grew, such state and local government subsidies had trouble keeping pace. Between 1980 and 1986, even though these subsidies grew at an annual rate of 10.6 percent, hospitals' losses on nonpaying patients rose to $6.9 billion. Thus, by 1986 government subsidies offset only 22.3 percent of all uncompensated care costs. Moreover, this larger uncompensated care burden was weighing more heavily on a subset of institutions—the traditional safety-net providers, urban hospitals, public hospitals, and major teaching hospitals (Prospective Payment Assessment Commission 1991).

In the late 1980s, the potential financial problems facing safety-net hospital providers became more difficult. During the entire decade of the 1980s and into the 1990s, hospital costs were growing rapidly. Over the 12 years between 1980 and 1992, for example, hospital expenses per adjusted admission grew at an annual rate of 10.0 percent—more than twice the general inflation rate (Figure 9.1).[6] Only once, in 1984, when Medicare implemented its prospective payment system (PPS) to control hospital payments, did this increase fall below 7.5 percent. This sharp cost growth had several negative implications for uncompensated care losses: (1) With hospital care becoming ever more expensive, it became increasingly difficult for people to afford insurance coverage; and (2) the treatment of people without coverage became a larger burden for hospitals. Added to this problem, government subsidies grew much more slowly. Between 1986 and 1992, state and local subsidy funds to hospitals increased from $2.0 billion to $2.8 billion—an annual rate of 6.0 percent. At the same time, uncompensated care costs rose from $8.9 billion to $14.9 billion—an annual rate of 8.9 percent. With government subsidies covering less than 19.0 percent of uncompensated care costs, the annual losses for such care reached $12.1 billion by 1992.

On the positive side, especially for those hospitals with a high proportion of privately insured patients, revenue growth through the 1980s was more than sufficient to support the costs that hospitals experienced (Figure 9.1). In fact, as discussed below, the excess revenue from private patients was sufficient, on average, to cover the losses from uncompensated care. In 1993, this trend of large increases in costs and revenues stopped. Revenues per adjusted admission increased by only 5.5 percent over the previous year—the smallest rise in decades. Cost growth similarly slowed, with expenses per adjusted admission increasing by 5.8 percent. This deceleration continued in 1994, with the increase in expenses per adjusted admission falling to 1.6 percent—well below

Figure 9.1 Annual Change in Total Hospital Revenues and Expenses per Adjusted Admission, 1980–94 (in Percent)

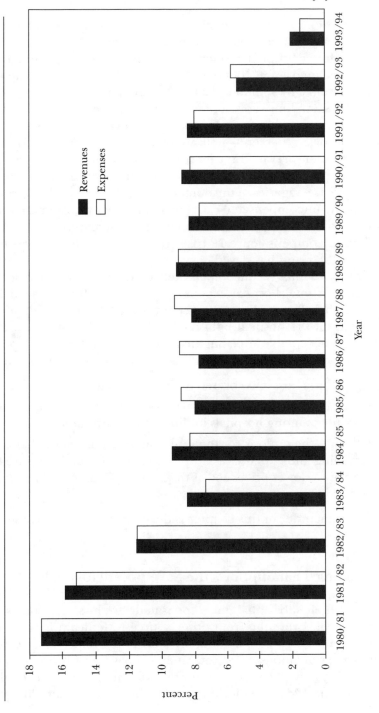

Source: Prospective Payment Assessment Commission analysis of data from the American Hospital Association Annual Survey of Hospitals.

general inflation. In fact, hospitals' success in keeping their costs below general inflation has lasted at least through 1996.

With slower hospital cost growth, the increase in uncompensated care costs declined as well. Between 1992 and 1994, uncompensated care costs grew from $14.9 billion to $16.8 billion, a rate of 6.1 percent per year. At the same time, government subsidies grew somewhat faster, at 7.1 percent per year. As a result, uncompensated care losses rose at an annual rate of 5.8 percent—well above the rate of inflation, but at a slower pace than prevailed for most of the previous two decades. Still, by 1994, hospitals were losing $13.5 billion on uncompensated care.

Despite the vagaries of uncompensated care costs and government subsidies, the uncompensated care burden borne by hospitals has been relatively stable. The proportion of total hospital resources used in providing uncompensated care rose from 5.5 percent in 1980 to 6.4 percent in 1986, and has stayed between 5.9 and 6.2 percent since then (Figure 9.2). Similarly, uncompensated care losses, which rose from 3.9 percent of total hospital expenses in 1980 to 4.9 percent in 1986, have stayed between 4.7 and 4.9 percent through 1994. It might appear, therefore, that the hospital industry has kept its uncompensated care burden at an acceptable level. But this apparent stability masks important differences among types of institutions and raises several questions:

- How have hospitals covered their losses on uncompensated care?
- Has this ability to finance uncompensated care been evenly distributed among hospitals in different circumstances?
- What is the outlook for the future in maintaining the balance in funding and expenses as hospitals face continued pressure from payors to lower prices and as the number of uninsured continues to grow?

The remainder of this chapter is devoted to analyzing these questions.

The Funding That Supports the Safety-Net Hospital

To support their substantial uncompensated care losses, hospitals must generate surplus revenue from other sources. Medicaid is an obvious source, because its purpose generally is to improve access to care for low-income populations. However, Medicaid payments historically have been below estimated costs of care for the patients covered. Through the first half of the 1980s, Medicaid payments hovered around 90 percent

Figure 9.2 Uncompensated Care Costs and Losses as a Percentage of Total Hospital Expenses

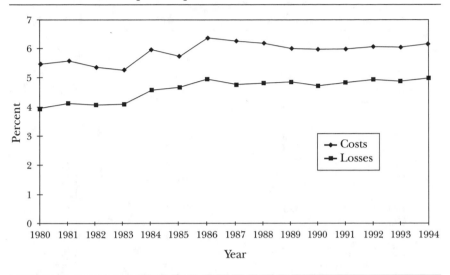

Source: Prospective Payment Assessment Commission analysis of data from the American Hospital Association Annual Survey of Hospitals.

of the costs of treating Medicaid patients (Table 9.3). Between 1986 and 1989, the ratio of Medicaid payments to costs fell from 88.2 to 75.8 percent.[7] This reflected a combination of rapidly rising hospital costs and expanding Medicaid eligibility that outstripped the availability of funds to pay for hospital care. The period from 1989 to 1992 saw a sharp increase in the Medicaid payment-to-cost ratio, primarily fueled by a vast influx of Medicaid disproportionate-share payments. This source of funding leveled off after 1992, but the sharp decline in hospitals' cost growth resulted in a continued rise in the payment-to-cost ratio. By 1994, this ratio had reached 93.7 percent, higher than at any time during the study period. At this rate, Medicaid payments probably exceed the marginal or added direct costs of treating Medicaid patients in most hospitals, but provide little in the form of excess payments to help subsidize the losses from uncompensated care. There is concern, however, that as states increasingly turn to Medicaid managed care it could result in lower payment-to-cost rates for those hospitals with the largest concentrations of such patients.

Medicare, the largest single source of hospital revenue, also has not been a consistently viable source to help support uncompensated

Table 9.3 Payment-to-Cost Ratios by Payor Category, 1980–94
(in Percent)

Year	Medicaid	Medicare	Private
1980	90.5	95.8	112.4
1981	92.9	97.2	112.1
1982	90.8	96.0	114.5
1983	92.0	96.8	115.5
1984	88.2	98.0	116.2
1985	90.4	101.1	115.6
1986	88.2	100.7	115.9
1987	83.0	98.2	119.9
1988	79.7	94.2	121.7
1989	75.8	91.4	121.6
1990	79.7	89.2	126.8
1991	81.6	88.4	129.7
1992	90.9	88.8	131.3
1993	93.1	89.4	129.3
1994	93.7	96.9	124.4

Source: Prospective Payment Assessment Commission analysis of data from the American Hospital Association Annual Survey of Hospitals.

care. Until PPS began in 1983, Medicare paid hospitals their costs, subject to certain limitations on allowed and covered services. For this reason, the Medicare payment-to-cost ratio was somewhat below 100 percent in the early 1980s, reflecting the 3–4 percent of costs that were not reimbursable (Table 9.3). With the implementation of PPS, the Medicare payment-to-cost ratio rose sharply, reaching 101.1 percent in 1985 and 100.7 percent in 1986.[8] Thereafter, as hospital costs rose and Medicare payments were more effectively constrained, the ratio of Medicare payments to costs fell to 88.4 percent in 1991. As with Medicaid, the decline in hospital cost growth has led to a rise in the Medicare payment-to-cost ratio in recent years. By 1994, the ratio had reached 96.9 percent—comparable with the level under cost-based reimbursement. But here, too, hospitals generated little in excess payments to cover the growing costs of uncompensated care.

These data show that hospitals, in the aggregate, have not been able to use Medicaid and Medicare to offset their uncompensated care losses. Two points are raised here, however. First, the aggregate flows of funds mask considerable variation across hospitals. Some hospitals receive subsidies through Medicaid disproportionate-share payments that tend to be targeted specifically toward major public hospitals. These subsidies can be substantial; total Medicaid disproportionate-share payments totaled $18.5 billion in FY 1994 (*Federal Register* 1994). Medicare also targets disproportionate-share payments to large urban hospitals with a high proportion of poor patients; these payments were estimated at $3.4 billion in FY 1994 (Prospective Payment Assessment Commission 1994). Second, the high rate of hospital cost growth between 1980 and 1992 made it next to impossible (and, moreover, inappropriate) for public programs with limited funds to keep up. But as cost growth has slowed more recently, without an equal reduction in payments, the payment-to-cost ratios for both Medicaid and Medicare have risen sharply, thereby lessening the added burden placed on excess private payments to cover the shortfalls from uncompensated care and from government programs. In fact, by 1997 the payment-to-cost ratio for Medicare may well exceed 100 percent.

Figure 9.3 Gains or Losses from Medicare, Medicaid, and Uncompensated Care as a Percentage of Total Hospital Expenses, 1980–94

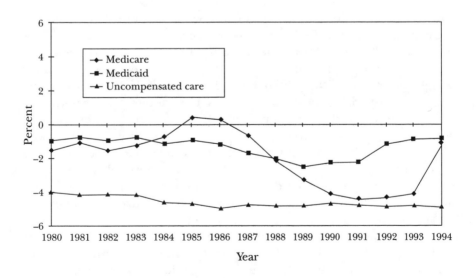

Source: Prospective Payment Assessment Commission analysis of data from the American Hospital Association Annual Survey of Hospitals.

To better understand the trends in net gains and losses from Medicaid, Medicare, and uncompensated care, they are shown separately in Figure 9.3. The patterns of revenue and cost were composed of four distinct trends between 1980 and 1994. Between 1980 and 1983, the pattern was fairly stable; uncompensated care losses were between 3.9 and 4.1 percent of total hospital costs, and Medicaid and Medicare losses were relatively level. Between 1983 and 1986, Medicare provided some surplus in the aggregate, as the initial PPS payments were set quite high and hospital cost growth paused. Meanwhile, both Medicaid and uncompensated care losses increased. From 1986 through 1992, uncompensated care losses were relatively stable, while Medicaid losses increased and then were offset by the jump in Medicaid disproportionate-share funding beginning in 1993. But Medicare went from providing gains equal to 0.3 percent of total hospital costs to losses of 4.4 percent. This occurred as Medicare restricted the growth in hospital payments, while hospital costs continued to grow at their historically rapid rate. In the final period, 1992–94, losses from uncompensated care and Medicaid remained fairly stable, but Medicare losses decreased from 4.4 to 1.2 percent of total hospital costs.

The Critical Role of Private Patient Revenues

Not surprisingly, surplus payments from private patients have been the primary source of help for hospitals to pay for uncompensated care losses during the 1980s. In 1980, payments from private patients exceeded costs by 12.4 percent (Table 9.3). As late as 1986, the payment-to-cost ratio for private payors was still at 115.9 percent. In the second half of the decade, even with costs rising, hospitals were able to generate private payments sufficient to expand the surplus. While hospital expenses per adjusted admission rose at a rate of 8.6 percent between 1986 and 1992, the ratio of payments to costs for private payors rose from 115.9 percent to 131.3 percent. With this influx of additional revenues, hospitals were able to expand services to the poor, despite escalating costs, and still keep total margins—revenues minus costs—above levels that had been achieved prior to the early 1980s.

The importance of the private payor surplus can be seen most clearly in Figure 9.4. In the top segment of the figure, the surplus of private payor payments relative to total hospital expenses are shown, and the bottom segment shows the losses from nonpaying patients and the shortfalls from Medicaid and Medicare as offset by a slight surplus from other government payors, again as a percentage of total hospital

Figure 9.4 Losses from Public Payors and Uncompensated Care versus Gains from Private Payors as a Percentage of Total Hospital Expenses, 1980–94

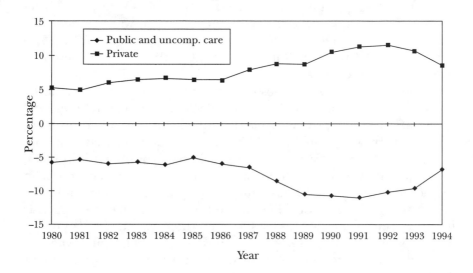

Source: Prospective Payment Assessment Commission analysis of data from the American Hospital Association Annual Survey of Hospitals.

expenses.[9] The inverse relationship between these two trends is quite clear. This strongly reinforces the theory that, at least through the early 1990s, hospitals had the ability to adjust the revenue flow from privately insured patients to compensate for losses they incurred in treating government and uninsured patients (or vice versa). This phenomenon has been labeled "cost shifting." Although cost shifting is inconsistent with a competitive market, in which institutions price services to maximize profits, it is consistent with the hospital environment of the 1970s and 1980s that was dominated by not-for-profit and public institutions on the one hand and private insurance that had limited power to control usage or prices on the other hand.

As seen in Figure 9.4, private payors have provided gains that offset losses from the major public programs and uncompensated care. In 1980, losses from public payors and uncompensated care were equal to 5.8 percent of total hospital costs, whereas gains from private payors were equal to 5.5 percent of costs. In 1986, public and uncompensated

care losses were still 5.9 percent, whereas private payor gains had risen
to 6.6 percent of total costs. By 1992, losses from public and nonpaying
patients had risen to 10.3 percent of total costs, but private payor gains
had jumped to 11.8 percent.

After 1992, private payors became more resistant to payment increases. In fact, despite the sharp decline in cost growth between 1992
and 1994, the payment-to-cost ratio for private payors fell from 131.3
percent to 124.4 percent (Table 9.3). That is, the growth in revenues
from private patients was even less than the very small growth in hospital costs. Fortunately, total losses from uncompensated care and the
shortfalls from Medicare and Medicaid declined. To be sure, there still
is a sizable surplus of private payments available to cover other shortfalls,
but there is growing concern that if the number of uninsured continues
to grow and the downward trend in the private payor surplus continues,
the surplus that remains will be inadequate for the task. This problem
will become even more serious if the relatively favorable payments from
Medicare and Medicaid decline in the future. This may be especially
true for some hospitals. There is ample evidence that the size of the
private payment surplus varies quite substantially by hospital type and
location and is directly related to the proportion of an institution's
patients that are privately insured. As the overall surplus shrinks, it has
a disproportionately negative impact on institutions that are important
safety-net providers and have a limited private patient census.

Distribution of Uncompensated Care Burden across Hospitals

Both the burden of uncompensated care and the ability to generate
funds to support that care vary considerably across hospitals (Table 9.4).
Hospitals located in large urban areas (metropolitan statistical areas with
populations of one million or more) devoted 6.2 percent of their total
resources to uncompensated care in 1994, compared with 5.1 percent
for rural hospitals. Except for public major teaching hospitals (facilities
with at least 25 residents for every 100 beds), there was little difference
among teaching categories. For that group of hospitals, 17.6 percent of
their total costs were used to provide uncompensated care. Hospitals that
received Medicare disproportionate-share payments provided a larger
share of their care to nonpaying patients, especially in large urban areas.
And the uncompensated care share for urban government hospitals was
14.2 percent compared with 4.6 percent for private voluntary hospitals
and 4.0 percent for proprietary hospitals.

Table 9.4   Share of Total Hospital Costs by Payor Category, by
Hospital Group, 1994 (in Percent)

Hospital Group	Uncom- pensated Care	Medicaid	Medicare	Other Government	Private
Large urban	6.2	16.5	35.7	1.6	37.0
Other urban	5.4	12.4	42.1	1.7	36.3
Rural	5.1	12.6	46.9	1.2	32.3
Major teaching, public	17.6	36.4	17.8	5.8	19.1
Major teaching, nonpublic	5.1	16.2	34.7	1.2	38.8
Other teaching	4.7	11.9	41.3	1.3	38.1
Nonteaching	4.8	10.7	44.9	1.3	36.6
Disproportionate-share, large urban	7.7	21.1	33.4	2.2	33.0
Disproportionate-share, other urban	6.1	14.8	40.0	2.0	34.9
Disproportionate-share, rural	6.0	16.4	45.0	1.7	29.3
Nondisproportionate-share	4.0	7.7	44.5	1.0	40.1
Voluntary	4.6	12.8	40.4	1.3	38.2
Proprietary	4.0	11.1	45.7	0.9	37.5
Urban government	14.2	28.4	26.0	4.2	24.5
Rural government	5.9	13.7	46.2	1.1	31.1

Source: Prospective Payment Assessment Commission analysis of data from the American Hospital Association Annual Survey of Hospitals.

Note: Disproportionate-share hospitals identified according to Medicare payment rules.

Not surprisingly, the groups hospitals that served the largest share of Medicaid patients were the same ones that provided the largest share of uncompensated care. Uncompensated care and Medicaid combined accounted for 54 percent of the total costs incurred by the public major teaching group during this period. In contrast, groups of hospitals that focused on treating Medicare patients had the smallest uncompensated care and Medicaid patient populations. The share of total costs accounted for by private payors did not vary as much, but these payors are crucial in providing the surplus funding to support the safety net. For most groups, the private payor share has been between 30 and 40 percent, with public major teaching hospitals (19.1 percent) and urban government hospitals (24.5 percent) constituting important exceptions.

Because the gains or losses from each payor depend not only on the number of patients, but on payors' payment policies, it is important to examine the pattern of those gains and losses for different groups of hospitals. As might be expected, public major teaching hospitals bear the largest uncompensated care burden in terms of loss (Table 9.5). Also, Medicare disproportionate-share hospitals bear a larger uncompensated care burden in the aggregate than other hospitals. Proprietary hospitals bear the smallest burden. Proprietary hospitals also had the smallest Medicaid losses among the ownership categories. Voluntary hospitals, on the other hand, had the largest Medicaid losses.

Medicare provides additional payments to teaching and disproportionate-share hospitals, and this special treatment is reflected in the

Table 9.5   Gains or Losses by Payor, by Hospital Group, 1994 (in Percent)

			Gains or Losses as Percent of Total Costs			
Hospital Group	Total Gains	Uncom-pensated Care	Medicaid	Medicare	Other Government	Private
Large urban	4.2	−4.8	−1.7	−1.9	0.2	9.0
Other urban	6.5	−4.7	−1.4	−3.6	0.2	13.0
Rural	5.9	−4.7	−1.3	−3.7	0.5	12.5
Major teaching, public	2.3	−8.0	−0.5	−0.3	0.9	6.5
Major teaching, nonpublic	3.8	−4.7	−1.7	−1.1	0.2	7.3
Other teaching	5.4	−4.6	−1.2	−2.9	0.1	10.8
Nonteaching	6.1	−4.5	−1.7	−3.7	0.2	13.1
Disproportionate-share, large urban	3.5	−5.6	−1.7	−0.8	0.2	8.3
Disproportionate-share, other urban	6.9	−5.1	−1.5	−2.7	0.3	12.9
Disproportionate-share, rural	6.0	−5.7	−1.5	−3.4	0.3	13.7
Nondisproportionate-share	5.6	−3.9	−1.1	−4.3	0.2	11.7
Voluntary	4.9	−4.5	−1.7	−2.9	0.1	10.6
Proprietary	12.3	−4.0	−0.6	−0.7	0.3	16.1
Urban government	3.2	−6.7	−1.1	−1.8	0.7	8.7
Rural government	5.3	−4.6	−1.1	−4.3	1.0	11.7

Source: Prospective Payment Assessment Commission analysis of data from the American Hospital Association Annual Survey of Hospitals.
Note: Disproportionate-share hospitals identified according to Medicare payment rules. Other governmet gains include government subsidies in excess of uncompensated care costs for individual hospitals.

pattern of Medicare losses.[10] Major teaching hospitals have much lower Medicare losses than the other groups, and disproportionate-share hospitals located in large urban areas, which receive the bulk of disproportionate-share payments from Medicare, also fare considerably better than average. Proprietary hospitals generally do not have characteristics that are accorded special treatment by Medicare, but they have held their cost growth well below that of other hospitals and so have smaller Medicare losses.

Voluntary hospitals that make up the majority of the safety-net institutions had losses on government payors and uncompensated care that totaled 9.1 percent of their total costs. This compared with a much lower rate of 5.3 percent for proprietary hospitals. The voluntary hospital loss rate was remarkably similar to that for urban government hospitals and rural government hospitals.

The overall financial status of hospitals in each group depends on their ability to offset losses from public payors and uncompensated care with gains from private payors. Hospitals in large urban areas have smaller gains from private payors than hospitals in other areas, and they fare worse overall, as represented by the total gains shown in Table 9.5.[11] Similarly, major teaching hospitals (public and nonpublic) have smaller gains from private payors and lower total gains. This pattern holds across all of the hospital groupings that have been examined. Of note is proprietary hospitals' 16.1 percent gain from private payors. This large gain, the result of an above-average private payor share and a high payment-to-cost ratio from those payors, combined with the smallest loss from public payors and uncompensated care, yields a 12.3 percent total gain for this group—almost twice as high as for any other hospital category.

The Effect of Increasing Financial Pressure on the Distribution of Uncompensated Care

The increasingly price-competitive nature of the healthcare marketplace raises concerns about hospitals' ability to provide care to the poor in the future. Indications are that private payors, which traditionally have provided the funding that has underwritten hospitals' losses from care to the poor, are continuing to resist payment increases. Thus far, hospitals have responded by maintaining a slower rate of cost growth that would have been unthinkable just a few years ago—the fourth quarter of 1996 was the tenth of the past 13 quarters in which the increase in expenses per adjusted admission has been at or below the general rate of inflation.

Figure 9.5 Change in Hospitals' Uncompensated Care Losses, by
Change in Private Payor Payment-to-Cost Ratio, 1992–94

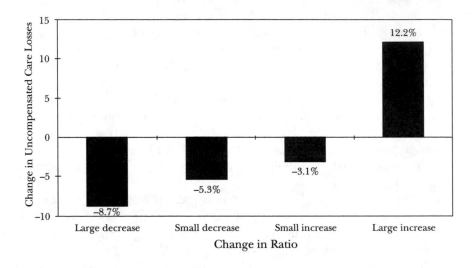

Source: Prospective Payment Assessment Commission analysis of data from the American Hospital Association Annual Survey of Hospitals.

Continued payment pressure may have other effects on hospitals, however. Of particular concern is the likelihood that hospitals faced with a declining surplus from private patient care will cut back the amount of services made available to those who cannot pay. An early example of this serious potential problem can be seen when comparing the changes in uncompensated care provided by hospitals that experienced the largest decline in private payor surplus with those institutions where the decline was more modest. When hospitals are grouped by the change in their payment-to-cost ratio from private payors between 1992 and 1994, a distinct pattern emerges (Figure 9.5). Hospitals that experienced the largest decrease in that ratio (10 percent or more) reduced their uncompensated care losses as a percentage of their total hospital costs by an aggregate 8.7 percent. Hospitals with large increases in the surplus *increased* their uncompensated care losses by 12.2 percent. Overall, uncompensated care losses as a percentage of total hospital costs decreased by 2.7 percent between 1992 and 1994. That is, hospitals with the highest declines in private payor surplus had declines in uncompensated care costs more than three times the average.

The hospitals that were most affected by the increased pressure from private payors, moreover, were the hospitals for which private payors accounted for the largest share of costs. These hospitals tended to be those with the lowest uncompensated care burdens before the declines. This trend indicates that growing price pressure from private payors may lead to a further concentration of nonpaying patients, and an increase in the corresponding losses among hospitals that already serve the highest proportion of those patients, straining further the safety net that provides care to the uninsured.

A Worst-Case Scenario

In November 1995, the Council on the Economic Impact of Health System Change developed a series of projections, assuming a tightening in the eligibility for Medicaid coverage and a continued decline in employer-sponsored health insurance coverage.[12] Under a worst-case scenario, it was assumed that Medicaid enrollment would be frozen at 1995 levels and the number of people with employer-sponsored insurance would decline in accordance with the downward trend in the employer-sponsored insurance rate from 1989–93 (Thorpe 1995). That is, fewer Americans would be insured through the employment market and none of the people in the increasing number of uninsured would be eligible for Medicaid coverage. Under such assumptions, if hospitals were willing to provide the increased uncompensated care required, it would result in net uncompensated care costs of $34.4 billion by 2002. This would translate into an increase in these unreimbursed costs of approximately $20 billion from 1995. If this situation were allowed to develop, and even if hospitals continued to generate the net surpluses from private patients as they have in the recent past, net margins (profits) would fall to −5.4 percent in 2002. The situation would be even more serious if the negative trend in net private patient surplus were projected to continue.

Because continued large negative margins are not possible, a more likely result would be sharp reductions in the availability of care in most institutions for those who cannot pay. This would leave the most "hard-core" safety-net hospitals with free care burdens not seen since the early 1960s. It also raises the very real possibility that millions of people in need would not receive care. Of course, new government programs could be developed to fill the gap, but they would have to be quite large—and this seems politically untenable in the current environment.

Although this illustration is a worst-case scenario, the negative pressures on each of the key factors that affect the availability of free care for the uninsured are very real. Price competition in the health sector is likely to continue, as is tightening in the eligibility for Medicaid coverage and reductions in the amount of employer-sponsored insurance and a less generous payment system from Medicare. It is hard, therefore, to imagine that the problems confronting the uninsured will not be worse in the future.

Conclusions

Safety-net healthcare providers have generally been the institutions that provide the bulk of care to the poor and receive the majority of their support from government funds. However, there also exists a "hidden safety net" composed of private hospitals that have provided substantial amounts of free care over the years. This free, or uncompensated, care has been supported primarily by private payors whose payments for care have exceeded the cost of that care. Public hospitals, too, have relied on these private patient subsidies to help them fulfill their broader social missions. Recently, private payors have become much more price conscious and have forced hospitals to lower their cost growth. Indirectly, this price competition has also put pressure on the amount of free care these institutions make available. This price pressure, therefore, threatens to weaken the hidden safety net for patients who lack the financial capacity to pay the high cost of healthcare. The question for the future is, "Even if government subsidy payments continue, what will happen to the broad availability of free care if the private payor subsidy amount is cut back?"

These trends leave us with a difficult balancing act. On one side, the increased pressure from private payors has been in response to growing concern about the rise in healthcare costs—an issue that dominated a presidential campaign in 1992 and has loomed large in the policy arena ever since. Curbing the rapid growth of government healthcare spending is also at the center of attempts to balance the federal budget, and has become a central issue in state and local finance as well. On the other side, the American people have expressed a desire to maintain access to healthcare for the entire population. Fulfilling this desire, however, will require either new programs to cover the uninsured, expanded categorical spending, or an increased willingness and ability of both public and private insurers to pay more than necessary for the care received by their insured. Assuming that this nation does not create some form of expanded coverage for the uninsured in the near future, it will become increasingly important to more carefully evaluate subsidy payment policies and improve the accuracy with which funds are targeted that have the express purpose of helping those most in need.

Notes

1. These studies are referred to by several authors in this volume.
2. Prospective Payment Assessment Commission analysis of data from the American Hospital Association Annual Survey of Hospitals.
3. Ibid.
4. Care to those who cannot pay is commonly referred to as charity care, whereas care not paid for by those who are held responsible for these costs is called bad debt. Although these two terms can differ greatly in their relevance to social policy, in practice it is difficult to distinguish between them. Hospitals rarely have information that would allow a definitive conclusion as to the patient's ability to pay, and different hospitals have different policies in this regard. Consequently, we refer to the two amounts together as uncompensated care.
5. In this analysis, it is not possible to distinguish between government subsidies to cover uncompensated care and subsidies for other purposes, such as the training of physicians and other health personnel. Therefore, we have counted all government subsidies reported by each hospital as offsets to uncompensated care, up to the total amount of uncompensated care costs reported by the hospital. Government subsidies above this amount are counted as other revenues.
6. This analysis includes revenues and expenses from all sources, including both inpatient and outpatient care and nonpatient care. Adjusted admissions are a weighted average of inpatient admissions and outpatient visits, with outpatient visits weighted by the ratio of outpatient revenues per visit to inpatient revenues per admission; this yields a measure of inpatient admission equivalents provided by hospitals during the year.
7. The payment-to-cost ratio shown in Table 9.3 reflects the extent to which a type of payor *group* (e.g., Medicaid) provides hospitals with payments sufficient to cover the cost of care for its patients. If payments exceed the cost of care, the payment-to-cost ratio is greater than 100 percent; if payments are less than costs, the payment-to-cost ratio is less than 100 percent. These ratios include all services provided to patients in each group in all hospital-based settings (i.e., inpatient, outpatient, and any applicable post-acute care).
8. Note that the Medicare payments and costs presented in this analysis are for all patient care provided by the hospital, including both inpatient and outpatient care and other hospital-based services. Because the PPS applied initially only to inpatient operating costs (and since 1991 also to inpatient capital costs), the effect of changes in its policies would be only partially reflected in these numbers.
9. Gains or losses as a percentage of total costs isolate the importance of each payor to hospitals' overall financial status. That is, if hospitals had Medicaid

losses of 0.8 percent in a given year, they would experience a total loss of 0.8 if they had exactly broken even on all other payors combined.

10. Again, note that Medicare losses referred to here include both inpatient and outpatient payments and costs. Also, these losses reflect all costs reported by hospitals, including some that are not allowable under the Medicare program.

11. Total gain is equal to net revenues from all sources (including nonpatient care activities) as a proportion of total hospital expenses. It differs somewhat from the total revenue margin often used to describe hospital financial performance in that it is a proportion of total expenses, rather than total revenues.

12. The Council is a nonpartisan organization supported by a grant from the Robert Wood Johnson Foundation and is administered by the Institute for Health Policy, the Heller School, Brandeis University.

References

Federal Register. 1994. 59 (83) May 2: 22677.

Levit, K. R., H. C. Lazenby, B. R. Braden, C. A. Cowan, P. A. McDonnell, L. Sivarajan, J. M. Stiller, D. K. Won, C. S. Donham, A. M. Long, and M. W. Stewart. 1996. "National Health Expenditures." *Health Care Financing Review* 18 (1): 175–214.

Prospective Payment Assessment Commission. 1991. *The Trend and Distribution of Hospital Uncompensated Care Costs, 1980–1989.* Technical Paper I-91-04. Washington, DC: The Commission.

———. 1994. *Medicare and the American Health Care System.* Washington, DC: The Commission.

———. 1995. *The Relationship of Hospital Costs and Payment by Source, 1980–1991.* Washington, DC: The Commission.

———. 1996. *Medicare and the American Health Care System.* Washington, DC: The Commission.

Thorpe, K. E. 1995. "The Combined Impact on Hospitals of Reduced Spending for Medicare, Medicaid and Employer Sponsored Insurance." Unpublished manuscript, Council on the Economic Impact of Health System Change. Waltham, MA.

III

Changes in Hospital Ownership and Care for the Uninsured

10

The Impact of Hospital Conversions on the Healthcare Safety Net

David Shactman
Stuart H. Altman

Introduction

One of the many structural changes now occurring in the American healthcare system is the conversion of hospitals from not-for-profit (NFP) to for-profit (FP) status. These conversions involve the transformation of billions of dollars in charitable assets and potential changes in access to health services, both of which may impact the healthcare safety net and the availability of care for the poor and uninsured.

But the nature of this impact is not simple to discern. There is the potential for both positive and negative implications from hospital conversions, only some of which directly impact the poor and uninsured. For example, expenditures on teaching and research differ widely among NFP and FP hospitals, but do not directly relate to safety-net issues. This chapter identifies and analyzes three major areas in which conversions may affect access and provision of care for the poor and uninsured:

1. The provision of charity care and community benefits
2. The provision of local health services
3. The price of health services

This work was supported by a grant from the Robert Wood Johnson Foundation.

In each of these areas there are trade-offs that must be considered. Opponents of conversions contend that NFP hospitals provide greater amounts of charity care, community benefits, and an array of important community services that often lose money, such as AIDs clinics, trauma centers, and neonatal intensive care units. Clearly, the provision of charity care directly affects the healthcare safety net, as do all of these services to some extent. If these services are likely to be reduced as the result of a conversion, then public policies that regulate or even discourage conversions might be appropriate.

Supporters of conversions contend, however, that the amount of charity care and community benefits provided by FP hospitals, when added to taxes they pay plus grants from foundations spawned by conversions, exceed the community benefits provided by their NFP counterparts. If that is the case, poorer communities might derive a net benefit from conversions, and public policy that encourages conversions might be appropriate.

How do we reconcile these opposing views? What can we conclude about the likely impact of hospital conversions on the poor and uninsured? The following three sections of this chapter addresses these three specific areas, and the final section offers concluding remarks and policy recommendations.

The Provision of Charity Care and Community Benefits

There are basically three ways by which conversions can affect the flow of charity care and benefits to the poor and uninsured: the direct provision of charity care and other services to members of the community; the portion of taxes (if any) paid by the successor FP that benefit the health needs of the community; and the proceeds of grants from foundations, created by conversions that fund community health needs.

The rising incidence of hospital conversions has been a fairly recent phenomenon, and studies do not exist that compare the provision of charity care and community benefits pre- and postconversion. Hence, it is not possible to cite empirical evidence or give a definitive answer to this question of relative provision of community benefits. As a proxy for such evidence, the overall behavior of NFP and FP hospitals as it relates to the provision of charity care and community benefits was examined.

Measuring Community Benefit

The issue of the relative provision of charity care and community benefits by NFPs and FPs has frequently appeared in the literature. Researchers have used a variety of definitions and methodologies to study these questions, and comparing their results is difficult. Because of this, advocates for both NFPs and FPs have been able to state widely divergent conclusions and find apparent support for their positions in the literature.

National versus State Studies

One reason for divergent conclusions is that some studies compare the behavior of NFP and FP hospitals within the same state, while other studies make comparisons using aggregate national data. Several prominent organizations analyzing aggregate national data (e.g., Prospective Payment Assessment Commission 1995, 1996; Gray 1986) found relatively small differences between NFPs and FPs in the provision of charitable care. These studies are discussed in more detail in the next section. But, as Lewin, Eckels, and Miller (1988) point out, aggregate data may be deceiving. Most FPs are concentrated in 13 states. These states have leaner Medicaid eligibility rules and fewer public hospitals than states chiefly populated by NFPs. As a consequence, Lewin, Eckels, and Miller found that the amount of charity care FP hospitals provide relative to total revenue is high compared with national averages, but low in relation to the amount provided by NFPs within the same states. They conclude that comparisons based on national aggregate data are misleading.

Charity Care and Bad Debt

Charity care is the most basic component in the provision of community benefits. Some researchers measure charity care by "charges" or potential revenue foregone. Criticisms of this approach focus on the ambiguity of charge data and suggest that a better measure of value is actual cost. Studies that measure by charges overstate charity care relative to those that measure by cost, and they overstate charity care for higher-margin hospitals (i.e., those hospitals having higher charges relative to cost). Researchers often use a cost/charge ratio to adjust data based on charges.

The direct provision of charity care, where no payment is expected, is often combined with bad debt as a measure of uncompensated care. The issue here is what type of patients incur bad debt expenses? If bad debt is incurred mostly by patients who are actually able to pay, but whose account is poorly managed by the hospital, that would hardly constitute charity. But if these are primarily services to low-income patients, it is quite another matter. The manner in which bad debt is classified is a nontrivial issue because it has been estimated that the level of bad debt far exceeds that of pure charity care. A study by the state of Maryland showed that 59 percent of bad debt was from individuals who were uninsured (Frank and Salkever 1994). Sanders (1995) references a 1988 study by Lewin, Eckels, and Miller in stating that more than 50 percent of NFP bad debt in a Florida study was from individuals earning less than 150 percent of the poverty level. Some hospitals simply classify any care that is unreimbursed as bad debt.

Hence, charity care will be underestimated if bad debt is excluded, but will be somewhat overstated if all of it is included. Not withstanding the potential for overstatement, the inclusion of bad debt with charity is herein encouraged as a measure of uncompensated care.

Losses from Medicare and Medicaid

Many analysts recognize that losses from public programs (mainly Medicare and Medicaid) represent an important form of community benefit for which hospitals do not receive full and fair compensation. Although both FP and NFP hospitals participate in these programs, the relative extent of their participation is not the same. The Prospective Payment Assessment Commission (ProPAC) estimates that, in 1994, losses from Medicare and Medicaid represented 1.7 and 2.9 percent, respectively, of the total costs incurred by NFPs, but only 0.6 and 0.7 percent of the total costs incurred by FPs (Prospective Payment Assessment Commission 1996). It must be recognized, however, that higher losses from these programs may reflect relative cost efficiency as well as relative patient mix.

Teaching and Research

The additional cost of teaching and research also are often included as community benefits. Many hospitals, including FPs, provide these services and do not receive full compensation. But from a national perspective, the overwhelming amount of teaching and research is performed either in NFP or public institutions.

Lower Prices

Some analysts have argued that lower prices charged by NFPs constitute a benefit to the community. They contend that NFPs do not fully exploit their market power to maximize revenues and, as a result, the benefit of lower prices inure to consumers. This is discussed in greater detail in the section "The Price of Health Services," below.

Losses from Providing Unprofitable Services

Many hospitals provide services that either consistently lose money or that tend to attract patients that are at higher risk for expensive services and who are more likely to be unable to pay. Examples of such services are AIDS clinics, burn units, and neonatal intensive care units.

Other Community Services

Finally, hospitals provide other services to communities such as education, screening, and community outreach. There may be reasonable justification for including these in total benefits, but these services are often unbilled and difficult to quantify. Moreover, they are sometimes used as marketing tools and occasionally are revenue producing. For these reasons, they are often excluded.

Taxes

Tax exemptions given to NFPs and tax payments made by FPs can have a significant impact on the healthcare safety net. Researchers and policymakers have questioned whether the community benefits provided by NFPs equal or exceed the value of the tax exemptions they receive. If they do, then NFPs provide added value to the community, much of which often benefits the poor and uninsured. If not, however, the taxes foregone could presumably be better distributed by the government and could be used to strengthen the healthcare safety net.

In comparisons of FPs and NFPs, researchers also disagree about whether tax payments made by FPs constitute community benefits. Advocates of FPs contend that taxes paid are for the public benefit, and that all tax payments should be counted when comparing the two ownership forms. Other analysts point out that taxes remitted to local communities, such as property taxes, have much more relevance to a community than federal income taxes, which have little local impact and may vary greatly from year to year. In terms of the healthcare safety net, few taxes directly impact services for the poor and uninsured, with the exception of those specifically earmarked for such services such as a premium tax to support a free care pool.

The Value of Foundations Spawned from Conversions

To determine the impact of conversions on the healthcare safety net, the value of charitable foundations that are spawned from conversions must be considered. New foundations formed as a result of conversions now have assets in excess of $5 billion (McDermott 1996), and annual grants from these foundations can have a significant benefit on community health services. Often these foundations target a substantial portion of their grant-making portfolio to poor and underserved populations.

The emergence of charitable foundations that has resulted from conversions is such a recent phenomenon that the combined activities of these foundations have not been summarized or analyzed in the literature. Indeed, many of these foundations are still in the process of determining their structure and mission. In addition, the recent history of the legal treatment of conversions has been inconsistent. Some communities have been successful in capturing the full fair market value of charitable assets when a NFP is sold or transferred, while others have not. Cases of abuse and personal enrichment in this area have now become common in the literature.[1] Furthermore, some states have carefully regulated the future use of charitable foundation assets, often limiting such use to provision of health services, particularly for the poor. Other states have permitted funds to be used outside the health area for such activities as arts, education, and a variety of other social and cultural activities.

For states to evaluate the full impact of a conversion on poor and underserved communities, the endowment and mission of any charitable foundation spawned from the conversion must be considered. It is important to note that state regulators can have an enormous impact on the amount and specific use of these assets.

From this discussion, it is evident that a widely accepted standard for community benefit would help inform researchers and policymakers about the relative contribution of various hospital types. There currently exists three well-known studies in this regard (e.g., Catholic Hospital Association, the Kellogg Foundation, and the Voluntary Hospital Association). However, no standard has been widely accepted, and until this happens, comparisons of studies employing different methodologies will be difficult.

Empirical Studies of Charity Care and Community Benefit

Twenty studies of comparative community benefit, virtually all of those found in the literature, were examined and have been summarized below. Studies comparing hospitals within states are presented separately from those based on national aggregate data because of questions regarding the methodological accuracy of using aggregate data. Within those classifications, the summary begins with studies that use the narrowest descriptions of community benefits (charity care only) and proceeds to those that are the most inclusive. An exception is the discussion of two industry-supported reports at the end of the within-state studies.

Studies Comparing Hospitals within States

Among those within-state studies that measured charity care separately from bad debt, the U.S. General Accounting Office (GAO) study is perhaps the best known (U.S. General Accounting Office 1990). The GAO studied hospitals in five states classified by both ownership and teaching status. They found that NFPs provided more charity care than FPs, but that the lion's share was provided by public and major teaching hospitals. Not-for-profit nonteaching hospitals provided more charity care than FPs, but the amount of charity care they provided was highly variable and often concentrated in a few hospitals. The GAO estimated that 57 percent of NFP hospitals provided less pure charity care (at cost) than the value of their tax exemption (counting federal and state income tax only). The GAO also compared charity care plus bad debt (charges) and found that 15 percent of hospitals provided less than the value of their tax exemption (counting federal and state income tax only). The GAO recommended that government consider policies to encourage NFPs to increase their provision of charity care.

Wolfson and Hopes (1994) studied seven NFP hospital systems in Florida in 1992. They included only pure charity care (at cost) as benefits and counted federal and state income, property, and sales tax. They found that six of the seven systems studied received tax savings well in excess of their provision of charity care.

Kane (1994) studied NFP and FP hospitals in Virginia. She counted pure charity care (at cost), losses on Medicare and Medicaid, and net costs for teaching and research as community benefits. Measuring benefits as a percentage of revenues, she found that NFPs provided more community benefits than FPs. Not-for-profit charity care exceeded FPs (3.7 to 1.7 percent), NFP losses on teaching and research exceeded FPs (1 to ≈ 0 percent), and NFP losses on Medicare and Medicaid were slightly less than that of FPs (1.1 to 1.16 percent). However, taxes paid by FPs were 8.4 percent of revenues. If one includes FP taxes in the measurement of community benefits, FPs provided nearly double the amount of total benefit. Kane concluded that states should consider requiring greater value for tax-exempt status.

Among those within-state studies that included both pure charity care and bad debt, Lewin, Eckels, and Miller (1988) examined NFP and FP hospitals in five states. They included charity and bad debt (at cost) as total community benefit. In four of the five states, they found that benefits provided by NFPs exceeded those provided by FPs by 50–90 percent. Only in California, where Medicaid eligibility is relatively inclusive and public hospitals are prevalent, did benefits of NFPs exceed FPs by only a small margin. These results, however, used combined data from all NFP hospitals (both public and private) and, hence, did not accurately reflect differences that exist between private NFP and private FP hospitals. The authors did present separate measures for the three hospital types in Tennessee, comparing the market share of each (statewide) to the share of total community benefits provided (statewide). They used the share of total hospital expenses (statewide) as a proxy for market share. They found that public hospitals had a market share of 21 percent but provided 30 percent of the total community benefits. Private NFPs provided community benefits at nearly equal proportions to their market share (61 percent market share, 62 percent of total benefits), whereas FPs had an 18 percent share of the market but provided only 8 percent of total community benefits. The authors concluded that private NFPs provided substantially more benefits than private FPs, and that consistent standards of comparison were needed to better inform policymakers.

Clement (1994) studied NFPs in California from 1980–81 through 1986–87. Included in her measure of community benefit were charity and bad debt (at cost), net cost of teaching and research, price discounts below FPs, below cost services *not* including Medicare and Medicaid, and net income (surplus). She estimated the value of tax exemptions by counting federal and state income tax and property tax. She found that the level of uncompensated care (charity plus bad debt) was less than benefits from tax exemptions, but that total community benefits exceeded estimated tax exemptions by three to four times. Clement also found much variability, reporting that 25 percent of hospitals failed to meet a wide variety of hypothetical minimum benefit standards. She concluded that the requirement of minimum standards for provision of benefits should be considered.

Gray (1991) compared NFPs and FPs in five states during 1981–83. He counted charges (not costs) for charity and bad debt. He found that, in four of the five states, benefits provided by NFPs exceeded those of FPs by 50–150 percent. Only in California did he find virtually no difference.

Two studies were performed in central Florida by private consultants, one supported by the NFP industry and the other supported by FPs (Healthcare Management Decisions 1995; Parker et al. 1995). Not surprisingly, they had opposite conclusions, even though both studies were based on the same 1993 data. In their measurement of total community benefit, Healthcare Management Decisions counted only pure charity (at cost) net of payments made on behalf of charitable care. Measuring tax, they counted federal and state income tax, sales tax, property tax, and Florida intangible property tax (state indigent care tax apparently was not included). They found pure charity care was 2.2 percent of NFP revenues and 0.6 percent of FP revenues. Comparing benefits to taxes, they found that only one of six NFPs provided a level of community benefits in excess of its tax exemptions.

Parker et al. (1995), using the same data but a different methodology, measured total community benefit by including charity care and bad debt (at cost), losses on Medicaid, net cost of education and research, and contributions to state indigent care pool (payments received on behalf of charitable care apparently were not netted out). For measurement of taxes they included federal and state income tax, property tax, and sales tax. Adjusting their figures to measure total benefits as a percentage of staffed beds, they found that NFPs provided 9.4 percent and FPs 5.3 percent. Computing community benefit plus taxes paid as a percentage of net revenue, they found that NFPs provided 8.8 percent and FPs 7.6 percent.

These two studies are presented last among the within-state studies, because they were performed by paid consultants, and they illustrate the difficulty in comparing studies that employ different methodologies.

Studies Comparing Hospitals Using Aggregate National Data

The remaining studies reviewed in this section use aggregate national data that may produce misleading findings as described above. The ProPAC reports on hospital statistics in this area are based annually on American Hospital Association (AHA) data. The 1993 and 1994 ProPAC data from 1995 and 1996 reports include charity care plus bad debt (at cost, with payments made on behalf of uncompensated care netted out), and the amount is expressed as a proportion of total costs. A summary of ProPAC's 1993 and 1994 data is presented in Table 10.1.

In 1994, the uncompensated care/cost ratio for private NFPs was 4.4 percent compared with 3.7 percent for FPs.[2] However, when gains and/or losses from Medicare and Medicaid are added to uncompensated care, the proportion of losses sustained by NFPs is considerably greater (9 percent of costs versus 5 percent of costs, for an 80 percent difference in the ratios).

Table 10.1   Gains or Losses by Payor, by Hospital Group, 1993 and
1994 (in Percent)

	Medicare		Medicaid		Uncompensated Care		Total	
Hospital Group	1993	1994	1993	1994	1993	1994	1993	1994
Not-for-Profit	−4.3	−2.9	−1.4	−1.7	−4.4	−4.4	−10.1	−9.0
For-Profit	−4.5	−0.7	−1.0	−0.6	−3.5	−3.7	−9.0	−5.0

Source: ProPAC 1995, 1996.

This observation must be tempered, however, with a consideration
of costs. Losses sustained for uncompensated care were approximately
the same for both ownership forms in 1993 and 1994. However, when
gains and/or losses from Medicare and Medicaid are added to uncompensated care, the difference in losses sustained (as a percent of total
costs) widened considerably (from a 12 percent difference in 1993 to an
80 percent difference in 1994). Because prices for Medicare and Medicaid services are highly regulated, one could assume that the widening
differential was due largely to the success of FP hospitals in lowering their
cost in response to market pressures. Hence, the inclusion of Medicare
and Medicaid losses in the measurement of comparative community benefits makes a significant difference, but part of that difference reflects
differences in cost.

Sanders (1993) used aggregate national data in a study of 595
Catholic hospitals in 1987. She included charity and bad debt (at cost)
and losses from Medicare and Medicaid in total benefits. She identified
wide disparities among hospitals and found that 75 percent of hospitals
provided only 38 percent of charity care (charity and bad debt only). This
disparity narrowed somewhat when losses from Medicare and Medicaid
were included. She suggested consideration of policies that would better
relate tax exemption to provision of community benefits.

The AHA examined aggregate national data comparing public,
private NFP, and FP hospitals in 1983 and in 1982 (AHA from Gray
1986). The AHA measured charges (not costs) for charity and bad
debt expressed as a percentage of total revenue. They found that the
ratio of benefits provided and revenues was 11.5 percent for public
hospitals, 4.2 percent for private NFPs, and 3.1 percent for FPs. In 1982,
public hospitals also provided the most benefits, but the level of benefits
provided by private NFPs and FPs was nearly equal. The AHA studies
have been questioned, however, because of low survey response.

The Office of Civil Rights (Rowland 1986), using aggregate national data from 5,800 hospitals in 1981, measured uninsured admissions as a percentage of total admissions. They found that public, private NFP, and FP hospitals accepted 16.8, 7.9, and 6 percent of uninsured admissions, respectively.

Several other studies not summarized individually were reviewed. Herzlinger and Krasker (1987) reported that NFP hospitals did not provide benefits worthy of their tax exemption. But Arrington and Haddock (1990) disputed the validity of those findings. Healthcare Management Decisions (1994) studied hospitals in Tampa Bay and reported findings similar to their central Florida study. However, they are not independent researchers, but paid consultants for the FP industry. The Voluntary Hospital Association studied Virginia hospital data from 1994 and Florida data from 1993 (Voluntary Hospital Association and SunHealth Alliance 1995a,b). They did not measure community benefits comparably to other studies that were reviewed, and they also are not independent, but represent the NFP industry. A summary of conclusions from all the above studies is outlined below.

- Not-for-profit hospitals provide significantly more charity care and community benefits than FPs. This is particularly evident when hospital types are compared within states and when a reasonably broad definition of benefits is employed.
- Despite the significant differences in benefits provided, there are wide variations in the provision of charity care by NFP hospitals. Public hospitals and NFP major teaching hospitals provide a disproportionately large share of community benefits, and a significant number of NFP hospitals provide very few community benefits at all.
- In general, the total amount of NFP contributions that are generally accepted as community benefits (charity, bad debt, losses from public programs, and net expense of teaching and research) often exceed the value of the tax exemption.
- If FPs include the amount of tax they pay as community benefits, they generally would be found to provide more community benefits than NFPs.

None of these studies considered the impact of new charitable foundations on the provision of community benefits. The annual amount of new foundation grant money, and how that money is spent, must be factored into any estimate of the net benefit or detriment to a community from a prospective conversion.

The Provision of Health Services

All hospital mergers and acquisitions, regardless of whether they involve different ownership forms, have the potential to consolidate and thus reduce the provision of health services. Currently, there is an oversupply of inpatient hospital beds, and some service reductions can be appropriate and cost efficient. Nevertheless, there may be economic incentives to reduce services that are needed by the poor and uninsured.

For example, the largest potential saving from hospital mergers comes from closing an entire hospital facility (The Advisory Board 1996). Although many factors are involved in the decision to close a hospital, there are greater economic incentives to close an older, inner-city hospital that serves many uninsured and public paying patients as opposed to a newer, suburban hospital with higher paying privately insured patients.

In addition, there are economic incentives to consolidate or close money-losing services. Often these services lose money because they attract lower paying public patients or the uninsured. Hence, services such as 24-hour emergency rooms, AIDS clinics, and neonatal intensive care units all tend to be money-losing services that disproportionately impact the poor and uninsured.

Hence, the healthcare safety net can be affected negatively by mergers, and state policymakers should be vigilant about the continued provision of services after a merger, whether or not the merging partners are FP or NFP institutions. An additional question, in regard to this chapter, is whether mergers involving conversion of ownership form are any more likely to reduce services than those in which ownership form remains the same.

Opponents of hospital conversions often contend that access to important services is more likely to be reduced when hospital ownership changes from NFP to FP status. Several reasons are commonly given to support this claim. First, FP hospitals have to be concerned primarily with profitability and the return to their stockholders, so they have a greater incentive to reduce unprofitable services. Second, FP management is less likely to be constrained by local ties in closing facilities and reducing employment. And third, FP management, not being subject to the control of local community board members, has greater freedom of action to terminate or reduce services and employment.

Those who support conversions often deny these claims, pointing out that FP hospitals often can access capital to upgrade existing facilities and to purchase new services that were previously unaffordable.

Supporters of conversions also cite cases in which NFP hospitals would have closed altogether without the availability of a FP partner. Furthermore, they contend that FPs are more responsive to the market, bringing in services that are demanded and terminating those services that are duplicated elsewhere and which NFPs have often maintained at inefficient operating levels.

Conversions are such a recent phenomena that we do not have empirical evidence of whether, or to what extent, access to services are changed postconversion. There is anecdotal evidence that service provision has been reduced by FPs postconversion (Greene 1995). Shortell et al. (1996) found reductions of nontraditional services postconversion. And, as mentioned above, evidence exists that hospital consolidation in general often results in consolidation of services. Furthermore, it is generally recognized that FPs have stronger economic incentives and fewer regulatory and administrative restraints in regard to closing facilities and reducing unprofitable services.

Recent legislation enacted in a few states reflects the concern of public policymakers with potential service reductions. For example, California (California Assembly Bill 3101, 1996) and Nebraska (Nebraska Bill 118, 1996) both enacted legislation in 1996 empowering regulators to consider the future provision of services in approving or rejecting proposed conversions.

Therefore, although statistical evidence is lacking, the incentive for potential service reductions following conversions is recognized, and the concern among policymakers is evident. Nevertheless, conversions provide a means to reduce overcapacity and duplication of service that is necessary to make the healthcare system more efficient. Communities must be concerned with the value of the services lost, who lost them, and the potential cost of using the next best alternatives. Policymakers will have to evaluate these issues on an individual basis and assess the potential impact of such changes in service provision, particularly as it affects poor and underserved communities.

The Price of Health Services

Although not as important as charity care and provision of health services, prices are a third way in which conversions might affect the healthcare safety net. Many lower income citizens are insured through public programs such as Medicaid, and some cannot afford healthcare services at any price. But access to care for some of the uninsured may be affected, at the margin, by the price of health services, and the capacity of public programs to provide health services to the poor is impacted by the price of providing those services. Hence, if FP hospitals have higher prices than NFPs, access to affordable healthcare may be diminished by conversions. If, on the other hand, FP hospitals are more cost efficient, and pass efficiency savings on to purchasers, conversions could make health services more affordable.

Many researchers in the 1980s examined price differences between NFP and FP hospitals. Although these studies had substantial methodological differences, most concluded that FPs priced their services higher than their NFP counterparts. But virtually all of these studies relied on data that were collected when the healthcare environment was substantially different.

There are indications that the ability to sustain higher prices is more difficult in today's competitive marketplace. One piece of evidence is the declining ability of hospitals to recover their losses from public payors by increasing their prices to the privately insured—a practice known as cost shifting. In 1992, hospitals (overall) received $1.31 for each dollar of care provided to private payors. But by 1994, the private pay ratio slipped to $1.24, indicating that the ability to sustain higher prices from private payors was diminishing (Prospective Payment Assessment Commission 1996).

One study in California measured price discounts given by hospitals as a percentage of their total asset value (Clement 1994). The difference in this measure between NFP and FP hospitals declined from 14.4 percent in 1980–81 to only 1.6 percent in 1986–87, indicating that high private pay charges, from which discounts were calculated, could not be sustained.

Other recent studies, however, indicate that price differences still exist. Parker et al. (1995) found that case mix adjusted inpatient charges of FP hospitals in central Florida in 1993 were 14 percent higher than those of their NFP competitors. The Voluntary Hospital Association and SunHealth Alliance (1995a) analyzed all Florida hospitals in 1993 and found that case mix adjusted inpatient charges of FP hospitals were 9.9 percent higher than those of NFPs. The Voluntary Hospital Association also conducted a study in Virginia (Voluntary Hospital Association and SunHealth Alliance 1995b) and found that case mix adjusted inpatient charges for FP hospitals in 1994 were 30 percent higher than those of their NFP counterparts. One must consider, however, that the authors of these three studies worked for or represented the NFP industry and were not independent researchers.

An examination of operating margins also reveals that price differences likely still exist. Table 10.2 shows payment/cost ratios by payor group and by ownership status for 1993.

Note that the differences in payment/cost ratios between voluntary and proprietary hospitals for Medicare and Medicaid are small, but the difference increases substantially in the case of non-price-controlled private payors (1.408 versus 1.277). Because differences in operating cost should not vary greatly by type of payor, one could assume that this difference is mostly an indication that FPs have higher prices for services in the private paying market.

The ability to maintain higher prices is becoming increasingly more difficult in the marketplace, particularly in areas where competition is the strongest, such as California. Overall, however, there is evidence that FP prices are still somewhat higher than those of NFPs. These higher prices could, on the margin, reduce affordability of care and should be considered along with other factors in evaluating the impact of hospital conversions.

Conclusion

There is no simple answer as to whether hospital conversions are a benefit or detriment to the healthcare safety net. This chapter has examined three areas in which conversions can impact healthcare for the poor and uninsured: the provision of charity care and community benefits, the provision of healthcare services, and the price of healthcare services.

The provision of charity care and community benefits directly impacts care for the poor and uninsured. On the whole, NFP hospitals provide significantly more charity care and community benefits than FPs,

Table 10.2 Payment-to-Cost Ratio by Payor Group by Ownership Category, 1993

Category	Medicare	Medicaid	Private	Total
Total Government	0.891	1.041	1.314	1.038
Total Voluntary	0.894	0.888	1.277	1.042
Proprietary	0.900	0.905	1.408	1.080

Source: Prospective Payment Assessment Commission.

and this should be a concern to policymakers. However, individual cases vary considerably, and when comparisons include proceeds from new charitable foundations and the ability to pay taxes, the impact on the safety net from any particular conversion is not a foregone conclusion.

Access to health services, particularly services that are unprofitable or that attract public paying patients, can be reduced or eliminated as a result of any merger or acquisition. This can have a negative impact on poor and underserved communities. Whether mergers and acquisitions that involve conversions to FP status are more likely to result in such service reductions is not known. But profit incentives and corporate structure provide reasons for concern in this area, and recent regulatory actions by some states reinforce these concerns. Nevertheless, FP investment also has the potential to enhance service provision and to improve cost efficiency by eliminating service duplications. Effective state regulation can be employed to ensure maintenance of services as well as other community benefits.

The level of hospital prices can affect access to care for uninsured individuals and the capacity of public programs to serve the health needs of the poor. Overall, there is evidence that FP hospitals have had, and continue to have, higher prices than their NFP counterparts. However, as markets become more competitive, these price differentials have narrowed.

It is apparent that conversions can have a considerable impact on the healthcare safety net, but that impact may vary widely from case to case. Because we are focusing on the provision of public goods, the private market, left to itself, may not yield the optimum provision of such goods. Therefore, this may be an appropriate area for state government intervention. If states legislate a process of preconversion submission and review, they will have the capacity to evaluate the potential impact of a conversion on the poor and uninsured, as well as on other members of the community. In that way, state health officials can approve those conversions that offer a net benefit to the community and deny, or renegotiate the terms of, those conversions that do not.

Notes

1. See, for example, Rissman (1995); Bell, C. (1996); Bell, J. (1996); Fox and Isenberg (1996); Meyer et al. (1996); Shactman and Altman (1996).
2. If one does not adjust for payments made on behalf of uncompensated care, the figures are 4.5 and 4.0 percent for NFPs and FPs, respectively. These are figures that have often been cited in the literature and the popular press.

References

The Advisory Board. 1996. *The Rising Tide.* Washington, DC: The Board.

Arrington, B., and C. Haddock. 1990, "Who Really Profits from Not-For-Profits?" *HSR: Health Services Research* 25 (2): 291–304.

Bell, C. 1996. "Ohio Blues Must Take Steps to Prove Deal's Fairness." *Modern Healthcare* 26 (26): 100.

Bell, J. 1996. "Vigilance is Needed to Protect Charitable Assets." *Modern Healthcare* 26 (25): 74.

Clement, J. 1994, "What Do We Want and What Do We Get from Not-for-Profit Hospitals?" *Hospital & Health Services Administration* 39 (2): 159–76.

Fox, D., and P. Isenberg. 1996. "Anticipating the Magic Moment: The Public Interest in Health Plan Conversions in California." *Health Affairs* 15 (1): 202–9.

Frank, R. G., and D. S. Salkever. 1994. "Nonprofit Organizations in the Health Sector." *Journal of Economic Perspectives* 8 (4): 129–44.

Gray, B. 1991. "The Performance of For-Profit and Nonprofit Health Care Organizations." In *The Profit Motive and Patient Care*, 90–110. Cambridge, MA: Harvard University Press.

———. 1986. "Access to Care and Investor-Owned Providers." In *For-Profit Enterprise in Health Care*, 97–126. Washington, DC: National Academy Press.

Greene, J. 1995. "Are Foundations Bearing Fruit?" *Modern Healthcare* 25 (12): 53–68.

Healthcare Management Decisions. 1994. *Tax-Exempt Benefits of Selected Tampa Bay Hospitals.* St. Petersburg, FL: Healthcare Management Decisions, Inc.

———. 1995. *Community Benefits and Tax-Exempt Status of Central Florida Hospitals.* St. Petersburg, FL: Healthcare Management Decisions, Inc.

Herzlinger, R. E., and W. S. Krasker. 1987. "Who Profits From Nonprofits?" *Harvard Business Review* 6: 93–106.

Kane, N. M. 1994. "Nonprofit Hospital Status: What Is It Worth?" Unpublished document, Harvard School of Public Health, Cambridge, MA.

Lewin, L. S., T. J. Eckels, and L. B. Miller. 1988. "Special Report: Setting the Record Straight—The Provision of Uncompensated Care by Not-for-Profit Hospitals." *New England Journal of Medicine* 318 (18): 1212–15.

McDermott, C. 1996. "The New 'Conversion' Health Foundations: Preliminary Results of GIH [Grantmakers in Health] Survey." Presented at the Council on Foundations Annual Conference, Atlanta, GA, 23 April.

Meyer, H., T. Hudson, J. E. Cain, S. L. Carr, and D. Zacharias. 1996. "Selling . . . Or Selling Out." *Hospitals & Health Networks* 70 (11): 21–46.

Parker, Hudson, Rainer, and Dobbs. 1995. "Analysis of Central Florida Hospital Community Benefits: Community Hospitals Compared to Investor-Owned Hospitals." Atlanta, GA: Parker, Hudson, Rainer, and Dobbs.

Prospective Payment Assessment Commission. 1995. *Medicare and the American Health Care System: Report to the Congress.* Washington, DC: The Commission.

———. 1996. *Medicare and the American Health Care System: Report to the Congress.* Washington, DC: The Commission.

Rissman, C. 1995. "Converting to For-Profit Health Care: What Advocates Should Know." *States of Health* 5 (8): 1–7.

Rowland, D. 1986. "Hospital Care for the Uninsured: An Analysis of the Role of Proprietary Hospitals." In *For-Profit Enterprise in Healthcare,* edited by B. Gray. Washington, DC: National Academy Press.

Sanders, S. M. 1993. "Measuring Charitable Contributions: Implications for the Nonprofit Hospitals Tax-Exempt Status." *Hospital & Health Services Administration* 38 (3): 401–18.

———. 1995. "The 'Common Sense' of the Nonprofit Hospital Tax Exemption: A Policy Analysis." *Journal of Policy Analysis and Management* 14 (3): 446–66.

Shactman, D., and S. H. Altman. 1996. "The Conversion of Hospitals from Not-For-Profit to For-Profit Status." Report to the Council on the Economic Impact of Health System Change, Waltham, MA, 30 December.

Shortell, S. M., E. M. Morrison, S. L. Hughes, B. Friedman, J. Coverdill, and L. Berg. 1996. "The Effects of Hospital Ownership on Nontraditional Services." *Health Affairs* 5 (4): 97–111.

U.S. General Accounting Office. 1990. *Report on Nonprofit Hospitals and the Need for Better Standards for Tax Exemption.* Washington, DC: The Office.

Voluntary Hospital Association and SunHealth Alliance. 1995a. *Florida Hospital Industry Analysis.* Washington, DC: Voluntary Hospital Association and Charlotte, NC: SunHealth Alliance, Inc.

———. 1995b. *Virginia Hospital Analysis.* Washington, DC: Voluntary Hospital Association and Charlotte, NC: SunHealth Alliance, Inc.

Wolfson, J., and S. L. Hopes. 1994. "What Makes Tax-Exempt Hospitals Special?" *Healthcare Financial Management* (July): 56–60.

11

Hospital Ownership Form and Care of the Uninsured

Bradford H. Gray

In the absence of universal health insurance, hospitals have financed and provided a great deal of service to the poor and uninsured, with estimates of hospitals' uncompensated care now more than $16 billion annually (Weissman 1996). This is a state of affairs for which the largely not-for-profit (NFP) hospital industry bears some historical responsibility, having developed and successfully marketed in the 1930s an ideology that extolled "voluntarism" rather than governmental activity as a "generic, heroic political ideology, set against incursions of 'socialized' medicine" (Stevens 1989, 170). Although the industry has long abandoned this policy stance, a legacy lives on in public expectations that hospitals will serve people who lack means to pay. Hospitals are implicitly expected to raise revenues to cover the costs of services for the uninsured. The major source of such funds has been from charges to insured patients.

Considerable controversy has surrounded this topic in recent years. Financing by cross-subsidization has been criticized as unfair to paying patients (Wikler 1988), as hidden taxation without accountability, and as a socially unjust way for society to treat people who lack means to pay for medical care. The viability of this mode of financing care has been brought into question by public policy strategies that rely heavily on managed care and competition to squeeze hospital costs, while policymakers have sought to control costs of public programs by reducing amounts paid to providers to levels that themselves require cross-subsidization

This work was sponsored by the Council on the Economic Impact of Health System Change.

(Prospective Payment Assessment Commission 1996). Anecdotal reports in the 1980s of uninsured patients being turned away from hospitals led not to legislation to increase coverage of the uninsured but to "antidumping" legislation to require hospitals to serve people needing emergency services, regardless of whether they have means to pay.

Hospital ownership form has been part of the controversy about the care to the poor and uninsured. On the one hand, there has been concern about the growth of the for-profit (FP) ownership form that is presumed to be responsive only to money demand. Serving the poor and uninsured is unwise in business terms, as attested by the negative relationship between hospitals' margins and the amount of uncompensated care they provide (Ashby 1991). On the other hand, the charitable activities of tax-exempt NFP hospitals have often seemed inadequate to critics (U.S. General Accounting Office 1990). The topic has become more urgent as the number of uninsured Americans has continually grown while large purchasers, including public programs and health maintenance organizations (HMOs), have introduced increasingly effective cost-containment methods.

The Significance of Ownership Form

American community hospitals are owned either by state and local governments (public) or by private organizations that are incorporated under state law as either FP or NFP corporations. Sixty percent of the 5,256 acute care hospitals enumerated by the American Hospital Association in 1994 were NFP, 26 percent were public, and 14 percent were FP (American Hospital Association 1994–95). These percentages are largely unchanged for the past 30 years.

This apparent stability conceals several significant changes and underestimates the extent to which the FP sector has grown. First, if measured in terms of beds rather than hospitals, the FP sector has almost doubled in size over the period, from 6 to 11 percent of acute care hospital beds between 1965 and 1994. Second, if one includes the approximately 400 psychiatric, alcohol and chemical dependency, and rehabilitation hospitals owned by FP companies and the 350 NFP and public hospitals that these companies manage, the FP sector accounts for almost 32 percent of U.S. nonfederal hospitals and approximately 23 percent of the beds.[1] The character of the FP sector has also changed in recent decades as independent proprietary institutions, which composed the FP sector prior to 1965, have mostly closed or have been acquired by investor-owned companies. This shift means that most FP hospitals are no longer run by owner operators, who were frequently doctors, but are now owned by parent corporations whose stockholders typically have no direct contact with the hospitals or their communities.

Public hospitals have a widely accepted role as safety-net organizations that serve the poor, and they commonly receive direct subsidies for that purpose. Not-for-profit hospitals are generally exempt from federal corporate taxes under Section 501(c)(3) of the Internal Revenue Service code; in addition, state and local governments generally grant such institutions exemptions from corporate, sales, and property taxes. Section 501(c)(3) exemptions are available to NFP organizations that are chartered for a small number of purposes—educational, religious, scientific, literary, or charitable (Simon 1987). Although exemptions of some teaching hospitals may have a basis in their educational and research activities, NFP hospitals are generally exempt as *charitable* organizations. This has shaped public expectations regarding issues such as care of the poor and the uninsured. For-profit organizations operate for the purpose of increasing the wealth of stockholders; this too has shaped public expectations regarding issues such as care of the poor and uninsured. For-profit hospitals pay corporate, property, and other taxes that are used by the government for public purposes, which could include some healthcare of the poor.

Ownership form has been a controversial matter in healthcare. There is even a meta controversy regarding why one might expect NFP organizations to behave differently from FPs. This question has been interpreted in two ways, with consequences for how the question is answered. We might call this the nominalist dispute.

Some advocates of investor ownership suggest that it is only the name or form of incorporation that differentiates FP and NFP hospitals, because all organizations face economic challenges and must show a positive bottom line if they are to survive. In this view, ownership form is a peripheral matter of little substantive importance.

This overstates the similarity of the forms, in my view, but it does point to some important common influences on institutional behavior. Economic performance is indeed important to both FP and NFP hospitals because both types rely heavily on retained earnings and debt for new capital outlays. The ability to borrow is closely linked to the organization's economic performance. The revenues of NFP hospitals, like those of FP hospitals, come overwhelmingly from payments received for services rendered. Although there are important exceptions, charitable contributions are not a major source of capital or operating funds for NFP hospitals. Given this set of circumstances, it is not surprising that NFP hospitals behave very much like a FP organization might be expected to behave.

Despite their similarities, FP and NFP organizations have important differences that begin with sources of capital. Differences first arise at the outset of operations: NFPs usually begin with capital raised from a mix of debt and donations or grants from private sources or government, whereas FPs begin with a mix of equity capital and debt. Equity capital provides special growth incentives. For organizations with growing earnings, equity capital can be much cheaper than debt. The higher the stock price in relationship to earnings, the cheaper the organization's access to equity capital.[2] High price/earnings ratios result from investors' expectations of future earnings; such expectations can be fed by a history of earnings increases, a pattern that is achieved more readily by way of acquisitions and mergers than by way of improved performance of a fixed set of hospitals or health plans.

Advocates of investor ownership commonly accompany their contentions about no real differences in operating styles and goals with the argument that the only real difference is in tax-exempt status, which in their view tilts what should be a level playing field. Estimates in the mid-1980s put the value of NFP hospitals' tax exemptions at approximately 5 percent of revenues (Copeland and Rudney 1990).[3] However, these estimates were rough or were based on questionable extrapolations from a small number of financially healthy institutions during a brief period when hospitals had unusually healthy bottom lines as a result of the early implementation of Medicare's prospective payment system.[4]

As a matter that differentiates FPs and NFPs, the tax-exemption issue has its own complexities. At certain points in their histories, many FP healthcare firms have enjoyed significant tax breaks designed to stimulate investment. Also, NFPs are not exempt from all taxes. They pay payroll taxes and, in some states, taxes levied by the state on hospital admissions or payments to government in lieu of taxes; in some locales NFP hospitals actually pay more taxes on average than do FPs because of their larger size and payrolls (see, for example, Parker et al. 1995).

In contrast to the view that bottom-line considerations force uniformity of organizational behavior is the view that ownership form involves much more than nominal and tax-related differences. Legal and economic analyses of NFP and FP organizations emphasize the absence of equity owners in the NFP form and the prohibition in NFPs of the distribution of profits to owners or other private persons (what Hansmann [1980] has called the nondistribution constraint). Also important is the related difference in internal accountability structures.

Managers of FP organizations are ultimately accountable to owners, who generally seek to maximize the value of their investments, whereas NFP managers are accountable to boards of trustees whose members lack an ownership stake and who may have a variety of values, motivations, and goals, including community service. Agency problems may exist on either the NFP or FP side, with managers pursuing their own interests as they define them, rather than focusing primarily on the interests of stockholders or the values of trustees. But FP healthcare companies use several devices to align the incentives of owners and managers. Senior executives commonly own substantial amounts of corporate stock, and companies often use large economic incentives to motivate executives toward corporate goals.[5]

Managers of NFP hospitals cannot ignore their organizations' economic well-being, but they are prohibited from sharing in profits. The governance structure of NFP organizations has no recognized obligation to maximize economic returns for owners, because there are no such owners. Moreover, whereas Wall Street closely watches the economic performance of publicly traded hospital companies and exacts stiff penalties for disappointing earnings, NFP hospitals are subject to public criticism when they seem to be more concerned with the bottom line than with service to the community.

All of this suggests that there are reasons to expect both similarities and differences in the performance of hospitals of different ownership forms regarding service to the poor and uninsured. What is the empirical evidence?

Ownership Form and Care of the Poor

Much of the knowledge about hospital services for the poor and uninsured is in the form of accounting data about uncompensated care, generally defined in accounting terms as deductions from gross revenues for bad debt and charity. The imperfections of uncompensated care as a measure of service to the "poor and uninsured" are obvious. Many of the poor are not uninsured, and the bad debt component of uncompensated care does not arise only from service to the poor. In addition, the measure does not take account of governmental subsidies to institutions (primarily public hospitals) that serve the poor.

National uncompensated care numbers based on American Hospital Association surveys show only slightly higher levels of uncompensated care in NFP than in FP hospitals, a pattern that has been quite persistent for many years (Ashby 1991). Uncompensated care data for 1994 showed

NFPs at 4.5 percent of revenues and FPs at 4.0 percent (Prospective Payment Assessment Commission 1996).

Public hospitals provide much higher levels of uncompensated care than do either NFPs or FPs and clearly play an important role in caring for the poor and uninsured. Many of these institutions receive direct governmental subsidies for this purpose, which enhances their ability to provide such services. Indeed, the amount of uncompensated care that public hospitals provide, *net of government subsidies,* is similar to that provided by other hospitals (Ashby 1991). For example, Ashby (1991) reports that for 1988–89, urban public hospitals' uncompensated care costs were 13.4 percent of revenues, compared with 4.8 percent for NFP hospitals and 4.5 percent for FP hospitals. However, when the subsidies were included, the public hospitals' number was 4.8 percent, the same as that for NFP hospitals and slightly higher than that for FPs.

The picture of comparable NFP-FP behavior is based on national uncompensated care numbers that are included annually in reports by a neutral and respected source, the Prospective Payment Assessment Commission (ProPAC). It is widely cited as evidence that FPs and NFPs are not really different. But this picture may be misleading because of problems regarding the source of the data and because it ignores state-level differences.[6] Moreover, combining bad debt and charity into the single measure, uncompensated care, magnifies the similarity of ownership forms; there is evidence that the share of uncompensated care that is attributed to charity is much larger in NFPs than in FPs, even when uncompensated care numbers are similar (Buczko 1994).

The ProPAC data come from unaudited self-reports by hospitals, with substantial missing data problems, in the annual surveys by the American Hospital Association. Moreover, the amount of a hospital's bad debt and charity is influenced by the magnitude of its charges, and many studies have shown that FP hospitals have higher charges than NFPs.[7] A clue to the extent to which underlying differences in service to the uninsured may be concealed by numbers about uncompensated care comes from two studies done in the early 1980s. Rowland's (1984) analysis of data from a 1981 survey by the Office for Civil Rights showed that 6 percent of patients admitted to FP hospitals were uninsured, compared with 7.9 percent in NFP hospitals and 16.8 percent in public hospitals (see also Institute of Medicine 1986). Frank, Salkever, and Mullan (1990) analyzed data from the National Hospital Discharge Survey and found that approximately 4 percent of discharges from FP hospitals were uninsured, compared with approximately 6 percent of discharges from NFP hospitals and 11 percent from public hospitals.

Both studies found a similar pattern, but a smaller magnitude difference regarding services to Medicaid patients.

National data likely mute ownership differences. Not-for-profits are found in large numbers in all states, including many that have low levels of the uninsured and, therefore, proportionately low levels of need for hospitalization of the uninsured. For-profits are concentrated in states with growing populations and friendly regulatory environments; many of these states also have relatively high numbers of uninsured people.[8] In such states, NFPs tend to provide much higher levels of uncompensated care than do FPs; this is true for Texas, Tennessee, Virginia, and Florida where NFPs provide substantially more (in some cases twice as much) uncompensated care than do FPs.[9] Studies from California, however, show similarly low amounts of uncompensated care in FP and NFP hospitals, perhaps because of the large numbers of governmentally subsidized public hospitals in that state.[10] An inference that can be drawn from this pattern is that NFPs may be more responsive to unmet needs for medical care than are FPs; where the demand for uncompensated care is low, they may concentrate on other forms of community benefit or simply charge lower prices.

Not-for-profit and for-profit differences in uncompensated care could be due either to differences in being asked to serve such patients or to differences in willingness to serve. Both factors may be involved. Norton and Staiger (1994) found that ownership differences in uncompensated care were largely explained by the FPs having acquired or located hospitals in relatively high-income areas. For-profit hospitals are also more likely than NFPs to put pressure on physicians not to admit uninsured and Medicaid patients (Schlesinger et al. 1987), and physicians report conflict over the treatment of indigents more often in FP than in NFP hospitals (Burns, Anderson, and Shortell 1990). Finally, FP hospitals have been substantially overrepresented among hospitals that have been found by the U.S. Department of Health and Human Services to have violated the 1986 "antidumping" legislation that forbade hospitals from denying treatment to emergency patients and women in labor.[11]

Uncompensated Care and Tax Exemptions

From a policy point of view, the performance of FP hospitals may not be the most important standard of comparison for NFPs. Not-for-profit hospitals' performance could also be compared with the value of their tax exemptions. Not-for-profit hospitals are tax exempt as *charitable* organizations, which the Internal Revenue Service defines in terms of *community benefit*, not free care. The argument is sometimes made that the value of the community benefit activities, particularly uncompensated care, provided by a hospital should be at least equivalent to the amount of the "subsidy" that it enjoys by virtue of its tax exemptions.[12] The U.S. General Accounting Office (1990) conducted a study of California and New York hospitals in 1990 and found that approximately 20 percent were providing less uncompensated care than the value of their federal tax exemptions; when the narrower definition of "charity care" was adopted, almost 30 percent of New York NFP hospitals and almost 60 percent of California NFPs provided less than the value of their federal tax exemption.[13] Federal legislation was subsequently proposed, but not passed, to link exemptions to an uncompensated care requirement. Such linkages have been made in a few states (Potter and Longest 1994; Barnett 1996).

The connection between tax exemptions and uncompensated care raises several important issues. First, some policymakers and some FP advocates would define community benefit for tax-exemption purposes solely in terms of charity care for the poor. For policymakers, this would address an important problem (the uninsured) that lawmakers have not addressed more directly and it seems (misleadingly) to refer to something quite concrete and readily measurable.[14] The appeal for FP advocates is the narrow picture it presents of the value of NFPs and because the amount of uncompensated care varies widely among NFP hospitals (as it does among FPs), depending on a number of factors including hospital location. If charity care were the sole measure of community benefit for tax-exempt organizations, some NFPs would fail the test. Moreover, the acquisition of some NFP hospitals by FP companies would be of little community concern. Data on uncompensated care are being used in policy battles at the state level.[15]

A strong case can be made for a broader view of the meaning of community benefit. Schlesinger, Gray, and Bradley (1996) developed a more comprehensive set of measures derived from tax law, economic theories of NFPs, and the work of scholars and hospital associations regarding community benefit. The authors identified 30 different dimensions, including activities that create positive externalities (e.g., contracting with essential community providers, reporting bad clinical practices to appropriate authorities), minimizing negative externalities (e.g., shifting the burdens of cost containment to providers or patients' families), providing public goods (e.g., involvement in research and educational activities), minimizing the exploitation of informational asymmetries, and various forms of community involvement.

The research base with which to assess the overall community benefits of different types of healthcare organizations has serious inadequacies, and a full summary of available information is beyond the scope of this chapter. But a wide variety of indicators suggest that NFPs have substantial advantages from a broadly defined community benefit standpoint (Claxton et al. 1997; Gray 1997). For example, local governance is much more typical among NFP than FP hospitals; NFP hospitals are more likely to be located in urban areas with large numbers of poor and uninsured; NFPs are much more involved in research and education than are FPs; NFP hospitals offer a greater array of services including some that typically lose money; and NFPs are much less likely than FPs to undergo recurrent changes of ownership and control.[16]

The advantage of a broad definition of community benefit is that it more fully captures the benefits that might be provided by NFP organizations and that might be at stake, for example, when organizations consider converting to FP status (Gray 1997). A disadvantage of the broad definition is that it is not based in a common metric that can be quantified and compared across organizations.

The breadth of one's view of the community benefit issue bears on one other tax-related issue. In debates about ownership form and community benefit, FP companies and advocates often argue that FP companies meet their social responsibility fully by paying taxes that NFP and public facilities do not pay. The percentage of revenues paid by FP hospitals in taxes appears to be greater than the difference between the average NFP and the average FP in the amount of uncompensated care that is provided. This has led to suggestions that FPs provide more social benefit than do many NFPs.

The question of whether communities are better off with tax-exempt NFPs or tax-paying FPs depends on several factors. First, it depends on the definition of community benefit that is used. If one uses the narrow measure of uncompensated care, it is clear that some FPs have higher levels than do some NFPs. This is less true if better measures than uncompensated care or more comprehensive measures of community benefit were used. Moreover, it is important to bear in mind the issues that have already been discussed—that uncompensated care is not the same thing as care of the poor and uninsured, that uncompensated care numbers are influenced by the magnitude of hospital charges, that a variety of measurement issues affect reports regarding uncompensated care, and that the need for uncompensated care varies across states and locales. If major stakes are to be attached to the relative performance of FP and NFP institutions in serving the poor and uninsured, improvements in measurement and analysis are needed.

Second, although the payment of taxes by taxable entities is clearly a good and socially responsible thing, most taxes paid by healthcare organizations represent a flow of funds from healthcare to other purposes and from communities to state or federal governments. Most taxes paid by corporations to federal or state governments are spent for purposes other than healthcare,[17] while presumably raising the cost of healthcare to purchasers. As was noted above, NFP organizations are *not* exempt from taxes that are used substantially for healthcare, particularly the payroll taxes that are used for the Medicare program.

Notwithstanding these points, the degree to which NFPs were similar to FPs on some measures, particularly uncompensated care, was surprising to many observers as research evidence began to accumulate in the early 1980s. The publication of this information in professional journals and in the 1986 Institute of Medicine report *For-Profit Enterprise in Health Care* led to critical scrutiny and some tax-exemption reform at both the federal and the state level. It also led to a great deal of self-examination and efforts at improvement by NFPs themselves.[18]

In recent years, NFP hospitals have come under much additional pressure to serve the poor and uninsured as justification of their tax exemptions. Some hospitals have begun including such service in their budgets and making public reports of their community impacts. Comprehensive reporting on hospitals' community benefit activities may both improve the responsiveness of NFPs to community needs and increase public awareness of important activities.

Conclusion

To summarize, national numbers on uncompensated care show very little difference among hospitals of different ownership form. The bulk of uncompensated care is provided by a relatively small number of public hospitals and NFP urban teaching hospitals. However, when measures other than national uncompensated care data are examined, or when comparisons are made in states that have large uninsured populations and few public hospitals, FP hospitals provide less service to the poor and uninsured than do NFP and public hospitals. For-profits are also more active than NFPs in discouraging admission of Medicaid and uninsured patients and more often run afoul of the antidumping law.

Policymakers have been willing to provide subsidies to public and, occasionally, NFP hospitals that facilitate the provision of care to the uninsured. In principle, such subsidies could also be provided to FP hospitals, but the absence of a history of commitment to the poor and the lack of a structure for monitoring the use of such subsidies reduces the likelihood of subsidies to FPs to provide access for the uninsured.

Most available data on uncompensated care and other community benefit activities in NFP hospitals come from an era in which NFPs were under little governmental pressure to provide and document their "community benefit" activities. Not-for-profits are subject to moral suasion and to pressure by way of the criteria for tax exemption. Notwithstanding the financial pressures in an increasingly competitive healthcare system, it is possible that FP-NFP differences in uncompensated care will grow in future years (Campbell and Ahern 1993). Research on psychiatric hospitals has shown that public pressure on NFPs is associated with greater differences with FPs in care for indigent patients (Schlesinger 1995). Nevertheless, relying on hospitals' ability and willingness to provide care for poor people in medical need barely merits the appellation "safety net" as an alternative to universal insurance coverage.

Notes

1. Calculations are based on the FP numbers as reported in Federation of American Health Systems (1995) and American Hospital Association (1994–95). These numbers include independent proprietary hospitals.
2. At least six HMO companies have had price/earnings ratios in excess of 30 in recent years; HMO companies are generally far below that now (see Kaiser Family Foundation 1995).
3. Nancy Kane, in an HCA-funded study, concluded that the cost of tax exemption among Virginia hospitals was approximately 8.4 percent of revenues (see Kuttner 1996).
4. Not-for-profit hospitals' total margins fell from 7.6 percent of revenues in the first year of the prospective payment system (roughly 1984, although the prospective payment system was phased in in a rolling fashion) to less than 4 percent within three years (see Prospective Payment Assessment Commission 1995b).
5. In interviews at Humana in 1987, I was told that as much as 50 percent of the compensation of CEOs in Humana hospitals was in incentives tied to explicit economic goals set by the corporation. Columbia/HCA establishes local joint ventures that own hospitals or other facilities, with local doctors and executives as investors. Kuttner (1996) was told by a Columbia/HCA executive that hospital CEOs who fall short of the corporate goal of a 20 percent gross return on revenues are "regularly called to

corporate headquarters in Nashville to explain and are ordered to redouble their efforts."

6. It is also sometimes argued that including urban teaching hospitals in the comparison misleadingly improves the uncompensated care numbers of the NFP sector, because these institutions often provide large amounts of uncompensated care and very few of them are FP. This is true, but the compositional difference between the sectors is not accidental and is itself significant. The composition of the FP healthcare sector is, after all, a reflection of the acquisition strategies of investor-owned companies. Sectoral differences in service to the poor and uninsured are, in part, a reflection of those strategies.

7. For-profits have higher prices, which inflate the amount written off as uncompensated care (see Gray 1991; see also Lewin, Eckles, and Miller 1988).

8. For example, Connecticut (with approximately 11 percent uninsured) and Massachusetts (with approximately 13 percent uninsured) have had no FP hospitals until the past year, whereas Florida (approximately 23 percent uninsured) and Texas (approximately 26 percent uninsured) have large numbers of FP hospitals.

9. The 1986 Institute of Medicine report *For-Profit Enterprise in Health Care* makes this point and summarizes the relevant literature to that date. For subsequent evidence on this point, see Lewin, Eckles, and Miller (1988); see also Gray (1991) and Arrington and Haddock (1990). A more recent series of reports on Florida, Virginia, Georgia, and Tennessee for 1993 or 1994 show that FP hospitals provide much less than their proportionate share of charity or indigent care (using several different definitions); these reports, which were done by the Voluntary Hospitals of America, Inc. (1995) and by the Atlanta law firm Parker, Hudson, Ranier, and Dobbs, are based on excellent sources of data. Unfortunately, these reports do not distinguish between government and private NFP hospitals, with Parker et al. (1995) referring to all either as not-for-profits or voluntaries and with the Voluntary Hospitals of America using the conceptually more interesting term, community-owned hospitals.

10. See Sofaer, Rundall, and Zellers (1990). The Institute of Medicine (1986) report and the Lewin, Eckles, and Miller (1988) article make this point. See also Brotman (1995), which reports no ownership differences in "indigent care" expenses in Georgia, attributing it to a regulatory requirement that all hospitals devote at least 3 percent of revenues to indigent care; however, Brotman does not actually provide any data.

11. See Steiber and Wolfe (1993, 1994). The most recent of these reports found that whereas 14 percent of community hospitals were FPs, 29 percent of hospitals cited for violations were FPs.

12. This argument reflects a particular interpretation, not shared by all legal experts, of the rationale for NFPs' tax exemptions. For a discussion of such rationales, see Simon (1987).

13. The difference between uncompensated care and charity care is that the

former includes bad debt (which can be, but is not necessarily, related to the patient's ability to pay) and the discrepancy between a hospital's costs or charges and the amount it receives from public programs such as Medicaid and Medicare. Hospitals commonly must subsidize services provided to Medicaid patients; regarding Medicare, the Prospective Payment Assessment Commission (1996) contends that hospitals in the aggregate made money during the first six years of the prospective payment system, lost money for the next three years, and in the past two years again realized a profit, in large part because of reductions in cost.

14. Complexities include whether "charity" patients should have to be designated in advance or whether charity also includes patients who prove unable to pay their bills. In addition, because the costs of services such as a hospital stay can vary enormously from patient to patient, it makes more sense to measure the extent of charity care in dollar terms rather than in terms of numbers of patients. However, requiring the documentation of the costs of the services provided to any particular patients—as opposed to the hospital's *charges* for such services—could be quite onerous, perhaps requiring the establishment of a new cost accounting system. But measuring uncompensated care in terms of *charges* would make the amount of charity care an organization provides a function, in part, of the size of the gap between the hospital's costs and its charges (see Lewin, Eckles, and Miller 1988).

15. As an example of the politics of this, a 1995 report by the consulting firm, Healthcare Management Decisions, Inc., for Columbia/HCA contended that several southwest Florida hospitals provided less community benefit than the value of their tax exemptions. The only community benefit that was counted, however, was the hospitals' "charity care" deduction from revenue; even other tangible measures (losses on Medicaid payments, unreimbursed educational costs) were ignored. An independent study of the same topic by a consulting firm hired by the Association of Voluntary Hospitals of Florida using a broader (though still relatively narrow) measure of community benefit, concluded that voluntary hospitals (defined to include both public and NFP hospitals) provided much larger amounts of community benefits than did FP hospitals, and substantially more than the value of their tax exemptions.

16. Much of this evidence is reviewed in Institute of Medicine (1986) and Gray (1991). See also Alexander, Lewis, and Morrisey (1985); Norton and Staiger (1994); LeBlanc and Hurley (1995); Prospective Payment Assessment Commission (1995a); Luft and Greenlick (1996); Veloski et al. (1996).

17. Less than 10 percent of federal spending from general revenues goes to healthcare, and less than 20 percent of state spending goes to healthcare.

18. Projects on the development and implementation of better community benefit standards were undertaken in the late 1980s by the Catholic Health Association, the American Hospital Association, the Voluntary Hospitals of America, and a Kellogg Foundation–sponsored project carried out at New York University with the cooperation of a significant group of hospitals.

References

Alexander, J., B. Lewis, and M. Morrisey. 1985. "Acquisition Strategies of Multi-hospital Systems." *Health Affairs* 4: 49–66.

American Hospital Association. 1994–1995. *Hospital Statistics.* Chicago: The Association.

Arrington, B., and C. C. Haddock. 1990. "Who Really Profits from Not-for-Profits?" *HSR: Health Services Research* 25: 290–304.

Ashby, J. 1991. *The Trend and Distribution of Hospital Uncompensated Care Costs, 1980–89.* Washington, DC: Prospective Payment Assessment Commission.

Barnett, K. 1996. *Community Benefit Law and California Hospitals: Opportunities and Challenges of SB 697.* Berkeley, CA: Western Consortium for Public Health.

Brotman, B. A. 1995. "Hospital Indigent Care Expenditures." *Journal of Health Care Finance* 21: 76–79.

Buczko, W. 1994. "Factors Affecting Charity Care and Bad Debt Charges in Washington Hospitals." *Hospital & Health Services Administration* 39 (2): 179–91.

Burns, L. R., R. M. Anderson, and S. M. Shortell. 1990. "The Effect of Hospital Control Strategies on Physician Satisfaction and Physician-Hospital Conflict." *HSR: Health Services Research* 25: 527–58.

Campbell, E. S., and M. W. Ahern. 1993. "Have Procompetitive Changes Altered Hospital Provision of Indigent Care?" *Health Economics* 2: 281–89.

Claxton, G., J. Feder, D. Schactman, and S. Altman. 1997. "Public Policy Issues in Nonprofit Conversions: An Overview." *Health Affairs* 16: 9–28.

Copeland, J., and G. Rudney. 1990. "Federal Tax Subsidies for Not-for-Profit Hospitals." *Tax Notes* 46: 1565.

Federation of American Health Systems. 1995. *Directory of the Federation of American Health Systems.* Washington, DC: The Federation.

Frank, R., D. Salkever, and F. Mullan. 1990. "Hospital Ownership and the Care of Uninsured and Medicaid Patients: Findings from the National Hospital Discharge Survey, 1979–1984." *Health Policy* 14: 1–11.

Gray, B. H. 1991. *The Profit Motive and Patient Care.* Cambridge, MA: Harvard University Press.

———. 1997. "Conversions of HMOs and Hospitals: What's at Stake?" *Health Affairs* 16 (2) 29–47.

Hansmann, H. 1980. "The Role of Nonprofit Organizations." *Yale Law Journal* 89: 835–901.

Healthcare Management Decisions, Inc. 1995. *Community Benefits and Tax-Exempt Status of Central Florida Hospitals.* St. Petersburg, FL: Healthcare Management Decisions, Inc.

Institute of Medicine. 1986. *For-Profit Enterprise in Health Care.* Washington, DC: National Academy Press.

Kaiser Family Foundation. 1995. "Sherlock Company P.U.L.S.E. Report." In *Marcus Welby Goes to Wall Street.* Menlo Park, CA: The Foundation.

Kuttner, R. 1996. "Columbia/HCA and the Resurgence of the For-profit Hospital Business." *New England Journal of Medicine* 355: 362–67.

LeBlanc, A. J., and R. E. Hurley. 1995. "Adoption of HIV-Related Services Among Urban U.S. Hospitals: 1988 and 1991." *Medical Care* 33: 881–91.

Lewin, L. S., T. Eckles, and L. Miller. 1988. "Setting the Record Straight: The Provision of Uncompensated Care by Not-for-Profit Hospitals." *New England Journal of Medicine* 318: 1212–15.

Luft, H. S., and M. R. Greenlick. 1996. "The Contribution of Group- and Staff-Model HMOs to American Medicine." *Milbank Quarterly* 74: 445–68.

Norton, E. C., and D. O. Staiger. 1994. "How Hospital Ownership Affects Access to Care for the Uninsured." *RAND Journal of Economics* 25: 171–85.

Parker, Hudson, Rainer, Dobbs. 1995. *Analysis of Central Florida Hospital Community Benefits: Community Hospitals Compared to Investor-Owned Hospitals.* Atlanta, GA: Parker, Hudson, Rainer, and Dobbs.

Potter, M., and B. Longest. 1994. "The Divergence of Federal and State Policies on the Charitable Tax Exemption of Nonprofit Hospitals." *Journal of Health Politics, Policy, and Law* 19: 393–410.

Prospective Payment Assessment Commission. 1995a. *Comparison of HMOs Across Paper Types.* Washington, DC: The Commission.

———. 1995b. *Medicare and the American Health Care System: Report to the Congress.* Washington, DC: The Commission.

———. 1996. *Medicare and the American Health Care System: Report to the Congress.* Washington, DC: The Commission.

Rowland, D. 1984. "Hospital Care for the Uninsured: An Analysis of the Role of Proprietary Hospitals." Paper delivered at the annual meeting of the American Public Health Association.

Schlesinger, M. 1995. *Mismeasuring the Consequences of Ownership: External Influences and the Comparative Performance of Public, For-Profit, and Nonprofit Organizations.* Working paper 204, Program on Non-Profit Organizations. New Haven, CT: Yale University Press.

Schlesinger, M., J. Bentkover, D. Blumenthal, R. Musacchio, and J. Willer. 1987. "The Privatization of Health Care and Physicians' Perceptions of Access to Hospital Services." *Milbank Quarterly* 65: 25–58.

Schlesinger, M., B. H. Gray, and E. Bradley, 1996. "Charity and Community: The Role of Nonprofit Ownership in a Managed Health Care System." *Journal of Health Politics, Policy, and Law* 21: 697–751.

Simon, J. G. 1987. "The Tax Treatment of Nonprofit Organizations." In *The Nonprofit Sector: A Research Handbook*, edited by W. W. Powell. New Haven, CT: Yale University Press.

Sofaer, S., T. G. Rundall, and W. L. Zellers. 1990. "Policy Changes Affecting Deductions from Revenue in California Hospitals, 1981–1986." *Hospital & Health Services Administration* 35: 191–206.

Steiber, J., and S. M. Wolfe. 1993. *Patient Dumping Continues in Hospital Emergency Rooms: An Updated Report on the Department of Health and Human Services' Enforcement of the Federal Patient Dumping Law.* Washington, DC: Public Citizen's Health Research Group.

———. 1994. *Update on "Patient Dumping" Violations.* Washington, DC: Public Citizen's Health Research Group.

Stevens, R. 1989. *In Sickness and in Wealth: American Hospitals in the Twentieth Century.* New York: Basic Books.

U.S. General Accounting Office. 1990. *Nonprofit Hospitals: Better Standards Needed for Tax Exemption.* Washington, DC: The Office.

Veloski, J., B. Barzansky, D. Nash, S. Bastacky, and D. Stevens. 1996. "Medical Student Education in Managed Care Settings: Beyond HMOs." *Journal of the American Medical Association* 276: 667–71.

Voluntary Hospitals of America, Inc. 1995. *Florida Hospital Analysis.* Irving, TX: Voluntary Hospitals of America, Inc.

Weissman, J. 1996. "Uncompensated Hospital Care: Will It Be There If We Need It?" *Journal of the American Medical Association* 276: 823–28.

Wikler, D. 1988. "The Virtuous Hospital: Do Nonprofit Institutions Have a Distinctive Moral Mission?" In *In Sickness and in Health: The Mission of Voluntary Health Care Institutions,* edited by J. D. Seay and B. C. Vladeck, 138–39. New York: McGraw-Hill.

12

The Role of Investor-Owned and Not-for-Profit Organizations in Providing Healthcare to the Poor and Uninsured: A Perspective

Thomas A. Scully

Introduction

The issue of caring for those who cannot afford to pay for themselves is important today because the traditional methods of support may become a thing of the past. The cost of care for most of the poor historically has been paid by government, through Medicaid and, to a much lesser extent, Medicare as well as through direct subsidies to public and private hospitals and clinics. These sources are shrinking. President Clinton has proposed that Medicaid spending fall by $59 billion over seven years compared with baseline spending. In 1996, both the U.S. Senate and the House proposed reducing Medicaid spending growth by $72 billion over six years. State and local governments also have reduced overall health spending and spending on healthcare for the low-income population, in particular. Government's ability, if not its willingness, to bear these costs has declined.

Historically, the number two source for financing healthcare for the poor and uninsured was the "invisible" transfer system, more commonly referred to as cost shifting, whereby those who could pay for their care

This work was sponsored by the Council on the Economic Impact of Health System Change.

were charged more than it cost so that healthcare providers could cover the costs of caring for those who could not afford to pay for all or any of the care they received. While a minority argues that cost shifting never existed, conventional wisdom holds that cost shifting does indeed exist, and there is reason to be concerned that it is shrinking.

Why is cost shifting shrinking? It is shrinking because hospitals and other providers have been transformed from price setters to price takers. Employers and insurers are increasingly unwilling to be the silent partners of healthcare providers in the cost shifting and transfer scheme. Not long ago, insurance companies essentially were funnels used to direct money from employers to providers. More recently, as the cost of healthcare skyrocketed, corporations began to view employee benefits, especially health coverage, as cost centers that should be managed in the same way that other parts of their businesses are managed. This change in corporate behavior has contributed to the growing dominance of managed care organizations. A major consequence for providers is that they must compete against one another for precious contracts and plan enrollees. This competition has reduced provider revenues, payment-to-cost ratios, their margins, and threatened their ability to cover the cost of caring for those unable to pay for themselves.

The Changing Healthcare Market

The market for healthcare is changing at a dizzying pace. Many types of treatment that were traditionally performed in hospitals are moving rapidly to outpatient clinics, ambulatory surgical centers, and even physicians' offices. As a result of these and other changes, a growing number of health policy analysts are suggesting that the days of the inpatient acute care hospital as we know it are limited, that in short order it will be a small intensive care vestige on a larger integrated healthcare delivery system.

The types of health plans from which employers and individuals can choose also are changing dramatically. In the past, the choice was almost exclusively the fee-for-service, see any doctor you want, indemnity and major medical health plan. Today the market is flooded with options: health maintenance organizations (HMOs), preferred provider organizations, point of services, and independent delivery systems. Also, providers rendered care that was paid for directly by insurers and individuals. It is now possible for employers and individuals to purchase the full range of services from provider-sponsored organizations.

In addition, it seems that the nature and structure of the mixed healthcare economy also is changing. Where once the only health insurance available was from not-for-profit Blue Cross and Blue Shield plans, today commercial insurers and for-profit HMOs play a central role in paying for healthcare. Some of the "blues" have converted their tax status from tax exempt to tax paying. Many more are contemplating it. And Columbia/HCA has made an offer to purchase Ohio Blue Cross.

In the hospital world there appear to be major changes as well. The trade press regularly reports on the purchase of hospitals by investor-owned management companies. According to the American Hospital Association, in 1994, just under 14 percent of acute care hospitals, 719 out of 5,229, were investor owned, down 1 percent from the high of just under 15 percent in 1987. In 1994, 11.2 percent of acute care hospital beds were in investor-owned hospitals. This is up just 0.4 percent from ten years earlier. It is possible that dramatic changes in what had once been a stable relationship have occurred in the last two and one-half years, the period for which official data are not available. The best estimate is that fewer than 50 hospitals nationwide have converted over this time period. This represents only approximately one-half of one percentage point—so the structural change is, in fact, overstated.

There are other developments that have raised concern for the future of not-for-profit providers and health plans. These providers in some areas are being asked to make taxlike payments to local governments to cover the cost of services that these municipalities provide—police, fire, etc. Hospitals are often one of the largest, if not the largest, landowners in a community. Exempting hospitals from property taxation is a very large subsidy to one of the largest revenue-generating enterprises in many communities. Similarly, some states, such as Texas, have enacted laws that require tax-exempt hospitals to provide a minimum level of community benefits or charity care. Texas set the level at four percent of total costs. Finally, the value of the federal nonprofit tax exemption is called into question periodically, not just for not-for-profit hospitals, but for all tax-exempt organizations. The question that is raised is whether the amount of benefits provided to the community by the organization are at least as great as the value of the tax exemption received.

Why the Concern?

Regardless of some indications to the contrary, there is concern that the tax-exempt status of not-for-profit healthcare providers and health plans is threatened, either as a result of being acquired by an investor-owned company or because the traditional tax treatment of not-for-profit health plans and healthcare providers may be limited or cease altogether.

And, with respect to providing care for the poor, there is concern that the loss of tax-exempt providers may mean that the motivation and financial wherewithal to provide free or low-cost care may also disappear. It also means, some believe, that the hospitals that bear the greatest burden for caring for the poor and uninsured will face severe financial challenges, and, if they do not survive (unless government accepts the responsibility), hospital care will be less available to those in poor areas. Finally, there is the view that conversions of hospitals from tax exempt to tax paying will reduce the community benefits that have historically been provided by tax-exempt hospitals.

Is the Concern Justified?

This section details the three concerns. The first concern is that investor-owned hospital management companies have selectively avoided owning facilities in inner city, rural, or other poor areas. Although the majority of hospitals in central cities are tax-exempt facilities, there are important exceptions. And, with respect to rural areas, the evidence contradicts the argument. Two large companies—Community Health Systems and Health Management Associates—almost exclusively purchase or build hospitals in rural areas. Columbia/HCA, Tenet Healthcare, and OrNda HealthCorp increasingly reach out to buy both inner city and rural hospitals as they build regional, not just metropolitan, networks.

There is no way to prove or disprove definitively the theory that tax-paying hospitals avoid inner city and poor areas. A clearly logical alternative to the purposeful avoidance theory is the argument that the location of tax-paying hospitals today is mostly an accident of history. Many urban hospitals began either as public poor houses or religious missions. At a time when little effective medical care existed, these institutions cared for the physical needs of the poor. Over time, hospitals, sometimes major institutions, grew from these roots.

Most tax-exempt hospitals were built after World War II with funds from the Hill-Burton Act. The earliest private investor-owned hospitals, on the other hand, were in rural areas, mainly in the West and South, where doctors, needing a place to practice, built small hospitals. The later expansion of tax-paying hospitals also occurred primarily in these areas, because this is where the population was moving and because, as funds from the Hill-Burton Act tapered off, new capital was needed to build facilities in the South and West. There was little demand for building inner-city hospitals in the Northeast and Midwest. Only recently, as some city and county governments have faced major financial difficulties, have they even considered getting out of the hospital business and selling community facilities to investor-owned providers. So, faster growth of investor-owned facilities in suburban areas of the South and West is due largely to population growth and timing—not avoidance.

The second concern is that tax-paying hospitals behave differently than tax-exempt hospitals, at least with respect to caring for the poor and uninsured. Considerable evidence exists that investor-owned hospitals care for the poor and uninsured at about the same level as tax-exempt hospitals. The current report of the Prospective Payment Assessment Commission (ProPAC) (1996) indicates that in 1994 tax-paying hospitals, on average, provided uncompensated care (defined as charity care, bad debt, and the Medicaid shortfall) equal to 4 percent of total costs. This compares very favorably with tax-exempt private hospitals, which provided uncompensated care equal to 4.5 percent of total costs (or rural government-owned hospitals, which provided uncompensated care equal to 4.6 percent of total costs). Not surprisingly, urban government hospitals significantly exceeded all other types of hospitals in the provision of uncompensated care. On average, they provided uncompensated care equal to 6.7 percent of total costs. It is hard to argue, based on this data, that tax-paying hospitals are an outlier when it comes to uncompensated care. More recently, independent researchers at Boston University, in a study published in *Health Affairs*, found that when investor-owned companies purchased not-for-profit hospitals, indigent care did not drop; in fact, it increased by a small amount after the purchase. This is shockingly inconsistent with general perceptions and undermines one of the very reasons tax-exempt status is conferred—to service uninsured patients.

There is also a legitimate debate about whether all tax-exempt hospitals are fulfilling the obligation they assume when they accept the exemption. In 1993, Texas enacted a law requiring tax-exempt facilities to provide charity care at least equal to 4 percent of patient care expenditures. A recent analysis by *Modern Healthcare* magazine sheds some light on a cloudy subject. The analysis showed that, as widely believed, accounting practices vary greatly with respect to reported uncompensated care. Although charity care in Texas was reported to have increased between 1992 and 1994 by 51 percent, from $347 million to $566 million, *Modern Healthcare* reported that "many hospital executives say that the considerable increase doesn't necessarily reflect true growth in dollars. Instead, executives [of tax-exempt hospitals] say they're keeping better track of charity care spending."

It is not surprising that the analysis found that these hospitals provide less charity care, because there is no charity care requirement for tax-paying hospitals. Again, accounting conventions are the culprit. Before the 1993 law, there was no great incentive for hospitals, regardless of tax-paying status, to report uncompensated care costs. Tax-paying hospitals, which seem to have a somewhat greater incentive to make a strong effort to collect unpaid bills, sometimes have reported some or all charity care as bad debts. On the other hand, because the 1993 law changed the incentive for tax-exempt hospitals, what previously had been bad debt may now be reported as charity care, because as *Modern Healthcare* quoted a Texas lawyer saying, "that's because not-for-profits have 'the attorney general breathing down their throats,' which gives them the incentive not to pursue bad-debt cases to meet charity care levels."

There seems to be three lessons in this. First, hospitals respond to incentives—but not always as intended. Second, not much is known about the facts of uncompensated care. Variation in accounting practices obscures any facts. Third, whether called charity care or bad debts, all types of hospitals provide considerable care to patients who do not pay.

The third reason that concern exists about conversions is that other community benefits, in addition to uncompensated care, may decline. No one knows the extent of the value of community benefits provided by hospitals. These benefits take on myriad or innumerable forms. Some hospitals offer prenatal classes or well-baby clinics. Others go into public schools as part of antismoking or antidrug efforts. Still others participate in health fairs or provide recreational facilities for the community. Although hard facts do not exist, there is no reason to believe that tax-paying hospitals do not also provide free care, health education classes, and other opportunities that are significant community benefits, and they do this while they pay taxes.

It may be that the most important characteristic distinguishing tax-paying from tax-exempt hospitals is that the former pay taxes. Property taxes are a concrete benefit to the local community. Income taxes go to both the state and the federal governments. The value of these taxes is easily quantified. In 1994, the last year for which data are available, these hospitals paid taxes totaling nearly $3 billion. And it is worth noting that these taxes were paid only by investor-owned hospitals that realized a profit. This group of hospitals, according to ProPAC data, are at the greatest risk of losses. Twenty-nine percent of investor-owned hospitals had negative margins in 1993. This compares with 22.2 percent of tax-exempt hospitals, 27.5 percent of rural government hospitals, and 20.9 percent of urban government hospitals. At the same time, investor-owned hospitals provided uncompensated care equal to nearly $4 billion—excluding contractual allowances for Medicare, which equaled another $10 billion.

Conversions of hospitals to tax-paying hospitals also generate significant community benefits. When an investor-owned hospital management company purchases a public hospital, the proceeds of the sale go into the city's or county's treasury and reduce the tax burden on all citizens of the jurisdiction. A tax-exempt community hospital conversion often results in the establishment of a community foundation governed by a community board. When Tulane University Hospital was converted to an investor-owned institution, Columbia/HCA established a foundation for teaching and research, funded with $130 million. In Wichita, Kansas, the conversion of Wesley Medical Center resulted in a $350 million foundation. In 1995 this foundation distributed $18 million in the community.

Conversions often have other significant community benefits. When Universal Health Services bought McAllen Medical Center in McAllen, Texas, it brought with it $50 million in capital. What had been a hospital with limited services became a facility with a full range of services, including a new neonatal intensive care unit. The converted hospital established a perinatology residency program and set up a $1 million foundation to fund nursing education. McAllen is in Hidalgo County in south Texas, eight miles from the Mexican border. Each month, nearly 100 "drop-in" deliveries for Mexican mothers are performed, free of charge. The hospital has improved, service to the community has improved, and Universal Health Services is investing in a new hospital in another nearby community with similar demographics.

When Quorum Health purchased St. Anthony's Hospital (a Catholic facility in Columbus, Ohio) in 1992, it was in financial disarray. Had Quorum not purchased it, it would have closed. The company infused capital into the hospital, introduced more efficient management, and worked closely with the medical staff to improve the quality of every aspect of the hospital. Recently, the hospital, now known as Park Medical Center, received a rating of 92 out of a possible 100 points on an evaluation by the Joint Commission on the Accreditation of Hospital Organizations (JCAHO). In 1991 JCAHO had found the hospital deficient in 21 different areas, including record keeping, quality of care, and physician credentialing. Quality and community service have now improved.

Conversions of tax-exempt hospitals to tax-paying hospitals, it is often argued, leads to resources being taken out of the community. There is ample evidence that conversions lead to better care, better management, and more investment in the community. In the hundreds of conversions nationwide, trustees are yet to be found who, four or five years later, felt that they had made a mistake for their community.

Conclusion

This chapter has tried to put into perspective, if not to rest, the concern that the conversion of health plans and healthcare providers from tax-exempt hospitals to tax-paying hospitals will reduce the care available to the poor and uninsured. Nonetheless, I share the larger concern that healthcare must be available for the poor and uninsured. I believe that member companies of the Federation of American Health Systems are well positioned to continue to meet their commitment. Hospitals that are able to respond to increasing pressure to reduce health spending by providing high-quality care with lower costs will be most able to continue to fulfill their community responsibilities. From St. Joseph's in Omaha, Wesley in Wichita, and Presbyterian in Oklahoma City to Michael Reese in Chicago, Miami Heart in Miami, and the University of Southern California Medical Center in Los Angeles, they continue to be strong and supportive members of communities of all sizes and makeup throughout the nation.

This does not mean that the financing and availability of care for the poor and uninsured are not issues that need continually to be addressed. On the contrary, the pressure to find a rational, long-term solution is growing. The Federation of American Health Systems will continue work to develop creative solutions to these problems, while its member hospitals continue to be good citizens and good neighbors in the communities they serve.

Reference

Prospective Payment Assessment Commission. 1996. *Medicare and the American Health Care System: Report to the Congress.* Washington, DC: The Commission.

IV

The Search for Solutions I: The Road Is Paved with Incremental Reforms at the Federal and State Levels

13

Less Is More: After the Clinton Plan, Let's Think Small

Henry J. Aaron

Introduction

The chapter that follows introduced a volume containing several papers by academics, public opinion experts, and government officials presented at a Brookings Institution conference that examined the lessons of the Clinton administration's monumentally unsuccessful effort to win approval of its national insurance plan. It was written in the summer of 1995 and reflected two sentiments, each of which combined what I think was cool and accurate appraisal with intense emotion.

The first sentiment was disappointment at the extreme ineptitude of the entire Clinton health reform effort. Despite comprising a highly talented team, the Clinton administration made virtually every mistake possible. The effort is, in some ways, reminiscent of the way the United States blundered into and out of Vietnam, an enterprise examined earlier in a Brookings Institution study, entitled (with no irony!), *Vietnam: The System Worked.*

The Clinton health reform initiative—I believed then and still believe now—definitively ended six decades of efforts to complete the social insurance edifice whose foundation and main structure were laid with enactment of the Social Security Act of 1935. It is inconceivable that any president for the foreseeable future will raise the banner of national health insurance. The political catastrophe that the Democratic

This work originally appeared in *The Problem That Won't Go Away: Reforming U.S. Healthcare Financing*, edited by Henry J. Aaron. © 1996. Reprinted by permission of The Brookings Institution.

Party experienced in 1994, to which the entire health reform episode contributed significantly, will stand like a political skull and cross bones warning any administration that trying to assure universal coverage carries lethal risks.

The second sentiment is one of bug-eyed fascination at the developments that have unfolded since the failure of the Clinton health plan and that show every indication of continuing for the indefinite future. The United States is embarked on a revolutionary course, creating a healthcare system unlike any that has ever existed here or abroad. Consolidation among providers both horizontally (hospital mergers and the formation of enormous physician groups, for example) and vertically (linkage of physicians to hospitals and of hospitals to insurers, for example) is transforming the delivery system. New contracting modes are transforming the financial incentives facing providers and patients alike.

Advocates of these reforms hold out great hopes that these new institutions will greatly increase efficiency. They believe that these private contractual relationships—which constitute a form of private regulation—will break the back of excessively rapid growth of healthcare spending and will squeeze out low-benefit uses of medical procedures while preserving high-benefit uses. Critics point to the steadily increasing numbers of the uninsured and the threat that these numbers will rise still more in the future. They warn of the squeeze on provider budgets that is narrowing the capacity of providers to provide uncompensated care.

Underlying the essay that follows is a belief that, in large measure, the optimists and the pessimists are both right. The healthcare system that is emerging will be leaner and more efficient than the flabby delivery nonsystem that it is replacing, although of course it will exhibit errors of judgment by private managers and may entail infuriating bureaucratization. But it will also be a meaner and less compassionate system in which people get only the care they or their employers or the government program for which they qualify pays for. For a long time, foreigners have looked down on a U.S. healthcare system that, as they saw it, permitted acutely ill people to go entirely without care. That image contained elements of truth. The uninsured have received less care and, too often, inferior care. But the foreign image was largely false because the uninsured were the beneficiaries of pervasive cross-subsidies. I fear that the foreigner's image may become more of a reality than it ever has been before.

The great question—the answer to which, as a financially comfortable and well-insured person, I am largely immune—concerns how the nation will respond to the emerging lack of access to care that will afflict millions of people. I express the view in what follows that the nation will find such lack of access—if, indeed, it occurs—repugnant and unacceptable, that it will react by demanding that actions be taken to provide such access, and that, in due course, the assurance of universal access to healthcare will return to the national political agenda and win approval. But it seems clear, when and if the issue reemerges, changes in healthcare technology, the healthcare delivery system, and the prevailing financial arrangements will assure that it will do so in a form unlike that in which it has been discussed over the past six decades.

Lessons from the Past

Generals revisit great battles to improve strategy and tactics. For similar reasons, practical politicians and scholars of public policy will revisit the debate over the Clinton health plan. What did planners do right? How can the mistakes of that experience be avoided in the future? In addition to creating a superlative teaching tool for future study, the Clinton plan and the failed effort to enact it did something far more—they definitively ended the healthcare financing debate as it was then known.

This debate began six decades ago and has flared up sporadically since. The prospect that the federal government should orchestrate some combination of public and private actions to bring about universal coverage has been part of the "unfinished agenda" of the political left at least since enactment of the Social Security Act in 1935. The Committee for Economic Security, which designed the Social Security Act, had believed in national health insurance but did not recommend it. They feared that doing so would have doomed its principal recommendations for a new old age retirement system and for unemployment insurance. President Harry S Truman advanced a proposal for national health insurance, but he was narrowly elected and confronted a Congress that had no interest in acting on his proposal. Many saw the enactment of Medicare and Medicaid in 1965 as the first step in resuming the unfinished journey to national health insurance. Presidents Nixon and Carter also advanced proposals to extend universal coverage to the nonelderly and, in addition, to control growth of medical costs. For various reasons, these efforts failed and nothing happened for the next 30 years after enactment of Medicare beyond marginal expansions in Medicaid coverage and the introduction of new methods of paying hospitals and physicians under Medicare. The passage of nearly 30 years without further major action might have been read as a bad omen for ultimate success, but many advocates of national health insurance saw it as evidence that ultimate success, which they never doubted, was that much closer. President Clinton's proposal to provide all Americans with health insurance "that is always there" and to slow the growth of healthcare spending was thus part of an historical mission that Democrats had been striving to complete for more than half a century.

That mission, it is now apparent, will not be completed in a form recognizable by traditional advocates of national health insurance. For reasons that in prospect seemed evident to some and in retrospect seem clear to most, President Clinton had no real chance to win congressional acceptance of a single bill transforming the financing of American healthcare. To begin with, he was politically weak. Elected by barely two-fifths of voters and having run behind most congressional Democrats in contested elections, he had little leverage with members even of his own party. Second, changes in congressional rules and in methods of financing and managing congressional campaigns that weakened party discipline had diminished the capacity of a president to force through costly and complex legislation important to most members of Congress. Third, and most important, no legislation remotely approximating the size and complexity of the Clinton health reform plan had ever been enacted in the United States except during war or major depression. Unlike earlier legislation that created land grant colleges or retirement pensions, the proposed legislation to reform healthcare financing would not fill a vacuum—after all, approximately 85 percent of nonelderly Americans already had insurance and one-seventh of the U.S. economy was devoted to producing healthcare services (Employee Benefit Research Institute 1994; Prospective Payment Assessment Commission 1995; and author calculations using data from *Survey of Current Business*). Thus, health reform required the reconstruction of entire industries, putting jobs and investments at risk, and confronting most Americans with the prospect of seeing familiar and comfortable arrangements for gaining access to a life-or-death service radically transformed. As Charles Schultze observed, it was as if the president had proposed to remake an entity as large as all of France in a single piece of legislation. The legislation affected the vital interests of hospitals, physicians, other health providers, medical device manufacturers, pharmaceutical companies, small businesses and large corporations, and organized labor. And since one goal of reform was to slow the growth of spending, the proposal had to reduce the expected incomes of these groups.

Four centuries ago, Machiavelli (1961, 51–52) captured the risks associated with large-scale reforms with a clarity scarce in Washington in 1993:

It should be borne in mind that there is nothing more difficult to arrange, more doubtful of success, and more dangerous to carry through than initiating changes in a state's constitution. The innovator makes enemies of all those who prospered under the old order, and only lukewarm support is forthcoming from those who would prosper under the new. Their support is lukewarm partly from fear of their adversaries, who have the existing laws on their side, and partly because men are generally incredulous, never really trusting new things unless they have tested them by experience. In consequence, whenever those who oppose the changes can do so, they attack vigorously, and the defense made by the others is only lukewarm. So both the innovator and his friends are endangered together. But to discuss this subject thoroughly we must distinguish between innovators who stand alone and those who depend on others, that is between those who to achieve their purposes can force the issue and those who must use persuasion. In the second case, they always come to grief.

The collapse of the effort to reform healthcare financing and the subsequent Republican electoral victory in November 1994 erased government-led reform of private health insurance from the national agenda for the foreseeable future. It now seems unlikely that any administration or Congress will take up this issue again in the way that President Clinton—or, earlier, Presidents Carter, Nixon, and Truman—did. They all saw the national government as the agent for enforcing universal national health insurance. The mechanisms varied, but all agreed on four key points: that universality was important, that the only way to reach that goal was a legal mandate requiring everyone to be insured, that only the federal government could enforce such a mandate, and that such a mandate was an acceptable instrument of social policy.

In the aftermath of the Clinton health plan and the 1994 Republican electoral victory, it is hard to find any major political figure who will advance these views. In the course of the political debate in 1994, the concept of universal insurance underwent an Orwellian transformation from its traditional meaning of essentially 100 percent coverage to 97 or 95 percent coverage, although such redefined "universality" would have left many of the prereform uninsured population still uncovered. The view that universal health insurance coverage is desirable but not vital has gained new respectability. The reason for the abandonment of universality as a goal was the realization, born of the complexity of the Clinton proposal, that the means necessary to achieve it were more than the country would tolerate. As Mongan (1996) discusses in a recent publication, the stages of erosion of the commitment to universal coverage stand as milestones in the demise of the Clinton plan.

Many commentators on the Clinton reform effort support the view that the administration, Congress, and the nation lacked the political consensus and the information to credibly describe the effects of any single bill to reform the U.S. healthcare system.

The only option available to the administration was to reach for goals far more modest than those it sought—the initiation of a *process* of change that would begin with modest, incremental steps to eventually achieve universal coverage and general reform. This approach would not have promised immediate cuts in federal healthcare spending, but, in the end, estimates of the Congressional Budget Office (1995) confirmed that the president's own proposal failed that test, at least for the first decade after enactment. Covering the costs of extended coverage would take all the feasible savings from reduced growth of spending and more besides. To contribute to deficit reduction, planners discovered, would take sizable tax increases, a step that in 1993 and 1994 seemed the political equivalent of public indecency. A strategy of small steps couched in a vision of longer term reform would not have made the giant strides toward reestablishing the conviction among the American people that limited government can achieve major social objectives. But the administration lacked the political resources to do more and, reaching for vastly more, squandered its limited capacity even to advance a small step toward its most cherished programmatic and political objectives.

Looking Forward

The events of 1993 and 1994 may have put proposals for government-guaranteed universal coverage and cost control in the "deep freeze," but they assuredly did not cool political interest in healthcare policy. The federal role in financing healthcare will remain a hot political issue for at least three reasons. First, the pressure to cut public spending to balance the budget means that Medicare and Medicaid will be in the legislative spotlight. These two programs represented 22 percent of projected federal government spending in the year 1996 (apart from interest on the debt), and the increase in spending on these two programs as a share of gross domestic product accounts for all of the projected increase in the federal deficit between 1996 and 2002.[1] Second, the retirement of the baby boom generation over the quarter century from 2010 to 2035 promises large additional increases in the cost of Medicare, which pays for acute care for the elderly and disabled, and of Medicaid, which pays approximately half of the national cost of long-term care. Third, a seemingly inexhaustible flood of new and costly medical technologies will continue to put financial pressure on everyone responsible for paying for health insurance, including not only federal and state governments, but also the private sector. Real healthcare spending has grown approximately 5 percent annually for more than four decades. Despite a recent slowdown in growth of healthcare spending, the forces that have pushed up costs for decades remain in place.[2]

For all of these reasons, healthcare financing as a national political issue will not go away. But the nature of the debate in the years after the demise of the Clinton plan will be altogether different from that of the past several decades. Public and private policy in the United States are combining to transform the healthcare financing system in ways that were not widely foreseen when the Clinton administration made healthcare reform its number one domestic priority. To understand the changes that are under way, it is necessary to recognize some key features of the current system.

A Brief Sketch of U.S. Healthcare Financing

Most Americans continue to enjoy rather good health insurance coverage. Some earn coverage at work. Others receive coverage through public programs, principally Medicare and Medicaid. Some of the uninsured pay for their own healthcare, but many receive "uncompensated" care. Indeed, uncompensated care is the balm that has made socially tolerable the abrasive fact that one nonelderly person in six is without insurance at any given time. The term "uncompensated" is really a misnomer. In fact, providers are generally compensated by "cross-subsidies" from those who pay for insurance for the covered population—companies that finance care for their employees and government programs that cover the aged and disabled—who have paid more than the full cost of the care for the patients they were covering.

The Demise of Uncompensated Care

That system has come under increasing pressure from two directions. First, the flow of cross-subsidies is drying up. Medicare, like private insurers, once paid more than full cost for hospital services. After a decade of slow increases in fees, Medicare now pays less than full cost,

as does Medicaid. Private companies, appalled at the rapid and unpredictable increase in the cost of insuring their employees, have begun to
negotiate aggressively for discounted prices from hospitals, physicians,
and other providers. One of the most important services provided by
many managed care organizations is just such aggressive bargaining. In
the simplest terms, each payor is trying to make sure that it pays just
for the services used by the people for whom it is responsible. Buying
services from preferred provider organizations can be characterized,
with some lack of charity but little inaccuracy, as a way to make sure that
one does not pay cross-subsidies. But if no payor provides cross-subsidies,
providers can render uncompensated care only to the extent that they
are prepared to render charity.[3]

Second, the number of uninsured has increased, stretching even
thinner any given capacity to finance uncompensated care. The population of uninsured was 24 million in 1980 and has risen since, to 31.3
million in 1985 and 41 million in 1994. This increase has occurred
although Medicare covers almost all of the elderly, and Medicaid coverage has increased from 21.8 million in 1985 to 33.4 million in 1993.
The proportion of Americans with private insurance coverage has fallen
from 83 percent in 1980 to 70 percent in 1991.[4] In 1984 Medicare moved
from paying hospitals based on estimated costs to prepayment based on
diagnosis at admission. Increases in these payments have been below
increases in actual costs and in 1993 covered approximately 89 percent of
cost. Medicaid reimbursements, as low as 76 percent of cost in 1989, now
cover an estimated 93 percent of cost. Medicaid and Medicare payments
to physicians average 60 percent and 73 percent of private payments,
respectively (Prospective Payment Assessment Commission 1995, 21).

All of these forces are likely to continue and intensify. Both short-
term deficit reduction goals and long-term cost projections make sizable
cuts in Medicare and Medicaid likely. Some savings may be achieved
through increased efficiency. Some savings will be achieved through further restraint on the growth of payments to providers; but this source of
savings will reduce the capacity of providers to provide uncompensated
care. Cost pressures on private payors will increase as well. The avalanche
of new and costly medical technologies shows no signs of diminishing
and may be increasing (Schwartz 1994). In addition, the average age
of the active labor force is increasing, adding further to medical costs.
For all of these reasons, private companies will have every reason to
bargain for discounts with unflagging zeal. And companies that provide
health insurance coverage and other fringe benefits to their workers
will have a continuing incentive to contract with other companies that

do not provide such fringe benefits for goods and services that parent companies once produced themselves. If the new suppliers do not have to return in increased cash wages all of the savings from the omitted fringe benefits, the contracting company can reduce costs.

Private Market Developments

Under the pressure of rising costs, private companies are transforming the organization of the delivery of healthcare in the United States. These changes, summarized under the vague term "managed care," encompass a variety of techniques that share one characteristic—someone other than the patient or the healthcare provider reviews the provision of healthcare to determine whether the right services are being provided and whether cost of provision is minimized. This agent has the power to influence patterns of care, staffing of hospitals, access to physicians, salaries and fees of providers, and other aspects of the delivery of healthcare.

One might think that insurers would always have performed at least some of these functions. Once they have enrolled clients, however, insurers have customarily paid bills and done little more. Furthermore, as employers increasingly have "self-insured," by paying all costs of healthcare for their employees, they intentionally used insurance companies or some other organization only to pay bills. The rapid growth of healthcare costs under such arrangements has led private companies to hire organizations to manage care. These intermediary organizations take many forms. Some are traditional health maintenance organizations (HMOs) that hire physicians or contract with physicians to provide services. HMOs exercise direct control over staffing, equipment and other facilities, and practice patterns of affiliated physicians. HMOs may allow enrolled members to secure service from physicians or other providers outside the HMO for an additional charge under so-called point-of-service plans. Independent practice associations are networks of physicians that agree to provide stipulated services to enrolled customers at a fixed periodic charge, but, unlike HMOs, typically pay physicians on a fee-for-service basis. In other cases, hospitals are affiliating with physician groups and offering services for preset fees. Profit-making companies have gotten into the business and have enrolled millions of patients.

These new organizations are forming with impressive speed. Most insured working-age Americans now receive care through an organization that uses at least some practices associated with managed care, and within a few years nearly everyone is expected to be under such arrangements. These developments are well advanced in selected areas. In Minneapolis and St. Paul, for example, three managed care plans enroll 75 percent of the area population. Similar trends are emerging in Boston. In fact, managed care companies are regulating patients' choice of physicians and access to treatment and medication with an aggressiveness that would surely evoke outrage and uproar if attempted by government.

As the number of surviving managed care plans falls, an old issue in economic policy will emerge—whether government should regulate an industry in which only one or a small number of companies controls the market. In such situations, the public has reacted in various ways. When so-called natural monopolies exist, which means that one company can supply, at lower cost than two or more companies can, all of a product that a market will buy, the customary reaction has been economic regulation to prevent the companies from charging excessive prices. Leading examples have been public utilities of various types. Even when natural monopoly does not exist, one or a small number of companies may come to control the market. In such cases, the traditional intervention has been antitrust enforcement.

Some health services are natural monopolies in most markets. Such services include many hospital-based diagnostic and therapeutic procedures. For hospital services in general, one hospital can satisfy all of the demands in many smaller communities, and the number of such communities is rising as modern technology lowers admissions and lengths of stay. In the case of healthcare plans, additional issues likely to provoke regulatory intervention arise. Is the general quality of care adequate? Is the plan providing adequate treatment for particular conditions? Are facilities located in areas that are convenient to residents of all parts of a community? Does the plan provide enough charity care? Are the inevitable errors of medical judgment adequately investigated and is corrective action sufficient? Will the community accept judgments of plan managers when the managers conclude that benefits from costly diagnostic or therapeutic procedures are so small for patients with particular conditions that these patients should be denied access to those technologies? As the number of health plans in a given community falls, issues such as these are likely to cause demands for government involvement in regulating the delivery of healthcare to reemerge.

These trends are playing themselves out in an era when the demand for curtailing the reach of government is in flood tide. The combination of trends in insurance coverage, of the curtailment of public programs to insure the poor, the elderly, and the disabled, and of the emergence and consolidation of powerful managed care organizations imply a period of great turmoil in healthcare financing. They will result, I believe, in pressures for a revived and heightened role of government. Three stages are likely.

Stage 1

In the first stage, the number of uninsured will rise and their access to care will decline because of continued private and public cost cutting. At the same time, the mass of the U.S. population will come increasingly to secure care through managed care organizations of one type or another. These organizations will compete aggressively to hold down costs and to increase enrollments, thereby giving themselves added leverage with providers. To keep down costs, these organizations will try to curtail services that produce small benefits relative to costs or that patients undervalue. In plain English, these organizations will ration care, husbanding savings so that their members can enjoy the fruits of new medical technologies and the growth of medical costs can be kept to a socially acceptable rate. People with high incomes or unusually strong tastes for medical care will retain the option of buying care through more costly organizations that do not ration care, but even this group will find that hospitals, whose staffing and equipment depend on the general availability of resources, will be more Spartan than in the past.

Stage 2

Popular discontent will grow as the numbers of uninsured increase and their choice of providers and access to care diminishes. The traditional method of dealing with problems of inequality and poverty in the United States has been one form or another of government assistance. This assistance could take the form of publicly supported clinics and hospitals. Or it could take the form once again of public support for measures to increase insurance coverage. At the same time, concern about the behavior of the few large managed care plans that will dominate most communities will cause government intervention to regulate health plans.

Stage 3

Healthcare delivery organizations will come to be seen as a type of public utility and be treated as such by governments. Governments will take steps to assure the delivery of healthcare to those who are uninsured or who, but for government policy, would be uninsured. Through this circuitous route, all Americans will achieve access to healthcare. Government will play a principal part in setting the policies of healthcare providers, although that role will differ from that envisaged by advocates of government-sponsored national health insurance and be far more extensive than that desired by its opponents. The course to this outcome will be much longer and more indirect than advocates of government-sponsored health insurance to ensure universal coverage ever imagined. In fact, the result may well be a collection of ad hoc prohibitions, mandates, standards, and subsidies quite different from the government role envisaged in past plans for national health insurance. This process will result in a system that is uniquely American but confirms that healthcare is too important for any modern society to permit many of its citizens to lack.

Postscript

Many readers may not find the vision of how healthcare financing arrangements will evolve that I have just outlined to be as probable as I do. They may doubt that insurance coverage will narrow, that access to care for the insured will waste away, or that health plans will ever achieve as much market power as envisaged. They may see other scenarios as more likely than the one sketched. Some may fear that a loss of access to healthcare by the poor may not cause the majority to intervene, because the poor have little political power. Others may hold, perhaps sensibly, that the current situation is so chaotic that any course is possible and none particularly likely. What is certain, however, is that the very events that make healthcare financing so dynamic will prevent it from leaving the center of the political stage for years, if not decades. For that reason more than any other, it behooves anyone interested in healthcare or American political life to examine the effort to reform healthcare financing that began so energetically in 1993 and ended so ignominiously in 1994.

Acknowledgments

I thank Joseph Milano for research assistance, Gary Burtless and Theda Skorpol for comments, and Joseph P. Newhouse for the citation to Machiavelli.

Notes

1. Author calculations based on Congressional Budget Office (1995, 58).
2. Between the first quarter of 1994 and the first quarter of 1995, real personal healthcare spending rose 5.1 percent. For further discussion of these issues, see Aaron (1994), and Huskamp and Newhouse (1994).
3. The issue is complicated by the distinction between average and marginal costs. Where overhead is significant, the additional cost for serving one more patient may be below the average cost of serving all patients. A hospital with half its beds empty, for example, can typically serve an additional patient at lower than average cost because the overhead costs are paid by those already using the facility. Underused facilities are therefore particularly vulnerable to demands for discounts by powerful buyers. As more and more buyers form groups to increase their leverage, the pressure on hospitals and other high-overhead operations becomes increasingly severe.
4. Author calculations based on data from Sorkin (1992, 172, 199); Prospective Payment Assessment Commission (1995, 5); and U.S. Department of Health and Human Services (1994, 246). See also Meyer and Silow-Carroll (1993, 4).

References

Aaron, H. J. 1994. "Thinking Straight about Medical Costs." *Health Affairs* 13: 8–13.

Congressional Budget Office. 1995. *The Economic and Budget Outlook: Fiscal Years 1996–2000.* Washington, DC: U.S. Government Printing Office.

Employee Benefit Research Institute. 1994. *Sources of Health Insurance and Characteristics of the Uninsured: Analysis of the March 1993 Current Population Survey.* Washington, DC: The Institute.

Huskamp, H. A., and J. P. Newhouse. 1994. "Is Health Spending Slowing Down?" *Health Affairs* 13: 32–38.

Machiavelli, N. 1961. *The Prince.* New York: Penguin Books.

Meyer, J. A., and S. Silow-Carroll, eds. 1993. *Building Blocks for Change: How Health Care Reform Affects Our Future.* Washington, DC: Economic and Social Research Institute.

Mongan, J. 1996. In *The Problem That Won't Go Away*, edited by H. Aaron. Washington, DC: The Brookings Institution.

Prospective Payment Assessment Commission. 1995. *Medicare and the American Health Care System.* Washington, DC: The Commission.

Schwartz, W. B. 1994. "In the Pipeline: A Wave of Valuable Medical Technology." *Health Affairs* 13: 70–79.

Sorkin, A. L. 1992. *Health Economics: An Introduction.* Lexington, MA: Lexington Books.

U.S. Department of Health and Human Services. 1994. *Health United States.* Washington, DC: The Department.

14

Incremental Health Insurance Coverage: Building on the Current System

Karen Davis
Cathy Schoen

$\mathbf{T}$he evolving U.S. healthcare system poses many uncertainties for American families' access to quality healthcare (Davis 1997). Given the trends in healthcare delivery today, the uninsured cannot wait for a national consensus on the broader issues of universal health insurance coverage or comprehensive reforms. Incremental reforms, however, can go a long way toward providing quality healthcare to the most vulnerable Americans. By targeting those populations at greatest risk and building on existing mechanisms through which Americans obtain health insurance, steps can be taken now to ease barriers to care and to provide a healthier foundation for the future.

Increased Risks for the Uninsured

Analyses of underlying economic structural change and longer-term wage, benefit, and employment trends lead to three main conclusions about health insurance for working families: (1) employment-based insurance has been eroding steadily over the past decade, (2) the erosion is likely to continue into the future, and (3) jobs are a less stable base for providing health insurance than they have been in the past. As of 1995, despite low unemployment and a growing economy, 5 million more people under age 65 were uninsured than in 1991 (40.3 million total uninsured), continuing the upward trend observed throughout the 1980s (Employee Benefit Research Institute 1996).

Studies of contributing factors to the increase in uninsured people point to an ongoing erosion of employment-sponsored coverage (Acs 1995; Bureau of Labor Statistics 1984, 1994). Not only have jobs moved out of industries that historically were likely to provide individual workers and their families with employer-paid coverage (such as manufacturing and construction), but employers have also generally decreased the share of premiums they will pay (Bureau of Labor Statistics 1996; see also Bureau of Labor Statistics 1984, 1994). Moreover, the steep decline in employer payments has come at a time of slow or stagnant real-wage growth for middle- and lower-income working families.

Medicaid expansions to children have partially offset this decline by offering subsidized coverage for children living in poor or near-poor families. Low-income adults, however, have had to rely increasingly on their own incomes for payment of insurance premiums as employer support dwindles. As health insurance coverage has become less affordable, the percentage of the working population covered by employment-based insurance has dropped, and the percentage of those who are uninsured has increased (Acs 1995; Bureau of Labor Statistics 1994).

Recent forecasts of coverage trends estimate that the number of uninsured will increase to 46 million by 2002 if Medicaid maintains modest growth, and considerably more if Medicaid coverage declines (Sheils and Alecxih 1996; Thorpe et al. 1995). In either scenario, analysts conclude that the long-term decline of employer-based coverage will continue, reflecting the underlying restructuring of the economy. The reductions mainly affect those at the middle and lower end of the income distribution. If stagnant wage growth continues for those in the bottom half of the income distribution,[1] lower-wage workers will find themselves even less able to afford coverage in the future.

One factor contributing to employers' reduced support of job-based group health benefits may well be the fact that individual employers and jobs have become a less viable base for health insurance than they were in an earlier era. Multiple jobs per family, more frequent job changes, an increase in part-time and contracted work, and a general movement of jobs away from manufacturing to the service sector tend to undermine the employment-based system that has traditionally linked premium payments to a worker's job status with a single employer. Whereas in the 1950s each working family was likely to have one full-time worker working for a single employer, in today's economy even individuals who work full time may be working multiple part-time jobs for different employers (Gardner 1996). Married-couple families today typically have two or more jobs. Nevertheless, employers have no ready means to coordinate family benefits equitably across different workplaces.

While the combined trends point to a rising number of uninsured people in the future, a parallel movement toward managed care may be reducing the availability of uncompensated care for those with no insurance. As managed care plans squeeze out the surpluses from care of those with private insurance (surpluses that have historically helped hospitals offset losses from care for the uninsured), access to free or subsidized care is increasingly at risk. The consequences of a person being uninsured in the future are likely to be even bleaker than in the past.

Moreover, managed care coupled with job-based coverage may contribute to discontinuity of relationships between patients and physicians. Whereas in the past changing one's job might mean changing a health insurance card, changing one's job or employment status today may well mean changing health system networks and physicians. For example, a recent survey of an employed population with employer-based coverage found that nearly half had been in their plans for less than three years, that three-quarters had changed plans involuntarily due to a change in plans offered or a change in jobs, and that half of those in managed care plans had had to change their physicians (Davis et al. 1995a).

Considered together, the market trends point to an increase in the number of uninsured low-income families at a time when resources for uncompensated care are decreasing. The risk of decreased access for those with poor and near-poor incomes heightens the need for incremental reforms. In addition, given the growing instability of employment-based coverage, such reforms must also seek out administrative bases that will be viable as the economy undergoes continuing restructuring in the next century.

Prioritizing Coverage

Tackling the problem of the uninsured in phases requires decisions as to who should be covered first. The following discussion reviews the merits of beginning with different vulnerable populations that can be served by incremental policy reforms.

Children

An argument can be made that any effort to reduce the number of uninsured people should begin with children. Indeed, the expansion of Medicaid over the last decade to include all children in families with incomes below the federal poverty level reflects the public concern for children's healthcare. Children depend on others to secure their future and have always had a special claim on society. Furthermore, an investment in the good health of children can yield dividends in terms of a more productive labor force in the future. Perhaps most compelling, children are also the least expensive of the uninsured to cover (Holahan and Rajan 1996).

Countering these arguments is the fact that children generally have access to care: Low-income children are already eligible for Medicaid, and most higher-income children have adequate private health insurance, typically provided by their family's employers. Of 70 million children under the age of 18, 10 million are uninsured, 17 million are covered by Medicaid or other public plans, and the remaining are covered by private plans (Fronstin and Rheem 1996). A new program covering all children would require the identification of funds to pay for the coverage of approximately 43 million children currently covered by private insurance—which could cost approximately $40–$50 billion—without providing any new coverage. The identification of sources to finance such a substantial investment is difficult; the diversion of funds from other children's programs or other investments that would also improve the lives of children—such as family income support, food stamps, education, or day care—is not easily justified. A lower-cost alternative would be to design an approach that covers uninsured children—while attempting to keep current insurance coverage for children in force—but this is easier said than done.

One targeted approach might be to expand Medicaid to include children in lower-income families who are least likely to already have private health insurance coverage or are least able to purchase such coverage. Some states—such as Florida, Maine, Minnesota, New York, Pennsylvania, Washington, Wisconsin, and Vermont—have expanded coverage for low-income children. Lessons learned from these states may be instrumental in the development of models for other states and the federal government.

Of the uninsured children nationwide, 3.5 million are in families with incomes below the federal poverty level, and 1.1 million are between the ages of 13 and 17, and, under current law, will be phased into

Medicaid coverage by the year 2002. The remainder of poor children presumably are eligible for Medicaid but are not yet enrolled. An additional 3.5 million children under age 18 are in families with incomes between poverty and twice the poverty level. Approximately 3 million uninsured children are in families with incomes above 200 percent of the federal poverty level (Holahan 1996).

Low- and Modest-Income Families

A second strategy is to expand health insurance coverage to low- and modest-income families—adults as well as children. Currently, Medicaid covers pregnant women up to 133 percent of the federal poverty level—but only during the course of pregnancy and only for pregnancy-related healthcare. Research documenting the importance of prenatal care for preventing low birthweight and infant mortality was important in the debate to expand Medicaid coverage for pregnant women (Institute of Medicine 1985). But the health needs of mothers do not end with pregnancy. Medicaid coverage of mothers, especially those in two-parent families and working women regardless of income, is quite limited (Holahan 1996). Moreover, low-income adult men are the least likely to have insurance coverage—half of poor men ages 18–64 are uninsured (Holahan and Rajan 1996).

Low-income uninsured people experience the greatest financial barriers to receiving needed care, are the least likely to get preventive care, and are the most likely to experience the harmful health consequences of being uninsured (Weissman and Epstein 1990). On the basis of sheer need for care, low-income uninsured people appear to have the greatest priority.

Of the 40 million uninsured, 23 million are poor or near poor, including 11 million poor adults and children, 7 million with incomes between 100 and 150 percent of poverty, and 6 million with incomes between 150 and 200 percent of poverty (Fronstin and Rheem 1996). Of those, 5 million are poor or near-poor parents of children, including 3 million poor or near-poor mothers (Holahan 1996).

Covering low-income families with children also has a strong rationale. Typically, health insurance coverage is family based. Healthy parents are important for healthy children. And the health of mothers, including mental health, is particularly important for the nurturing and support that children need.

Expanding Medicaid to cover low-income adults as well as children would promote family-based insurance coverage and also improve the continuity of coverage. Today, 15 percent of women who lose Medicaid coverage do so because their pregnancy has ended (Short 1996). Twenty-eight percent of women are on Medicaid for less than one year (Short 1996). Women enrolled in Medicaid may lose their eligibility when they become employed or experience an increase in earnings. When they do find employment, it is rare that such jobs provide health insurance. Thus, two-thirds of women leaving Medicaid become uninsured (Short 1996). If they were covered by a Medicaid managed care plan, loss of Medicaid can also mean loss of their current source of healthcare. Improving family coverage would reduce the turnover in Medicaid coverage and permit managed care plans and safety-net providers to continue serving this low-income population.

With the end of Aid to Families with Dependent Children (AFDC), rethinking Medicaid eligibility also makes sense. Some states (including Hawaii, Oregon, and Tennessee) have expanded coverage to poor families regardless of welfare or work status. Current requirements that states continue Medicaid coverage for individuals who would have been eligible under AFDC will be administratively complex. It is, then, an opportune moment to shift to an income-conditioned basis of eligibility rather than continuing the policy of tying Medicaid to welfare eligibility.

Unemployed Workers

Unemployed workers are another group at high risk of being uninsured. Thirty-two percent of unemployed adults are uninsured, and half are either currently uninsured or have been uninsured at some point in the last two years (Davis et al. 1995b), for a total of almost 2 million unemployed adults who are uninsured. Many unemployed workers are eligible to continue coverage under an employer plan through Comprehensive Omnibus Budget Reconciliation Act (COBRA) provisions, but few can afford to pay the premium at a time when income is reduced and prospects for new employment may be uncertain. Only approximately 20 percent of those eligible for COBRA coverage participate (Claxton 1996). For workers who are unemployed and temporarily uninsured, subsidies to help pay the premium could prevent a loss of coverage. For workers covered under managed care plans, financing premiums during this transition could also improve continuity of care.

Older Adults

Another rationale is to begin with those people with the greatest health problems. Disabled or chronically ill adults require extensive healthcare to maintain functioning or slow the progression of disease and disability. Research indicates that uninsured chronically ill people are far less likely than their insured counterparts to experience proper medical management of their conditions, and, consequently, they have worse health outcomes (Hafner-Eaton 1993; Bindman et al. 1995).

Furthermore, sick individuals are at greatest financial risk of incurring major medical expenses (Donelan et al. 1996). To obtain private coverage at an affordable rate can be especially difficult for this group, as policies that cover chronically ill people often entail paying very high premiums. In addition, private health insurance often excludes preexisting conditions.

Medicare is not available for those under age 65 and is therefore not an option for people forced into early retirement because of disability or other health reasons. Although Social Security gives older adults the option of initiating coverage at age 62, albeit with reduced benefits, Medicare has no comparable provision. Nor does Medicare cover spouses or other dependents under age 65. To permit older adults to purchase Medicare, on a subsidized or nonsubsidized basis, would be an administrative mechanism for helping this group of vulnerable adults.

Medicare also covers those who are permanently and totally disabled for two years or more. In practice, beneficiaries must first become eligible for Social Security Disability Insurance, which has a six-month waiting period, so the effective waiting period for Medicare is 2½ years. Removing this waiting period, or permitting disabled people to purchase Medicare on a subsidized or nonsubsidized basis, is another option.

The major disadvantage of beginning with older adults who experience serious health problems is that they are the most expensive to cover (Davis 1990; Stapleton, Kennell, and Iovanna 1993). With limited dollars, the targeting of older, sicker adults achieves the smallest reduction in numbers of uninsured—although it arguably makes the greatest contribution to fulfilling the major purpose of all insurance, which is reducing financial risks.

Building on Existing Administrative Mechanisms

One of the obstacles to the enactment of universal health insurance coverage was the complexity of creating new administrative mechanisms for covering the entire population and trying to fit these mechanisms to job-based coverage. In addition to the option of establishing a new program to cover all children, there are currently a range of insurance mechanisms that form a logical base from which to expand coverage incrementally. Medicaid currently covers low-income mothers and children. Employer plans are open to unemployed workers through COBRA. Medicare covers people age 65 and over, as well as those who are disabled for two or more years. Other options are also available: vouchers or tax credits to small businesses or people to subsidize the purchase of coverage through private offerings, such as the small business coalitions or purchasing cooperatives that have been developed in some cities; quasipublic options, such as state public employee health plans and the federal employee health benefits plan; and public options such as Medicaid and Medicare.

With any of these options, the basic unanswered questions are (1) who and how many people should be covered, (2) how much could and should the uninsured pay toward their own coverage, (3) how could expanded coverage to the uninsured be designed to minimize employers' dropping coverage for low-wage workers in response, (4) what would the expansion of coverage cost, and (5) how could expanded coverage be financed?

These questions deserve careful consideration. Despite the best of intentions, it is not likely that incremental policy reforms will achieve perfect equity. The current system of health insurance in the United States is a complex patchwork. Two families with the same income and characteristics are likely to have widely differing insurance coverage. A low-income woman with children may be covered by Medicaid in one state, but a comparable family in a neighboring state may be considered ineligible for Medicaid coverage. A working family earning $30,000 may have employer-financed health insurance, whereas a similar family working in a different industry or different-sized firm may not. Although one unemployed worker may have the option of continuing employer coverage under COBRA, another worker may not have the opportunity to enroll in COBRA because his or her former employer did not offer insurance coverage. Short of scrapping our current complex system and committing the financial resources to achieve universal coverage, these inequities are likely to persist.

An evaluation of alternative incremental options should be based on a pragmatic consideration of assisting those in greatest need, of building on feasible and simple administrative mechanisms, and of assuming constrained resources for expanding coverage. Ideally, an incremental approach would suggest a logical phasing in of coverage as experience is gained and as greater financial resources can be committed to a workable system.

A case can be made for any number of alternative approaches, but the key issue is who will pay. The rejection of employer-mandated health insurance coverage in the 1993–94 healthcare reform debate suggests that any additional financing for expanded coverage is most likely to come either from public funds or to some extent from the uninsured themselves. With public funding comes the requirement for public accountability of funds.

There continues to be a debate about whether public programs or private insurance plans are more effective in controlling costs. The evidence on administrative costs is fairly clear cut. Medicare and Medicaid average administrative costs of 2–4 percent, larger employer plans typically experience 10–15 percent, and the individual insurance market has the highest administrative costs (U.S. House of Representatives 1993). Few would dispute that Medicaid has the lowest provider payment rates, and the growth in Medicaid managed care brings to that program whatever efficiencies are available from capitated payment. Medicare also permits health maintenance organizations to participate, and that portion of Medicare is growing, although from a low base (Health Care Financing Administration 1996b). The hospital and physician fee-for-service portions of Medicare—the benefits at the core of any expanded insurance coverage—are growing at 5 percent annually (Congressional Budget Office 1996) and again start with substantial discounts to private insurance fees, including managed care plans that pay providers on a fee-for-service basis (Physician Payment Review Commission 1995).

With limited prospects for a major expansion of public funding, it is essential that incremental expansions target those most in need, allowing them an opportunity to purchase their coverage in the most economical way. This suggests focusing on the poorest and sickest in a way that builds on the existing Medicaid and Medicare public programs. The remainder of this chapter focuses primarily on those options that would build on this base.

Expanding Medicaid

Given the success of Medicaid in enrolling the most vulnerable populations in health insurance plans, including one-third in managed care plans, expanding Medicaid to cover other low-income people is a relatively quick and administratively feasible strategy. Options are discussed below.

Accelerated Coverage of Children Aged 12–18 in Families with Incomes up to the Federal Poverty Level

Currently, states are required to bring poor children into Medicaid one year at a time, so that all poor children will be eligible for Medicaid by the year 2002. The acceleration of this timetable would bring one million poor uninsured adolescents into the program more quickly. Costs of covering children are relatively low, and the potential long-term benefits are high. The teen years are a critical time when counseling, health education, and preventive care can influence long-term health behavior to form the foundation for healthier adult years.

Coverage of Parents of Medicaid Children

The coverage of women only during pregnancy or the coverage of children but not their parents creates particular problems, both for health plans organized for families and for continuous coverage. Short spells with and without coverage particularly undermine Medicaid managed care strategies that seek to get families into long-term relationships with regular sources of care and that require plans to be accountable for the health of families. Similarly, the short duration of welfare means high turnover and regular disruptions in coverage for plans that are paid in advance for longer-term care of enrollees. Even though Medicaid beneficiaries may find a minimum- or low-wage job that helps them leave welfare, they are still likely to have incomes below the poverty level and to work at jobs that do not provide health benefits. If states are given the option of covering poor parents of Medicaid children with federal matching, or mandating coverage, it would reduce turnover in enrollment, promote continuity in relationships with primary care physicians, and permit greater emphasis on preventive care.

Ideally, coverage would be extended to all parents of Medicaid children, but, if funds do not permit, this expansion could begin solely with the one million poor uninsured mothers (Holahan 1996). This would improve continuity of care for women in their child-bearing years and promote better family-centered healthcare.

Subsidized Purchase of Medicaid for Near-Poor Families

If Medicaid could be purchased on a subsidized or sliding-scale basis by low-income families above the poverty level who do not have access to employment-based health insurance coverage, it would encourage them to move into jobs or work increased hours and still keep their health insurance. At the same time, sliding-scale availability of Medicaid would make affordable coverage available to uninsured working families without forcing them to reduce work time so as to qualify for welfare assistance. To allow for the subsidized purchase of Medicaid would thus reduce the inequity in health insurance coverage between working and nonworking families and provide a stable source of coverage for those workers with a series of part-time, temporary, or seasonal jobs.

One issue that requires serious attention is the definition of near poor. Tighter eligibility limits, such as 150 percent of poverty, would cost less than making coverage available up to, say, 250 percent of poverty. Yet graduating a sliding-scale premium over a limited income range requires a very sharp increase—or, in economic terms, a very high marginal tax rate. For example, the poverty level for a family of four is approximately $16,000. A typical unsubsidized premium for family coverage would be approximately $6,000. If coverage were free to families under $16,000, but no subsidies were available above 150 percent of poverty ($24,000), up to 75 percent of the additional income earned over this income range would be consumed by the premium.

Another consideration is the substitution for current private coverage. Some have argued that Medicaid coverage of children "crowds out" private coverage (Cutler and Gruber 1996; Dubay and Kenney 1997). Yet few children with incomes above 150 percent of poverty are covered by Medicaid, and private coverage below this income range is rare (Dubay and Kenney 1997). Similarly, employer-provided coverage for near-poor adults is rare. For example, approximately 35 percent of adults and children with incomes between 100 and 150 percent of poverty are covered by employer plans. However, 53 percent of those with incomes between 150 and 200 percent are covered by employer plans, as are 75 percent of those between 200 and 300 percent. Clearly, the higher the income cutoff, the greater the risk that employers will drop private insurance coverage.

Making Medicare Available to Older Adults

One approach to ensuring the availability of health insurance to older adults is to give them the option of purchasing Medicare. The policy option of permitting adults under age 65 to purchase Medicare could be extended on a subsidized basis (Davis 1990).

Premiums for older adults could be based on expected average costs for older adults in average health. This would require additional federal revenues to subsidize the premium—if, as seems likely, the Medicare buy-in option attracts older adults in poorer health. Some higher costs of adverse risk selection may be offset by Medicare's lower administrative costs and provider payment rates.

The broadest option is to permit purchase of Medicare coverage by all older adults over, for example, age 55. This would expand the option of Medicare coverage to an estimated 7 million older adults between the ages of 55 and 64 who are not covered under an employer or former employer health insurance plan (Holahan 1996). Some subsidies would be required, if, as expected, relatively sicker older adults find this option attractive. Also, subsidies would be required to make coverage affordable for modest-income older adults by, for example, capping the premium contribution at a fixed percentage of income.

A more targeted approach would be to expand Medicare coverage first to spouses and dependents of Medicare beneficiaries. It is estimated that 0.6 million spouses and 0.3 million dependents of Medicare bene-ficiaries are either uninsured or purchase health insurance individually; they might opt for coverage under Medicare, if it were available and affordable (Davis 1990).

Another group for targeted buy-in expansions are those individuals who have retired early and receive Social Security cash benefits at age 62. Approximately 3.4 million individuals aged 62–64 are receiving Social Security cash assistance. Approximately 12 percent (0.4 million) of these individuals are uninsured, and approximately 17 percent currently pur-chase coverage from individual health insurance plans. To permit Social Security cash assistance recipients who are not covered under employer plans to purchase Medicare could extend coverage to an additional one million older adults (Davis 1990).

A still more limited step would be to eliminate the two-year waiting period for coverage of the disabled under Medicare at age 62. This would assist those older adults who must retire early for health reasons and who face sharply reduced incomes and high health expenses as they wait for health insurance coverage.

All of these incremental policy options would reduce the number of older adults at risk, but at a significant cost. Coverage of older adults is expensive because per capita costs are highest among this group. Moreover, the option of early buy-in to Medicare coverage might accel-erate the trend for employers to drop retiree health coverage (Pension and Welfare Benefits Administration 1995). Yet employers are cutting back on such commitments in any event; already only 33 percent of Medicare beneficiaries have employer-provided retiree benefits (Health Care Financing Administration 1995). As the baby boom population hits the 55–64 age range at the turn of the century, the number of uninsured older adults will become an increasingly serious problem.

In the context of broader options to address the financial solvency of Medicare, including raising the age of eligibility, to allow beneficiaries to buy in at an earlier age on a subsidized basis makes some sense. To be able to trade off higher premium contributions, for example, for those over age 65 with coverage options for those under age 65 would make it easier for people to pay for their out-of-pocket medical expenses over the course of their retirement.

Financing Options

All of these options require additional budgetary outlays at a time when budgetary pressures are particularly intense. To make precise cost estimates would require more sophisticated modeling of a specific plan. Yet some rough estimates are possible. The 1993 average Medicaid cost per covered AFDC child is $1,057, whereas the average Medicaid cost per covered AFDC adult is $1,959 (Liska et al. 1995). Those low-income children and adults not covered by Medicaid are in somewhat better health than Medicaid beneficiaries, suggesting that these averages represent the high end of per capita costs. As a rough rule of thumb, $1,000 per child and $2,000 per adult would be required to provide coverage under Medicaid to low-income families.

To apply these per capita costs to individuals below poverty would suggest that full coverage of all poor uninsured Americans (7.5 million adults and 1 million children aged 12–17) under Medicaid might add $16 billion annually to the program if all participated. To provide partial subsidies (say 50 percent) for the near-poor uninsured (up to 150 percent of poverty) would extend coverage to 5 million adults and 2 million children at a cost of approximately $6 billion. To go further to 200 percent of poverty would extend coverage to another 4 million adults and 1.5 million children at a cost of approximately $4 billion. The total price tag for covering all uninsured adults and children up to 200 percent of poverty, therefore, would be approximately $26 billion. More modest proposals could reduce this cost by limiting coverage to parents with children, excluding childless couples and single individuals, or by limiting coverage to mothers and children.

It is more difficult to make a rough estimate of the cost of opening Medicare to uninsured older adults. In 1994 the average cost of Medicare beneficiaries aged 65–74 was $3,300 per enrollee (Health Care Financing Administration 1996a). To extend coverage to one million uninsured older adults aged 62–64 would probably cost on the order of $3–$4 billion. Precise estimates would depend on the extent of adverse risk selection. Healthcare costs for all people aged 62–64 should be lower than for those of people aged 65–74; however, Medicare buy-in can be expected to attract relatively sicker people who do not have access to affordable private coverage.

Options for financing expanded coverage include earmarking budget savings from changes in disproportionate-share payments to hospitals under Medicare and Medicaid for this purpose (in FY 1997, approximately $4.4 billion annually from Medicare [Congressional Budget Office 1995] and $16.9 billion annually from Medicaid [Liska et al. 1995]); increasing tobacco taxes (in 1997, $10 billion annually, based on 1993 national health expenditure data [Congressional Budget Office 1995]); earmarking corporate taxes paid by for-profit health providers and plans; or assessing a 2 percent surcharge on managed care plans, employer health insurance plans (including Employee Retirement Income Security Act plans), and Medicare (approximately over $10 billion annually).

Trust Fund

Another way to limit budgetary outlays is to devote a fixed sum to a trust fund for expanding coverage to the uninsured and to establish a waiting list among eligible categories. For example, a $10 billion uninsured trust fund could be established from some of the sources suggested above, with priorities based on age (children first), gender (women first), income (poorest first), or health status (sickest first). Priorities could also restrict coverage for those with other options available to them, such as employer coverage. If partial, rather than complete, premium subsidies were provided, participation rates would depend on the extent of the subsidies. This "willingness to pay" would also limit enrollment by those who had free sources of care available to them through such programs as the Veterans' Administration health system or community health centers. To discourage employers of low-wage workers from dropping coverage, various disincentives could be designed, including taxing employers that do not cover workers (earmarked for the trust fund covering the uninsured) or excluding as an allowable business expense health insurance premiums for higher-wage workers when low-wage workers are underrepresented among those participating.

Summary

To reengage the issue of expanding health insurance coverage is a difficult task, both economically and politically. Yet to put expanded health insurance coverage back on the national agenda is especially urgent in the changing U.S. healthcare system. With the ongoing erosion of employment-based coverage, the strong opposition by small business to the concept of mandating employment-based health insurance coverage, and the fact that jobs are no longer as long lasting or stable as they once were, linking health insurance to employment may work even less well in the future.

Absent a new foundation on which to build toward universal coverage, more modest, pragmatic steps should be explored. Building on Medicaid and Medicare and, as necessary, subsidizing costs of coverage for the uninsured, the opportunity can be offered to broaden access to care at a time when market forces threaten to close doors previously open to the uninsured.

Note

1. For recent reviews of earnings trends, see Kodrzycki (1996) and Levy and Murnane (1992).

References

Acs, G. 1995. "Explaining Trends in Health Insurance Coverage between 1988 and 1991." *Inquiry* 32 (1): 102–10.

Bindman, A. B., K. Grumbach, D. Osmond, M. Komaromg, K. Vranizan, N. Lurie, J. Billings, and A. Stewart. 1995. "Preventable Hospitalizations and Access to Health Care." *Journal of the American Medical Association* 274 (4): 305–11.

Bureau of Labor Statistics. 1984. *Employee Benefits in Medium and Large Firms, 1983.* Bulletin 2213. Washington, DC: U.S. Government Printing Office.

———. 1994. *Employee Benefits in Medium and Large Firms,* 1993. Bulletin 2456. Washington, DC: U.S. Government Printing Office.

———. 1996. *Current Labor Statistics* (Table 25, p. 78). Monthly Labor Review. Washington, DC: U.S. Government Printing Office.

Claxton, G. 1996. *Reform of the Individual Health Insurance Market.* New York: The Commonwealth Fund.

Congressional Budget Office. 1995. *Reducing the Deficit: Spending and Revenue Options.* Washington, DC: U.S. Government Printing Office.

———. 1996. *Reducing the Deficit: Spending and Revenue Options.* Washington, DC: U.S. Government Printing Office.

Cutler, D. M., and J. Gruber. 1996. "Does Public Insurance Crowd Out Private Insurance?" *Quarterly Journal of Economics* 111 (2): 391–430.

Davis, K. 1990. Uninsured Older Adults: The Need for a Medicare Buy-in Option. Testimony before the Subcommittee on Health, Committee on Ways and Means, U.S. House of Representatives, Washington, DC.

———. 1997. "Uninsured in an Era of Managed Care." *HSR: Health Services Research* 31 (1): 641–50.

Davis, K., K. S. Collins, C. Schoen, and C. Morris. 1995a. "Choice Matters: Enrollees' Views of their Health Plans." *Health Affairs* 14 (2): 99–122.

Davis, K., D. Rowland, D. Altman, K. S. Collins, and C. Morris. 1995b. "Health Insurance: The Size and Shape of the Problem." *Inquiry* 32: 196–203.

Donelan, K., R. J. Blendon, C. A. Hill, C. Hoffman, D. Rowland, M. Frankel, and D. Altman. 1996. "Whatever Happened to the Health Insurance Crisis in the United States?" *Journal of the American Medical Association* 276 (16): 1346–50.

Dubay, L., and G. Kenney. 1997. "Did Medicaid Expansions for Pregnant Women Crowd Out Private Coverage?" *Health Affairs* 16 (1): 185–93.

Employee Benefit Research Institute. 1996. *Sources of Health Insurance and Characteristics of the Uninsured: Analysis of the March 1996 Current Population Survey.* Washington, DC: The Institute.

Fronstin, P., and E. Rheem. 1996. *Sources of Health Insurance and Characteristics of the Uninsured: Analysis of the March 1995 Current Population Survey.* EBRI Issue Brief No. 170. Washington, DC: Employee Benefit Research Institute.

Gardner, J. 1996. "Hidden Part Timers: Full-time Work Schedules, but Part-time Jobs." *Monthly Labor Review* 119 (9): 43–44.

Hafner-Eaton, C. 1993. "Physician Utilization Disparities Between the Uninsured and Insured: Comparison of the Chronically Ill, Acutely Ill, and Well Nonelderly Populations." *Journal of the American Medical Association* 269: 787–92.

Health Care Financing Administration. 1995. *Medicare: A Profile.* Washington, DC: U.S. Department of Health and Human Services.

———. 1996a. *Health Care Financing Review.* Medicare and Medicaid Statistical Supplement, Table 14. Washington, DC: U.S. Department of Health and Human Services.

———. 1996b. *Profiles of Medicare.* Washington, DC: U.S. Department of Health and Human Services.

Holahan, J. 1996. *Expanding Insurance Coverage for Children.* Washington, DC: The Urban Institute.

Holahan, J., and S. Rajan. 1996. *Medicaid Coverage of Low Income People.* Washington, DC: Kaiser Commission on the Future of Medicaid.

Institute of Medicine. 1985. *Preventing Low Birthweight.* Committee to Study the Prevention of Low Birthweight. Washington, DC: National Academy Press.

Kodrzycki, Y. K. 1996. "Labor Markets and Earnings Inequality: A Status Report." *New England Economic Review* (Special Issue): 11–25.

Levy, F., and R. Murnane. 1992. "U.S. Earnings Levels and Earnings Inequality." *Journal of Economic Literature* 30 (3): 1333–81.

Liska, D., K. Obermaier, B. Lyons, and P. Long. 1995. *Medicaid Expenditures and Beneficiaries: National and State Profiles and Trends.* Washington, DC: Kaiser Commission on the Future of Medicaid.

Pension and Welfare Benefits Administration. 1995. *Retirement Benefits of American Workers: New Findings from the September 1994 Current Population Survey.* Washington, DC: U.S. Department of Labor.

Physician Payment Review Commission. 1995. *Annual Report to Congress.* Washington, DC: The Commission.

Sheils, J., and L. Alecxih. 1996. *Recent Trends in Employer Health Insurance Coverage and Benefits.* Washington DC: The Lewin Group, Inc.

Short, P. F. 1996. *Medicaid's Role in Insuring Low Income Women.* New York: The Commonwealth Fund.

Stapleton, D. C., D. L. Kennell, and R. Iovanna. 1993. *Health Care Costs and Older Workers.* New York: The Commonwealth Fund.

Thorpe, K. E., A. E. Shields, H. Gold, D. Shactman, and S. H. Altman. 1995. *Anticipating the Number of Uninsured Americans and the Demand for Uncompensated Care: The Combined Impact of Proposed Medicaid Reductions and the Erosion of Employer-Sponsored Insurance.* Waltham, MA: Council on the Economic Impact of Health System Change, Brandeis University.

U.S. House of Representatives. 1993. *Health Care Resource Book.* Committee on Ways and Means. Washington, DC: U.S. Government Printing Office.

Weissman, J. S., and A. M. Epstein. 1990. *Falling through the Safety Net.* Baltimore, MD: The Johns Hopkins Press.

15

Incremental Reform: The Health Insurance Portability and Accountability Act of 1996

Gail R. Wilensky

Incremental reform, the unmentionable words of the 103rd Congress, is once again a concept that can be discussed in polite company. For those concerned about healthcare reform and frustrated by the experiences of 1993–94, there are several reasons to regard this change in attitude as a positive sign for the future.

The first reason is that incremental change is the way change driven by legislation generally occurs in the United States. Second, different populations among the uninsured are uninsured for different reasons, and attacking their problems serially and incrementally may be almost as effective as resolving them simultaneously. Third, the recent passage of the Health Insurance Portability and Accountability Act of 1996 (HIPAA) (P.L. 104-191) may have laid the framework for the development of an individually sponsored insurance system, a system that could complement the employer-sponsored insurance system that has dominated insurance coverage for the under 65-year-old population for the past several decades. Finally, the passage of the HIPAA, at the end of what can only be described as an unusually bitter and partisan congressional session, gives hope that the nation may be able to continue legislating at least some changes in healthcare, despite the expected continued contentiousness in the Congress.

Incremental Reform: The Way Change Occurs

Henry Aaron (in this volume) examines in detail why only incremental reform seems possible in the current political environment. Although

I agree with much of his thinking, I have a few thoughts to add on this subject.

Not only is incremental reform the only way healthcare reform is going to occur in the current environment, incremental reform is the way most social legislation has occurred, at least during the twentieth century. The one period that might arguably challenge this characterization occurred during the New Deal, particularly with the wave of legislation passed during the first Roosevelt term. But even then, with the pressures of the Depression and a nation in despair, it is unclear whether Roosevelt would have been able to pass (and sustain) legislation that had an effect comparable to the reorienting of a trillion dollar sector such as President Clinton was attempting to do with the Health Security Act. President Truman, who strongly advocated a national healthcare program that would certainly have qualified as nonincremental legislation, obviously was unsuccessful in passing this portion of his legislative agenda.

Although the nonincremental nature of the Health Security Act exacerbated its problems of passage, this legislation was doomed legislatively almost from its inception because of its reliance on employer mandates and global budgets (Wilensky 1994). Both are mechanisms that were designed to allow the Clinton administration to fund expenditures implicitly that it knew could not be funded explicitly (i.e., through increased taxes). Unfortunately for the legislation, employer mandates and global budgets, as well as the price controls that accompany them, are almost as much an anathema to conservative Democrats as to most Republicans. Without the support of conservative Democrats or a large number of Republicans in their place, there were never the numbers needed to pass this legislation in the House of Representatives or in the Senate. As it happened, the legislation became so unpopular by the end of the 103rd Congress that it never even came to a vote.

The Uninsured: A Heterogeneous Group

A second reason to support the rehabilitation of incremental reform strategies has to do with the characteristics of the uninsured themselves. Volumes have been written on the characteristics of the uninsured over the last 15 years (Wilensky 1984, 1988; Ries 1986; Swartz and Sulvetta 1986; Wilensky and Ladenheim 1987; Rowland et al. 1994; Swartz 1996), and, although it depends on precisely what time period and which characteristics are of concern, the basic distributional characteristics of the uninsured have stayed surprisingly constant over time.

The uninsured tend to belong to one of two different groups. The largest group, accounting for approximately two-thirds of the uninsured, are the working uninsured and their families. Most of these workers work for small firms or are self-employed and are not offered employer-sponsored insurance as part of their compensation package. A related group of the uninsured that has been growing in size are dependents of working insured people in which the worker is not offered dependent coverage or the dependent coverage is regarded as too expensive by the worker and is declined. Most of the working uninsured are lower middle income or middle income (two to four times the poverty level), although as many as 10 percent are high income.

The other important group of uninsured, the remaining one-third, are individuals who are poor or near poor. These individuals may work part time, or in some cases even full time, but more generally they are unemployed or out of the labor force for substantial periods during the year. For various reasons, such as family composition or change in family status, asset level, or state eligibility rules, these poor uninsured are not eligible for Medicaid or other public insurance.

Implications for Incremental Reform

It is useful to think about the uninsured in terms of the working uninsured and those who are poor or near-poor uninsured and generally not working, because, aside from a new national entitlement program (an idea that seems rather unlikely given our recent experience), the strategies for insuring them may differ.

Most of the working population have employer-sponsored insurance. This represents a use of the employees compensation package that would otherwise go to the employee as increased wages. It has long been recognized that the main driver for this form of insurance is the tax treatment of employer-sponsored insurance that allows workers to exclude employer contributions for insurance (as well as other fringe benefits) from their taxable income. Because individuals who purchase insurance on their own have to use after-tax income, insurance is a more expensive commodity for individuals who do not have access to employer-sponsored insurance; consequently, they are less likely to buy it. There are other reasons group insurance is generally less expensive than individual insurance, including lower selling costs and larger numbers of individuals to use in the pooling of risks. Considering these factors together, it is not surprising that those employees without employer-sponsored insurance, most of whom are not offered sponsored insurance, are much more likely to be uninsured.

For people who are poor or near poor, having employer-sponsored insurance is still important, but if the employee's contribution is of any significance, the individual may still not purchase insurance. More often, these individuals work for small firms that do not offer coverage, they work only intermittently, or they do not work at all. Any resolution of their coverage problems, given their income level, is more likely to require heavily or fully subsidized coverage or access to the direct provision of services.

The Health Insurance Portability and Accountability Act as an Example of Incremental Reform

Many people regarded the passage of the HIPAA mostly as a signal that healthcare reform could still proceed in the post–Health Security Act era rather than as a significant piece of legislation on its own. To be sure, it limited the use of preexisting condition restrictions and resolved the problem of "job lock," which is the fear that a worker or a family member with preexisting medical conditions would be forced to stay in a job because they may not be able to get health insurance from a new employer, at least for any preexisting condition. It also provided assurance that people who got sick would not have their health insurance canceled by guaranteeing the availability and renewability of health insurance coverage, at least for certain employees and individuals.

Although portability issues are certainly not trivial and were one of the main drivers of the so-called health insurance crisis of 1992–93, the estimates of the number of people who might be affected by the HIPAA tend to be rather small compared with the 37–39 million uninsured people. What has received much less attention are various other provisions of the HIPAA, one of which could have important ramifications for the working uninsured.

Besides portability-related provisions, the HIPAA includes the following provisions related to health insurance:

- a limited number of small businesses and self-employed individuals can contribute to medical savings accounts;
- long-term care policies are treated for tax purposes as are other health insurance policies; and
- an increase in the tax deduction for health insurance for the self-employed.

It is the latter provision that has the potential of laying the framework for tax-subsidized, individually purchased insurance for current and future workers who are uninsured.

Under the HIPAA, the self-employed will gradually be able to deduct up to 80 percent of their health insurance premium by 2006, as opposed to the 30 percent for 1996. By 2006, the self-employed will therefore have a tax deduction for health insurance comparable to or even better than most employees with employer-sponsored insurance. If this provision were made available to all workers or to any individual without employer-sponsored insurance or public insurance, it would equalize the currently inequitable tax treatment between those workers with employer-sponsored insurance and those without.

It may also be desirable to assure unsponsored workers access to a large group insurance pool because this would reflect the other main advantage that workers have with employee-sponsored insurance. A strategy that was included in the Dole-Packwood health insurance bill introduced in 1994 was to allow employers with fewer than 50 employees the option of purchasing insurance through the Federal Employees Health Benefit Plan, the plan the federal government offers its employees. A similar provision could be considered for people without access to employer-sponsored insurance.

By equalizing the tax subsidy associated with employer-sponsored insurance and opening up a large risk pool for individuals relying on individually purchased insurance, along with the other provisions of the HIPAA, the federal government would have removed most existing barriers to accessing insurance. This would not guarantee that the working uninsured would purchase insurance, but the majority of lower-middle-income and middle-income workers now have employer-sponsored insurance in which the employer has used the employees' compensation to buy insurance with the advantage of the tax deduction, and this would equalize the treatment between these groups. For those who are more comfortable with the use of government power to break down the barriers that prevent access to coverage rather than using the power of government to guarantee coverage, this would be an important step in the right direction. It would also provide some assurance that the erosion of employer-sponsored insurance and the increased interest of many workers in part-time entrepreneurial activities would not necessarily result in increased numbers of uninsured.

The Remaining Problems

If the tax deductibility provisions of the HIPAA were extended to all those without employer-sponsored or public insurance and an ability to access a group insurance pool were also made available, the most significant problems that would remain concern the poor and near-poor uninsured.

There are a variety of options that could be devised to cover the poor uninsured, such as expanding Medicaid to cover all of the poor, providing a vanishing low-income voucher to cover the poor and near poor, funding centers of care for poor people without insurance, funding block grants to states who could decide how best to care for their low-income populations, and so forth.

The most significant barriers to resolving the problems of the poor uninsured is that they are likely to cost more money or at least require more explicit funding than the state and federal governments currently spend. By removing some of the regulatory restrictions in Medicaid, it may be possible for the states to make somewhat better use of their funding than they can under current restrictions, but the increasing use of the waiver process by the Health Care Financing Administration to allow states expanded use of managed care for their Medicaid populations has probably captured most of the easy savings.

The issues this nation will have to face before it resolves the problems of the poor uninsured is how much more funding, if any, it is willing to spend on care for poor people, where and under what circumstances care should be provided, and which level of government should make these decisions. These have proved to be difficult decisions for the United States to make in the past and will undoubtedly continue to be difficult in the future, especially with the current focus on deficit reduction. In the meantime, steps can be taken to help the working uninsured that will be far easier for us to take. We should not scorn these steps just because they will not solve all the problems of the uninsured. We are a nation that resolves most of its problems incrementally. We need to remember that when it comes to the contentious and highly charged issues involving healthcare.

References

Ries, P. 1986. *Health Care Coverage by Age, Sex, Race and Family Income.* Hyattsville, MD: Advance Data, National Center for Health Statistics.

Rowland, D., B. Lyons, A. Salganicoff, and P. Long. 1994. "A Profile of the Uninsured in America." *Health Affairs* 13 (2): 283–87.

Swartz, K. 1996. "Who Owns the Problem of the Uninsured." *Inquiry* 33 (2): 103–5.

Swartz, K. and M. Sulvetta. 1986. *The Uninsured and Uncompensated Care: A Chartbook.* Washington, DC: National Health Policy Forum, George Washington University.

Wilensky, G. 1984. "Solving Uncompensated Hospital Care: Targeting the Indigent and the Uninsured." *Health Affairs* 3 (4): 50–62.

———. 1988. "Filling the Gaps in Health Insurance: Impact on Competition." *Health Affairs* 7 (3): 133–49.

———. 1994. "Health Reform: What Will It Take To Pass." *Health Affairs* 13 (1): 179–91.

Wilensky, G. and K. Ladenheim. 1987. "Financing Health Care for the Uninsured. Issues and Options." *Frontiers of Health Services Management* 4 (2): 3–31.

16

Can We Count on the States to Cover the Poor and Uninsured?

Trish Riley

Introduction

The importance of the states' role in implementing healthcare reform for the poor and uninsured cannot be underestimated. States remain closer to the problem of the uninsured and are experimenting with a variety of policy initiatives to provide them healthcare coverage. Because of this unique position, states can initiate successful incremental reform that results in expanded access to the uninsured. This is not to say that states accomplish these reforms without challenges, obstacles, and setbacks, but the overall effort has created reform, often with the assistance of foundations, federal waivers, and congressional support. Federal health reform is the promise of a feast, but state initiatives such as children's health plans, insurance reforms, purchasing alliances, expanded Medicaid eligibility, Medicaid restructuring through Section 1115 waivers, expansion of managed care to Medicaid beneficiaries including vulnerable populations, and strengthening the safety net are delivering real and needed sustenance to the uninsured.

Comprehensive Reforms and Access Initiatives

Lacking the needed resources to cover all the uninsured, states have launched initiatives since the mid-1980s to expand health coverage of at least some of the poor and uninsured, and these efforts continue today. By 1995, foreshadowing later federal action, 48 states had enacted small group or individual market insurance reforms, 21 states had enacted legislation to stimulate the development of purchasing alliances, and 43 states had specific programs in place, often designed as subsidies to make health insurance more affordable, to cover the uninsured. Twenty-seven states had established children's health plans, programs for uncompensated or indigent care existed in 31 states, and 16 states covered other uninsured groups (Intergovernmental Health Policy Project 1995). Six states, Hawaii, Florida, Massachusetts, Minnesota, Oregon, and Washington, had enacted comprehensive reforms designed to ensure universal coverage.

Major Medicaid Initiatives

Managed Care

In addition to initiatives to make health insurance more affordable and accessible, states embarked on efforts to expand Medicaid's reach to cover more of the poor and uninsured. Convinced that access to Medicaid eligibility did not guarantee access to care, and worried by double-digit growth in the Medicaid program, states moved aggressively to enroll Medicaid beneficiaries in managed care. They believed that, by providing a mandate for 24-hour, 7-day-a-week coverage, managed care would guarantee access to medical care, replacing the doctor shopping and the reliance on costly emergency room treatment that characterized fee-for-service healthcare. By negotiating capitation rates, states were able to reduce expenditures by 5 to 15 percent, compared with fee-for-service healthcare (Hurley, Freund, and Paul 1993). By 1995, as a result, 45 states and the District of Columbia enrolled at least one-third of their Medicaid beneficiaries in managed care (Kaiser Commission on the Future of Medicaid 1996b).

Expanding Medicaid Eligibility

Medicaid eligibility has been expanded as well, stimulated by the Omnibus Budget Reconciliation Act of 1989 in which Congress required the states to phase in coverage of children and pregnant women. By 1996, states were required to cover all children of age 13 and younger up to 100 percent of the poverty level, and children to age 6 and pregnant women up to 133 percent of the poverty level. But 34 states chose to move beyond federal mandates and expanded Medicaid to women and children up to 185 percent of the poverty level (National Governors' Association 1996).

Medicaid Waivers

Most recently, states have relied on Medicaid research and demonstration waivers (Section 1115 waivers) to reform state programs and expand access for the poor and uninsured. Section 1115 waivers were also critical components of the universal coverage legislation enacted in six states. Under the waivers, many states sought to use funds generated by savings from managed care and the recapture of the disproportionate-share payments to hospitals to expand coverage to the uninsured. Ten states are currently implementing Section 1115 waivers, six states have been approved but have not yet implemented the program, and ten states have proposals under review. Twelve of these approved waivers expand coverage and will, when fully implemented, insure 2.2 million people that were previously uninsured (Reichard 1996).

Period of Retrenchment

The states' appetite for reform was substantially greater than their capacity to implement those initiatives. Initial timetables for reform were often found to be overly ambitious as states confronted a changing policy environment after the 1994 election; the realities of federal policy barriers; and the need to build new eligibility and enrollment systems, data, and managed care capacities to achieve the promise of their reforms.

For Oregon, Washington, and Massachusetts, a linchpin of their reforms was a plan to require employers either to provide health coverage for their employees or pay into a pool to enable the state to do so. For this "play-or-pay" approach to succeed, all employers would need to participate. However, employers who self-insure cannot be subjected to state regulation and are governed instead by the Federal Employee Retirement Income Security Act (ERISA). States could not implement their play-or-pay proposals without congressional approval to waive current ERISA laws. Only Hawaii had been granted an ERISA waiver to mandate employer health coverage of employees, but that waiver was granted because Hawaii's law and practice predated the enactment of the federal ERISA law. Congress would not allow Oregon, Massachusetts, and Washington to waive ERISA requirements, thus slowing their progress toward universal coverage. Related setbacks during 1995–96 resulted in considerable retrenchment in state efforts to expand coverage to the poor and uninsured. For example, states experienced problems in implementing complex Section 1115 waivers, which in turn slowed efforts to expand coverage. Florida and Massachusetts failed to gain legislative support for Section 1115 waivers that would have expanded

Medicaid to some of the uninsured, and Tennessee experienced significant problems in its rapid conversion to managed care in an environment that had little managed care infrastructure in place. Citizen referenda and legislative action imposed tax caps in several states, which stymied the financing of access initiatives. Most important, the mood of states changed, and, on the heels of the failure of the Clinton health plan, public sentiment seemed to favor more incremental reforms. For the first time in nearly two decades, Republicans held a majority of governorships. Many of these governors had campaigned for smaller government and tax cuts. With Medicaid expenses growing rapidly, these governors also felt that unless they brought spending in this program under control, their capacities to fund other priorities such as education, jails, or crime prevention would be severely limited. At the same time, term limits were beginning to be felt in the 20 states that had enacted them. Several noted health leaders faced imminent retirement, worrying some that any progress on improving access for the uninsured would be slowed.

For example, one of the outcomes of the changing political climate was that, in Oregon and Washington, the legislatures repealed significant portions of their recently enacted health reforms; and Massachusetts, Minnesota, and Hawaii slowed their implementation timetable and reduced the scope of reforms.

Progress Amidst Setbacks

Despite this period of retrenchment, states have made considerable incremental progress. MinnesotaCare, a program that subsidizes coverage for low-income, uninsured families and single adults, had enrolled 93,000 by June 1996, bringing the state's rate of uninsured from 6.0 to 5.5 percent (Intergovernmental Health Policy Project 1996b) and meeting its target of cost containment, as spending grew only 6.2 percent. While repealing most of Washington's 1993 Health Services Act, the legislature expanded the Basic Health Plan, increasing subsidies for an additional 200,000 citizens. In August 1996, the program was covering 151,000 individuals. Since April 1995, Washington has provided coverage for certain employer groups, and 700 workers from 200 firms have purchased coverage (Intergovernmental Health Policy Project 1996b). Provisions in the reform that strengthened public health were retained and expanded, and $20 million was appropriated for its implementation.

Oregon and Hawaii both experienced far greater-than-anticipated enrollment in their health expansions, and both states have also experienced fiscal problems that could have an impact on future implementation activities. Oregon had expanded coverage in the Oregon Health Plan to 110,000 uninsured, and the once-controversial initiative to prioritize health services appeared to be meeting with success.

Hawaii's unexpectedly high enrollment resulted in a significant budget deficit and, in response, substantial restructuring of the QUEST program. The QUEST program pools low-income workers enrolled in the State Health Insurance Program, Medicaid women and children, and adults receiving general assistance in a managed care demonstration program. At its high point, enrollment peaked at 163,000. Following implementation of a cap on enrollment, restructuring of the subsidy program, and some benefit reduction, the program had stabilized with an enrollment of 147,000 (Intergovernmental Health Policy Project 1996a).

Florida's Health Security Plan, which would have expanded Medicaid managed care to cover the uninsured, received a federal Section 1115 waiver but stalled when the state legislature failed to provide needed support. However, Florida did launch the portion of its 1992 reforms, which created community health purchasing alliances designed to enable businesses with 1–50 employees to participate in the group health insurance market. As of June 1996, 76,000 employees and their dependents from 17,199 businesses were enrolled in one of nine available alliances, and the state reported prices that were on average 6 percent below comparable non-alliance-based plans (American Political Network 1996a).

Tennessee, despite considerable difficulty in launching TennCare, its Section 1115 waiver program, had succeeded in only two years in ensuring healthcare coverage for nearly all its citizens. Currently, Tennessee boasts that 95 percent of its citizens are insured and cites extensive efforts to provide the needed oversight of the program.

Finally, Massachusetts reinvigorated the enthusiasm of state initiatives to expand access by enacting significant health reforms in 1996. Funded largely through a tobacco tax, the Massachusetts reform will expand coverage to 150,000 uninsured children, increase coverage for workers who become disabled, and offer prescription drug coverage for 65,000 low-income adults. The state's Section 1115 waiver, which had been approved by the Health Care Financing Administration but not the state legislature, had planned to finance expansions through tax credits for small businesses, rather than a tobacco tax. The new Massachusetts law established a commission to consider the feasibility of tax credits and to examine the state's uncompensated care fund.

Successful Smaller-Scale Initiatives

Expanding Medicaid

Several states had also embarked on reform initiatives of a smaller scale that met with considerable success. In Rhode Island, for example, that state's Section 1115 waiver program, RIte Care, had expanded benefits and coverage for uninsured children and pregnant women at or below 250 percent of the poverty level and worked to create a health plan comprised of community health centers, organizations that had a long track record of serving the uninsured. An October 1996 analysis by the University of Delaware's Center for Applied Demography and Survey Research credited state insurance reforms, which included 100 percent tax deductions for small firms and self-employed, and Medicaid expansions for a reduction in Delaware's percentage of uninsured in the population from 14.8 percent in 1990 to 13.6 percent in 1995 (American Political Network 1996b).

Protecting the Safety Net

States continue to address the needs of the poor and uninsured by developing and supporting the providers who have historically served them, such as public and teaching hospitals and urban and rural health clinics. An unanticipated impact of Medicaid capitation was to remove critical direct payments to these providers without any guarantees that health plans would contract with them at rates that could sustain care to the uninsured. In response, when California launched its statewide Medicaid managed care program, some managed care plans were required to contract with public hospitals and clinics; Rhode Island and Massachusetts have supported the development of community health centers to form their own managed care plans; and Kentucky is limiting its Medicaid managed care contracting to two state university–led, nonprofit healthcare partnerships.

States are also embarking on efforts to expand care to medically underserved areas. Tennessee, through its TennCare program, is redirecting $50 million of graduate medical education payments directly to universities and holding them accountable to provide more primary care providers in underserved areas. Minnesota passed legislation in 1996 to create a Medical Education and Research Trust Fund that will be distributed with the goal of improving access to care. New York, Massachusetts, and other states are studying how to maintain funds to support uncompensated care pools in light of diminished revenues to those pools as payments are instead made directly to managed care organizations.

Future Incremental Reports

Clearly, to expand healthcare coverage for the poor and uninsured, state initiatives have been modified and progress has been slowed. But the issues remain inescapable for state governments. Medicaid, which covers 60 percent of the poor, is the second largest component of state budgets. The problems of the public safety net—public hospitals, health centers and teaching hospitals—which serve many of the uninsured, are visible every day to state policymakers. As mergers, acquisitions, and conversions from not-for-profit to for-profit status change the healthcare marketplace, and as managed care grows and once-reliable streams of revenues for state uncompensated care pools and safety-net providers diminish, states must grapple with their "community" responsibilities. States must act, albeit incrementally, both because they operate under balanced budget requirements and must keep their own health spending (for employees, Medicaid, and others) in check, and because they are visibly close to the problems of the uninsured. Unlike members of Congress, state legislators are more likely to see and know their uninsured constituents, in part because only nine states have full-time, year-round legislatures (Kurtz 1992). State legislators are more likely to know local providers than a member of Congress who is home less frequently.

Predictions that states would abandon efforts to expand healthcare access for the poor and uninsured abounded after the 1994 elections, but proved largely false. Twenty-eight states proposed to expand Medicaid eligibility in 1994–95, whereas only two sought to reduce it (American Public Welfare Association 1996) and nine states submitted Section 1115 waivers to reform Medicaid after January 1995, six of which proposed to expand coverage to at least some segment of the uninsured (Fiore 1996).

States are likely to embark on continued incremental reforms, including Medicaid restructuring through Section 1115 waivers, expansion of managed care to the elderly and disabled, modest expansions to cover more children, strengthening the safety net and addressing the affordability of private insurance. Currently, about half the states have some type of children's health plans, and a number of states are considering the creation or expansion of those plans. The governor of

Maryland announced a plan to continue healthcare coverage at state expense for certain legal immigrants denied Medicaid coverage by recent congressional action. Other states may follow suit.

In the next several years it may be that states will directly subsidize and support safety-net providers so as to ensure continued access for at least some of the uninsured. One possible indicator to support this claim is the finding that participation in Medicaid managed care by safety-net providers has increased substantially from 1994 to 1996. Fourteen states reported that public health departments contracted with managed care organizations in 1994. Twenty-five did in 1996. Similarly, federally qualified health centers contracted with Medicaid managed care plans in 19 states in 1994, but in 30 states by 1996 (National Academy for State Health Policy 1997).

States are likely to soon revisit the importance of essential community providers, especially if major commercial plans continue to restrict or eliminate Medicaid enrollment. In Florida and Pennsylvania, significant commercial plans have withdrawn from the Medicaid marketplace or submitted renewal proposals that were unacceptable to the state. It is unclear whether these business decisions were anomalies or a developing trend. Some states fear that major commercial plans, having reaped initial profits from Medicaid enrollment, may find these cost savings unsustainable over time and may withdraw from the Medicaid marketplace. Given Medicaid's increased reliance on managed care and the mergers of commercial plans, states may be challenged to provide capitation rates that ensure sufficient competition among high-quality plans for Medicaid's business. If so, states will be forced to create alternatives and may wish to develop the capacity of safety-net providers to participate in managed care arrangements.

The Challenge of Financing Incremental Reform

New Sources of Funding

In an era of tax caps and likely diminished growth in federal programs, will states be able to sustain their incremental reforms? States are clearly looking to new sources of revenue to support initiatives and, like Massachusetts, 27 states now tax tobacco. Also, 40 states are currently engaged in complex litigation on behalf of Medicaid to sue tobacco companies for damages resulting from smoking. States are also taking a more active role of oversight in the conversion of not-for-profit health insurers and providers to for-profit status, intent on capturing and retaining the value of those public goods for a public purpose. Not-for-profit hospitals and insurers were established for charitable purposes and reaped significant tax exemptions over their years of operation. The value of these public subsidies is significant as is the value of the public purpose such institutions serve to help cover and care for the uninsured. When such organizations lose their not-for-profit status, their assets should remain so as to continue to benefit the community. In 1996, California and Colorado enacted laws regulating the conversion of Blue Cross plans, and California and Nebraska passed similar laws regulating hospital conversions that, in part, ensure that public benefits are properly valued and retained for community service.

Some states are beginning to act in ways that reflect their roles as large purchasers. Collectively, states are responsible for more than $10 billion of health purchases for their own employees, $59 billion for Medicaid, and spend additionally on behalf of retirees, prisoners, and others for whom they provide healthcare coverage. Minnesota and Washington, for example, pool state employee benefit plans with nonstate purchasers, and other states have shown interest in a similar consolidation of their purchasing power.

Redirecting Spending for Long-Term Care

Where many states anticipate achieving their greatest savings so as to sustain new initiatives is in redirecting Medicaid's long-term care expenditures. State enthusiasm for Medicaid managed care came in large part from the perceived success in improving access, sustaining quality, and reducing costs for women and children under Medicaid. Buoyed by their experience and cost savings of 5–15 percent for Aid to Families with Dependent Children enrollees, states are rapidly moving to enroll elderly and disabled in Medicaid managed care. These populations account for 27 percent of Medicaid enrollees but make up 59 percent (Kaiser Commission on the Future of Medicaid 1996c) of the program's expenditures. Nineteen states enrolled elderly and/or disabled in Medicaid managed care in 1994, but by 1996, 35 states were doing so (National Academy for State Health Policy 1996) and more states will soon follow. Minnesota and Colorado have received the only Section 1115 waivers to allow the states to blend Medicaid and Medicare; the New England states are jointly developing a waiver proposal for these populations.

Because nearly all elderly Medicaid beneficiaries and many who are disabled also qualify for Medicare, it is difficult to coordinate acute and long-term care, and incentives exist for the programs to cost shift between programs. By better coordinating the two programs, states hope to improve the quality of care and yield significant Medicaid savings.

Slowed Growth of Medicaid Spending

Finally, the most significant incentives for states to revisit efforts to expand healthcare expansions for the poor and uninsured may result from the slowed growth in Medicaid expenditures and recent federal actions. For years Medicaid has experienced double-digit growth that state legislatures have come to anticipate. But in the first half of 1996, Medicaid growth was held at 2.5 percent and is expected to remain below 10 percent in the near future (Kaiser Commission on the Future of Medicaid 1996a). Pressure will be great for states that anticipated more growth to use expected savings for a number of competing priorities, but so may those funds be used for incremental healthcare expansions. In a speech to the American Association of Health Plans in September 1996, Secretary of Health and Human Services Donna Shalala signaled an interest in expanding Medicaid to cover low-income uninsured workers and uninsured children, noting the potential of Section 1115 waivers to accomplish that goal. Bruce Bullen, president of the State Medicaid Directors' Association, similarly warned that states will likely engage in efforts that will increase Medicaid spending. He noted that the recent low growth is in part due to state savings and in part brought on by states withholding action during the recent uncertainty over how Congress would deal with block grant proposals. For example, states were not as aggressive in using state funds for related programs to match Medicaid while the threat of a block grant remained. A block grant would likely have required states to maintain all levels of state funding while limiting the amount of federal dollars available (Bullen 1996). Thus, Bullen asserted, states had restricted intergovernmental transfers, but one can expect at least some additional Medicaid expansions through waivers and other state initiatives now that the block grant has not been enacted.

States will also feel pressure to respond to forces beyond their control that impact the stability of healthcare coverage. First, should insurers' predictions prove correct and should they seek health insurance premium increases in response to passage of the Kassebaum-Kennedy bill, states will need to revisit the issue of affordability of health coverage. Second, as workforce restructuring and employment practices contribute to a further decline in employment-based coverage, states will feel the pressure of the swelling ranks of the uninsured. Finally, by delinking Medicaid and welfare eligibility, but requiring that Medicaid eligibility track previous welfare standards, Congress may have complicated states' roles in reaching and enrolling the poor into the Medicaid program. Medicaid coverage will no longer be automatic with the receipt of welfare, and states will be free to have different income standards for each.

To implement these changes, states will need to develop new approaches to Medicaid eligibility and enrollment to ensure that all those eligible for Medicaid are enrolled in the program. As welfare reform triggers workforce participation, mechanisms to ensure transitional Medicaid coverage will need to be in place. States will be challenged to provide some continuity of healthcare coverage as welfare reform is implemented. Former welfare beneficiaries may become employed in low-wage jobs without health benefits, and the potential for increasing numbers of working uninsured must be confronted.

Conclusion

State efforts to expand health coverage to the poor and uninsured have been incremental, variable, but persistent. Retrenchment in the support of comprehensive reform has not spelled an abandonment of state initiatives. Like Sisyphus pushing the rock up the hill, state action is slow and difficult. But over the past 10 or 15 years, states have shown the capacity to develop workable programs to cover the uninsured. Where these experiments have met with failure, more often than not, states have learned from their mistakes and remedied problems. Where legislative support has weakened, reforms have been narrowed but not abandoned. But not all states are engaged in the effort to cover the poor and uninsured, and no state, no matter how credible and competent its program design, can finance coverage for the uninsured without help from the federal government. Nevertheless, states continue to move ahead with reform, often more quickly than formal research and evaluation. Even absent the analysis of evaluations under way to determine the effectiveness of reforms, nearly every state is actively engaged in at least some initiatives to expand access to the poor and uninsured, and no evidence exists to suggest this trend will end. At the very least, state innovation, no matter how small, will keep the issue of the uninsured visible in the public debate.

References

American Political Network. 1996a. *American Healthline* 5 (109).

———. 1996b. "Delaware: State Credits Managed Care for Drop in Uninsured." *American Healthline* 5 (130).

American Public Welfare Association. 1996. *State of State Medicaid Programs Fiscal Year 1995*. Washington, DC: American Public Welfare Association.

Bullen, B. 1996. Kaiser Commission on the Future of Medicaid, Capitol Hill Forum. 3 December.

Fiore, M. 1996. Personal communication.

Hurley, R. E., D. A. Freund, and J. E. Paul. 1993. *Managed Care in Medicaid: Lessons for Program and Policy Design*. Chicago: Health Administration Press.

Intergovernmental Health Policy Project. 1995. *Fifty State Profile: Health Care Reforms*. Washington, DC: George Washington University.

Intergovernmental Health Policy Program. 1996a. "Reform Revisited: HI, RI Waivers Meet Different Fates." *State Health Notes* 17 (236): 1.

———. 1996b. "Reform Revisited: States Realize Access, Cost Goals." *State Health Notes* 17 (234): 1.

Kaiser Commission on the Future of Medicaid. 1996a. Capitol Hill Forum. 3 December.

———. 1996b. *Medicaid and Managed Care*. Washington, DC: The Commission.

———. 1996c. *Medicaid Beneficiaries and Expenditures by Enrollment Group*. Washington, DC: The Commission.

Kurtz, K. T. 1992. "Understanding State Legislatures: Research & Commentary." In *Extension Remarks*, edited by L. C. Dodd. Boulder, CO: University of Colorado.

National Governors' Association. 1996. *State Medicaid Coverage of Pregnant Women and Children*. Washington, DC: The Association.

National Academy for State Health Policy. 1996. *Medicaid Managed Care: A Guide to States*, 3rd ed. Portland, ME: The Academy.

———. 1997. *Medicaid Managed Care: A Guide to States*, 3rd ed. Portland, ME: The Academy.

Reichard, J., ed. 1996. "Clinton's Creeping Incrementalism." *Medicine & Health* 50 (37): 1.

17

The State Health Agenda: Austerity, Efficiency, and Monitoring the Emerging Market

Raymond C. Scheppach

Introduction

With the demise of President Clinton's healthcare initiative in 1993, there was an expectation that the focus for extending coverage to low-income people would shift back to the 50 state capitals. However, the mood of the electorate shifted and the healthcare industry was undergoing enormous change. Although the states made incremental progress in increasing coverage during the early 1990s by implementing Medicaid Section 1115 waivers, by 1996 expansions ceased as the states' focus shifted to increasing the efficiency of delivering healthcare services. Essentially, states are now concentrating on reducing the rate of growth of Medicaid, reorganizing state healthcare agencies, and monitoring the changing healthcare marketplace to ensure that consumers have the information to make informed decisions. Only after the states convince the electorate that they are delivering healthcare services efficiently and the healthcare marketplace has stabilized will the states again shift their focus to expanding coverage for low-income people.

Given that Medicaid is the dominant government program for delivering healthcare services to the poor, the first two sections of this chapter provide an overview of the changing federal-state relationship in Medicaid. The next section summarizes the major two obstacles that states face in expanding healthcare coverage to low-income people, while the following section describes state challenges such as covering the working poor, the emerging problem of uncompensated care, and the problem of increasing costs. The remaining sections describe the new state fiscal realities and their impact on the healthcare agenda of the states. Recent action to expand coverage of low-income people during the 1992–96 period is also summarized. However, these sections also stress that this action slowed dramatically in 1996 as the state focus shifted to emphasizing efficiency through managed care, restructuring state health agencies, and monitoring changes in the healthcare industry.

The Recent Past

During the late 1980s and early 1990s, healthcare reform was a major issue at both the state and the federal levels. During this period, a number of states, such as Florida, Minnesota, Oregon, and Washington, enacted major legislative reforms to control healthcare costs, to expand coverage significantly, or to achieve both objectives. A large number of other states, including Colorado and Maine, were experimenting with more incremental reforms, such as creating high-risk pools or instituting malpractice reforms. When Bill Clinton was elected in 1992, much of the state action stopped, as the focus of healthcare reform shifted from the state capitals to the nation's capital. With the failure of the Clinton comprehensive healthcare reform initiative, many believed that the action would again shift back to the states. Yet, although states were willing to continue making incremental changes, particularly those interested in saving money, they were unwilling to substantially expand eligibility. Many of the states that had previously enacted major reforms either repealed them or failed to implement components of the initial legislation. Unfortunately, the window of opportunity for comprehensive healthcare reform was now closed.

National polls still place healthcare among the top issues of concern to Americans, but public officials are still skittish about proposing new comprehensive initiatives. The following factors may help explain their apprehension:

- There continues to be no national consensus on a vision of a reformed healthcare system. Moreover, no consensus is likely to be reached until a number of states are able to experiment with comprehensive solutions.
- With the federal deficit for 1996 having been reduced to only $107 billion, there is a growing national consensus to eliminate

the remaining deficit by 2002. This fiscal conservatism could preclude major expansions of healthcare eligibility and benefits at the federal level.

- Fiscal conservatism is not only a barrier to expanded healthcare benefits at the federal level, but also is a major obstacle at the state and local levels. Currently, states are more interested in reducing the rate of spending increases and cutting taxes than in expanding existing programs or creating new ones.

- There is considerable uncertainty regarding the future costs and structure of the healthcare industry. The rate of change in the structure of this industry will need to slow before major expansions in eligibility and benefits will again move to the top of the national agenda.

The bottom line is that, with the exception of Medicare, there will be few major healthcare initiatives enacted at either the federal or the state level over the next several years. The next several years will be a period of incremental change. The major themes at both the federal and the state levels will be austerity, increased efficiency, and monitoring the emerging healthcare market. These themes are a reaction to changes in the mood of the electorate across the nation. First, citizens are demanding that government spending increases be limited and that budgets be balanced. Second, voters want government programs to be run more efficiently. This means downsizing and consolidating agencies, implementing performance budgeting and value purchasing, and privatizing, where applicable. It also means making public programs more customer oriented. Third, the ideological debate that has raged between those who advocate a price-regulated healthcare industry and those who place their faith in a competitive market approach has been won by the proponents of a market-based system. Even states such as New York that traditionally have believed in regulation are shifting to a more market-based system. This means that both federal and state policymakers will need to monitor the emerging healthcare market to determine whether consumers are reaping the benefits of higher-quality and lower-cost healthcare.

The Federal Framework

What happens in healthcare reform in the states over the next several years will depend, to a large extent, on changes at the federal level. The Medicaid program, because of its sheer size—$93 billion in federal funds and $71 billion in state funds—dominates state-federal relations and often drives state health policy changes. The state matching share for Medicaid alone currently equals 19 percent of the average state budget (National Association of State Budget Officers 1996). This proportion of state budgets is second only to the 23 percent that states spend for all elementary and secondary education. Furthermore, Medicaid has been the source of many innovations over the last several years, with states both instituting value purchasing and expanding coverage under federal waivers. It is also true that the federal government provides another $4 billion through approximately 90 categorical health grants to states. These grants fund a broad system of healthcare programs, including rural health and maternal and child health programs. Changes to the funding levels or structure of these grants would also have an impact on state programs.

A Balanced Budget

Although politicians, ranging from congressional representatives to the president, historically have campaigned on the need to balance the federal budget, the events leading up to the 1996 presidential campaign have made it a top priority for the president and the 105th Congress. Not only is there a national consensus that the federal government should balance the budget, but there also is substantial political momentum to attain this goal in five years (i.e., by 2002). This debate will likely play out in two related but different legislative initiatives. First, Congress may pass the balanced budget constitutional amendment with sufficient votes to send it to the states for ratification. If this were to happen, a significant number of states would likely ratify the amendment within a year. However, it is questionable if it would be approved by the required 38 states. Second, eliminating the deficit by 2002 will be a major part of the 1998 budget debate as Congress adopts the budget resolution and enacts the reconciliation and appropriations bills that would implement the deficit reduction plan.

The current deficit is down to $107 billion for FY 1996, but this estimate is somewhat deceiving. Unfortunately, the baseline deficit path is back up again and, depending on the underlying growth of the economy, is in the range of between $140 billion and $160 billion over the next five years, even assuming a reduced annual growth rate in Medicaid of approximately 8 percent. Such a deficit, coupled with campaign promises by both the president and the Congress for a major tax cut, means that it will be difficult to attain a zero deficit in five years notwithstanding the national consensus to do so. If there is a willingness to make changes to the way the consumer price index (CPI) is computed, however, this would make the problem much more manageable.

Nevertheless, the debate on whether to balance the budget has subsided. Now the focus is on which programs to cut, not whether to meet the goal of a zero deficit. This will mean that the nation will be entering a new period of austerity at the federal level, which will likely affect state health programs in the following ways:

- There will be little money available to increase healthcare eligibility or benefits for any population group.
- There will be pressure to make cuts in the $4 billion for existing state categorical health grants. This is a very vulnerable portion of the federal budget because it is part of the domestic discretionary component that is appropriated annually.
- There will be a demand for efficiency changes in Medicaid and, perhaps, even some type of cap on the rate of growth.
- There will be significant pressure to reduce the rate of growth in Medicare spending.

Medicaid

During the 1980s and early 1990s, Medicaid grew dramatically with annual increases in a number of years of more than 20 percent. As of 1994, Medicaid was projected by the Congressional Budget Office to continue to grow approximately 10 percent per year over the next seven years. Such a high growth rate, coupled with the growing political imperative for a balanced budget, led Republicans during the 104th Congress to develop proposals to block grant Medicaid and devolve it to the states. The quid pro quo was that states would have much more flexibility to run Medicaid efficiently and to tailor the program to the needs of each state, while the federal government would have major budget savings. This was similar to the welfare proposal that eventually was enacted by Congress and signed into law by the president. In both cases, the federal entitlement to benefits for low-income people would be eliminated and replaced with various types of state guarantees. However, the divisions in Congress, the breakdown of support from some governors, and opposition by the president all contributed to the failure to enact a restructured Medicaid program.

As of late 1996, both the budget and the political dynamics around Medicaid changed dramatically. First, the rate of growth in Medicaid for

FY 1996 dropped to less than 4 percent. This was caused by a number of factors, including

- a significant decline in the rate of increase in healthcare prices in general;
- a reduction in the number of individuals receiving Aid to Families with Dependent Children (AFDC) and, therefore, receiving Medicaid as the unemployment rate dropped because of the strength of the economy;
- a slowing in the growth of the elderly and disabled populations with low incomes;
- a savings caused by the significant increase in the number of Medicaid recipients who are enrolled in managed care through federal waivers;
- a cap on the increase in the disproportionate-share hospital spending due to reforms enacted in 1991;
- aggressive fraud and abuse control efforts;
- a new political environment in states to hold the rate of growth in all expenditures down so as to make incremental tax cuts; and
- state action to shift some costs from FY 1996 to FY 1995 so as to build the base year that would be used to establish state-by-state allocations if a Medicaid block grant was enacted.

With respect to the changing budget outlook, few would argue that the growth in Medicaid will remain at 4 percent. This is because some of the reasons for the recent decline in the growth rate are cyclical, such as the strength of the economy, whereas others, such as some of the managed care savings, may produce a one-time reduction in costs. It is also doubtful, however, that Medicaid growth will return to the 10 percent previously projected by the Congressional Budget Office (1996). It is most likely that the baseline over the next five years will be in the 5 to 7 percent range. Although this lower growth rate projection will reduce the pressure on Congress to restructure the Medicaid program so as to accrue huge budget savings, some savings may still need to be achieved.

Concerning the changing political dynamic, President Clinton was reelected partially on a platform to oppose any major changes to the Medicaid entitlement. Given the president's opposition to entitlement changes and the fact that there are less potential budget savings from restructuring Medicaid, it is likely that Congress and the president will first look to some middle ground to make incremental changes to

Medicaid. This would mean developing a package of efficiency changes that the nation's governors could support, such as

- making managed care easier to implement by eliminating the need for a waiver;
- eliminating the "75/25" rule that restrains Medicaid participation to 75 percent of health maintenance organization enrollment;
- eliminating or modifying the Boren Amendment that prescribes Medicaid reimbursement rates;
- making federally qualified health centers an optional service to states; and
- providing states with more flexibility to implement home- and community-based waivers for long-term care.

The Congressional Budget Office rarely "scores" (i.e., estimates significant budget savings for) efficiency changes, so it is clear that both the president and the members of Congress will look for additional ways to generate budget savings in the Medicaid program. After incremental efficiency changes, it is most likely that they will look to cap disproportionate-share hospital payments for some states. Finally, the president, as well as some members of Congress, will advocate a cap on the per-beneficiary spending of each state. Although such an approach appears simple, it raises a number of efficiency and equity issues because the per-beneficiary spending of states differs dramatically, from $2,261 in Tennessee to $10,036 in New Hampshire (Kaiser Commission on the Future of Medicaid 1996). The differences in per-beneficiary spending reflect differences in disproportionate-share hospital payments, the mix of eligible populations (i.e., between acute care and long-term care), and the relative cost of healthcare in the state. In view of the political momentum for a balanced budget, further reductions in the long-term rate of growth in Medicaid will be debated during the 105th Congress.

Categorical Healthcare Grants

The federal government currently provides approximately $4 billion through 90 categorical healthcare grants to state governments (Advisory Commission on Intergovernmental Relations 1993). The largest grant is for maternal and child health, but there are a significant number that total less than $50 million to all states. Some of these grants require a state match, whereas others do not have this requirement. Because these grants fall within the nondefense discretionary spending category of the federal budget and are appropriated on an annual basis, they are easier than entitlements to cut. It is highly likely that the funding levels of these programs will be reduced so as to meet the budget targets. Whether budget cuts could be offset partially by consolidation of these programs to give states greater flexibility to meet their unique needs remains to be seen. States will continue to push for consolidation, however, particularly given the significant number of small categorical grants with their own administrative requirements that reduce the efficiency of the programs.

Obstacles to Comprehensive State Healthcare Reform

As with other public policy issues, there are times, such as in the late 1980s and early 1990s, when states have displayed leadership in healthcare reform, whereas there are other times, such as in the 1960s, when the federal government has taken the lead by enacting Medicaid and Medicare. One level of government can fill the policymaking void when other levels are unable to act because of a lack of political consensus or will. Most of the barriers to reform are transitory in that they depend on changing political attitudes or economic circumstances. Currently, however, there are two major structural realities that limit states from moving forward aggressively to reform healthcare. The first, which is a major obstacle, is the Employee Retirement Income Security Act (ERISA). The second, which is less important, is the employer-based model under which most individuals receive healthcare benefits.

ERISA

The ERISA was enacted in 1974 to place federal standards on pension plans and exempt employee pension plans from state regulations (Corporate Health Care Coalition 1995). Although it is unclear whether Congress intended to include health plans in this preemption, all court decisions have interpreted the law to cover self-insured health plans. States have been preempted from regulating these self-insured plans, and, by default, the federal government has chosen not to regulate this industry. Consequently, for all practical purposes, this industry is free from regulation. Whether or not the existence of ERISA has had a positive impact on the healthcare industry and ultimately on the ability of private employers to provide low-cost insurance is up for debate. Clearly, self-insured plans have been a major driving force for cost-effective healthcare. Many would argue that these plans have created the current changes in the industry, particularly the move toward managed care. It is also true, however, that these self-insured plans may have forced some cost shifts to the individual and small group markets, thereby raising costs and reducing the number of insured people.

Whether ERISA has been a benefit or a liability over the past 30 years is questionable. What is clear, however, is that ERISA creates a bifurcated system, part of which is under state jurisdiction and part of which is under federal jurisdiction. This means that neither the federal government nor the state governments sees healthcare as its responsibility and thus neither develops a comprehensive national vision of the healthcare system to guide regulation. Either the federal government or the state governments will need to take primary responsibility for healthcare reform, and states are unable to do so without Congress passing legislation that amends ERISA. Although the 104th Congress made major concessions to state government in the unfunded mandates and welfare reform legislation, it is extremely doubtful that the 105th Congress will change the ERISA legislation. Until that happens many states may be reluctant to take aggressive reform action.

Substitution of Public Coverage for Private Coverage

In the United States, healthcare is currently provided through both employment-based arrangements as well as the two major public programs of Medicare and Medicaid. If military health coverage and a few other small public programs are included, about one-third of the insured population receives healthcare through public programs and about two-thirds receive it through employment-based coverage. Although many of the working poor have access to employer-sponsored healthcare, increasing numbers may not choose to enroll because they are eligible for Medicaid at no cost. Furthermore, the number of employers willing to subsidize dependent care has been declining. Both factors contribute to the tendency for expansions in public programs to be merely substituted for employer-sponsored programs. This substitution of public coverage for private coverage complicates the goal of increasing healthcare coverage for low-income people.

The 1989 Medicaid expansions for children below age six and pregnant women with incomes at or below 133 percent of the poverty level greatly reduced the number of poor children who do not have health insurance. States have also continued to expand eligibility for Medicaid to people with higher incomes; 6 states now cover up to 200 or 300 percent of the poverty level and 34 states cover infants and pregnant women up to 185 percent of the federal poverty level (National Governors' Association 1996). Some recent surveys indicate that 66 percent of all workers and 51 percent of women workers with young children and family incomes between $10,000 and $20,000 are eligible for employer coverage (Curtis and Page 1996). Moreover, most of those eligible accept coverage. The percentage of children above the poverty level in employer-sponsored insurance plans, however, has declined from approximately 66 percent during the late 1970s to 63 percent in 1990 to 52 percent in 1993. Some researchers have suggested that this decline is the result of children moving to Medicaid. For example, researchers from The Urban Institute (Dubay and Kenney 1995) found that, among Medicaid recipients,

- 43 percent of children age ten and younger with incomes between 100 and 133 percent of the poverty level were eligible for employer-sponsored care; and

- 52 percent of pregnant women with incomes between 160 and 185 percent of the poverty level were eligible for employer-sponsored care.

Although the cost of this substitution as a percentage of the Medicaid budget is very small from a public policy standpoint, it points out the problems inherent in a system that is partially publicly funded and partially privately funded. Such substitution will complicate further Medicaid expansions.

State Challenges

The responsibilities for healthcare assumed by the various levels of government within the intergovernmental system are relatively rational. The federal government has major responsibility for the elderly (i.e., people above age 65), with the important exception of the lower-income elderly who are in nursing homes. It also shares responsibility for all low-income people with all states and even provides a higher federal share for poorer states. Given that neither the elderly nor low-income people are equally distributed across states, the federal government is in a unique position to redistribute resources from higher-income people through the tax systems to people in need who may be concentrated in lower-income states. This redistribution role is a proper role for the federal government. Except for the regulatory responsibilities associated with ERISA, the major responsibility to ensure that people receive high-quality healthcare resides with the states. The current state challenges are varied and run the gamut from increasing access to monitoring emerging healthcare markets.

Access

Healthcare coverage in the United States has been eroding over the past few years, due partially to increased competition in the global marketplace and the rise of service industries as the predominant basis of the U.S. economy. As of 1995, an estimated 40.6 million people in the United States, or approximately 15.4 percent, were without coverage for the entire year (Bureau of the Census 1996). The percentage of uninsured differs substantially among states, however, from a high of more than 20 percent in Arizona, California, New Mexico, and Texas, to the single digits of Hawaii, Iowa, North Dakota, Vermont, and Wisconsin (Advisory Commission on Intergovernmental Relations 1993). Such a lack of coverage continues to be a major public policy issue for states. Not only is total access a problem in most states, but there are increasing concerns with respect to two major components—the working poor and uncompensated care.

The Working Poor

Higher-income people generally receive healthcare benefits through their employers, whereas low-income people, especially women and children, have access to Medicaid. This does not include the elderly who receive care through Medicare. However, individuals and families with incomes above 100 percent but below 200 percent of the poverty level—often referred to as the working poor—often have lower coverage than the other two groups. There is a growing concern for these people from a fairness standpoint; they are working hard to make ends meet and are paying taxes but are receiving no healthcare subsidy, whereas those on welfare are receiving a rich package of healthcare benefits. Many of the nation's governors and state legislators are looking for more cost-effective ways, either under Medicaid or alternative approaches, to help this group through partial subsidies to receive healthcare benefits.

Uncompensated Care

Without universal healthcare coverage, there is a need for some ad hoc system to cover emergency and other healthcare services provided by hospitals and physicians for low-income people who are not eligible for Medicaid and are unable to pay. The following strategies have been used to address the problem of uncompensated care (Weissman 1996):

- disproportionate-share payment under both Medicare and Medicaid to urban and rural hospitals with a relatively high rate of uncompensated care;
- Hill-Burton Act payments to hospitals for charity care;
- direct subsidies by state and local governments to government-owned hospitals and not-for-profit hospitals;
- cost shifting to private payors to cover hospitals' costs for uncompensated care; and
- general assistance programs with medical benefits.

Due to the new budget realities of federal, state, and local governments, as well as competition-driven changes in the healthcare industry, all of these current sources of revenue are eroding. Medicaid disproportionate payments are now capped, public hospitals are being sold, and not-for-profit hospitals are being merged. Finally, managed care reduces the potential for cost shifts to the private sector for hospital uncompensated care. This burden of uncompensated care may worsen with the implementation of the new welfare reform law's restrictions on the eligibility of legal immigrants.

Costs

Although the rate of increase in healthcare prices has slowed recently to approximate the general rate in inflation as measured by the CPI, it is unclear whether this slower rate of growth will be sustained. Now that the debate on whether to move toward a deregulated market-based system or one that requires price controls has been won by advocates of the competition model, the public policy challenge is to help create a climate in which this competition enables consumers to access a cost-effective benefit package at a price that is relatively stable over time. Ensuring that the market works effectively requires the following:

- an entity that measures the quality of healthcare providers;
- readily available comparable information on benefits, costs, and quality of providers so that consumers can make informed decisions on competing plans and providers; and

- a sufficient number of providers in the local marketplace so that it is not dominated by one or several providers who are able to artificially increase prices or lower quality.

State Fiscal and Regulatory Climates

Not only is the federal government under political pressure to eliminate the deficit, but states are under similar pressure to reduce the rate of increase in state expenditures and to provide tax cuts. Although states raised taxes $45 billion over the time period 1988–94 so as to avoid major spending cuts, they have cut taxes more than $10 billion over the period 1994–96 (National Governors' Association and National Association of State Budget Officers 1996). Furthermore, for both 1996 and 1997, total state spending will grow only approximately 4 percent each year. This is dramatically below the 7.2 percent annual average growth over the 1979–95 period. Essentially, voters want state government to ratchet down the rate of spending increases and continue to cut taxes. They do not want expansions in existing programs or new programs nor do they want major cuts. Clearly, they want states to hold the line on spending. This is extremely unusual given the fact that the economy has been strong and thus state revenue growth has been high by historical standards. In the past, increased revenues were mostly spent. Recently, however, spending has been controlled, surpluses increased, and taxes cut. There is a similar situation on the regulatory front. The general regulatory climate in states is to review existing regulations and to eliminate and simplify, where appropriate.

Increased Access—State Action

Since 1990, states have increased healthcare coverage to approximately 1 million low-income people. They are using a number of incremental approaches to increase access, including optional Medicaid benefits to increase the coverage of children and pregnant women; Section 1115 Medicaid demonstration waivers; direct insurance subsidies; and direct care by way of clinics and other community health entities.

Optional Medicaid Benefits

Under current law, states are required to cover children up to age six and pregnant women up to 133 percent of the poverty level. Furthermore, for children age 6 and older, each year the age is increased by one year until all children up to age 18 at 100 percent of the poverty level are covered. States also have the option to cover infants and pregnant women up to 185 percent of the poverty level. Currently, 34 states have exercised the option to expand eligibility for infants and pregnant women up to 185 percent of the poverty level (National Governors' Association 1996). Another ten states have extended Medicaid coverage to children in families with incomes above 133 percent of the poverty level.

Section 1115 Medicaid Demonstration Waivers

Although states have had the option to apply for Section 1115 waivers for some time prior to 1992, only Arizona in 1981 and Oregon in 1991 have applied for statewide managed care waivers. When President Clinton was elected in 1992, being a former governor and sympathetic to the states' desire for flexibility, he encouraged the U.S. Department of Health and Human Services to work with the states to implement waivers to both generate budget savings and to expand coverage.

The demonstration waivers gave the states the ability to place large components of their Medicaid-eligible individuals in managed care plans. Under a revenue neutrality assumption, the savings could be used to expand coverage to other low-income people. During the ensuing four years, 36 states were granted waivers. Fifteen of these waivers allowed states to expand coverage. A total of 700,000 people who otherwise would not be eligible for Medicaid received coverage nationally under Section 1115 waivers (The Alpha Center 1996). A few of the programs have witnessed dramatic increases in the number of people covered who would not have been eligible under the traditional Medicaid program. For example, TennCare in Tennessee enrolled more than 330,000 new enrollees. Other large programs include the Oregon Health Plan with 145,000 new enrollees, Minnesota Care with more than 90,000, and Hawaii Quest with 45,000 (Kaiser Commission on the Future of Medicaid 1996). In terms of coverage in the individual states, the changes as a percentage of the nonelderly population receiving coverage have been dramatic, with TennCare at an additional 7 percent, Hawaii and Oregon at 4–5 percent, and Minnesota at 2–3 percent (Kaiser Commission on the Future of Medicaid 1996). Some of these programs, such as in Oregon and Vermont, have stopped covering people at 100 percent of the poverty level, whereas others, such as in Tennessee and Washington, have no limit on enrollment.

More recently, however, fewer states have applied for Section 1115 waivers that would expand coverage. Although Massachusetts is planning a major expansion of coverage, the Illinois waiver does not expand coverage. Kentucky has retracted its initial plan to expand coverage and, should New York receive its waiver, only a minor expansion would be made. Moreover, neither the Maryland nor the Oklahoma waivers expanded coverage. Finally, although Ohio's waiver allows it to expand coverage up to 100 percent of the poverty level, the state has yet to fund the option. These actions are consistent with the fiscal conservatism in states. Any budget savings from using managed care for Medicaid are now more likely to go back to the state treasuries rather than being used to expand care.

State-Funded Programs

In addition to expanding Medicaid, either by expanding optional coverage for pregnant women and children or by implementing Section 1115 waivers, some states have expanded coverage through independent programs. Most of these programs provide direct but partial subsidies of premiums for private insurance. Hawaii, Minnesota, Oregon, and Washington have been the leaders in using this approach to enhance coverage (Advisory Commission on Intergovernmental Relations 1993). Most of these programs use a sliding scale based on a share of the premium. From a budget perspective, however, it may be necessary to adjust the subsidy depending on the number of participants. For children's expansions, New York's child health plans have more than 105,000 children enrolled, and Pennsylvania's plan has been expanded to 50,000 enrollees.

Future Changes

Expansions in coverage during the 1980s and 1990s were comparatively small relative to the national average uninsured rate of 17 percent. Through Medicaid waiver expansions, Medicaid optional changes, and programs to provide private subsidies, more than 45 states have expanded coverage. Riley (in this volume) is correct in her assessment that states have made incremental progress in expanding coverage but is wrong in her assumption that it will continue in the near future; the new breeze of fiscal conservatism in the states will likely halt any significant expansion in the immediate future. Few states will expand coverage, and any expansions will focus primarily on children because they are of relatively low cost and high priority. Instead, states will be implementing the new welfare reform eligibility criteria for Medicaid and attempting to reduce Medicaid cost increases further through managed care.

The New State Health Agenda

In the short run the state focus has shifted away from enhancing coverage to responding to the new fiscal conservatism of citizens and the fact that the structure of the healthcare industry is changing dramatically. The emerging themes are containing costs, increasing efficiency, and monitoring the new healthcare marketplace. Only after states convince the electorate that they are delivering healthcare services efficiently and the healthcare marketplace has stabilized will states again shift their focus to expanding coverage for low-income people.

State Healthcare Agency Restructuring

Not only are states focusing on developing more value purchasing in Medicaid programs, but there is significant interest in making the various healthcare agencies more efficient through consolidation, downsizing, and restructuring.

During the 1980s, the level of healthcare spending and therefore the number of employees in state healthcare agencies grew very rapidly. By the early 1990s, most states had administrative bureaucracies that were both difficult to manage and inefficient because of the extensive fragmentation within and among state healthcare agencies. By the mid-1990s, voters were beginning to raise concerns regarding the effectiveness of government programs in general and the size of state healthcare spending in these agencies in particular. In response to these concerns, state governments evaluated the need for more integration, coordination, accountability, and customer orientation. Furthermore, the prior emphasis on measuring the success of a program based on inputs, such as the number of clients served or the number of providers participating, was giving way to a new focus on outcomes, such as a reduction in the infant mortality rate. Advances in information technology have also enabled these shifts in focus.

Current and future needs for major consolidation and integration of healthcare agencies are being driven by the need to increase government efficiency across the board, but also by a number of factors that are unique to this industry:

- The role of the state in Medicaid is changing from bill payor to value purchaser.
- The healthcare industry is changing dramatically, undergoing both vertical and horizontal restructuring that requires different types of monitoring.

- The new welfare reform law eliminates the coupling of eligibility between AFDC and Medicaid and gives states new options to establish eligibility.

A recent survey of states indicates that during the 1997 state legislative session, 9 states anticipate that state health agency restructuring will be a legislative issue, whereas 11 states indicate that the restructuring of the Medicaid agency may appear on the legislative agenda. Finally, 35 states indicate that the structuring of managed care regulatory, oversight, and monitoring responsibilities will likely be a major activity (Maralit, Orloff, and Desonia, forthcoming). At the same time that the healthcare industry is restructuring, states are launching health agency restructuring initiatives to enhance the effectiveness of programs and services and to ensure appropriate oversight of the newly emerging healthcare market.

The New Challenge of Making the Market Work

Not only are states focusing on the efficiency of delivering healthcare services, but the rapid change in the structure of the healthcare industry has also forced them to pull back from expanding coverage and to begin monitoring the rate of change. Specifically, states are developing an information base to determine the type and extent of future regulation.

Most of the sectors of the U.S. economy are market based. The healthcare industry is in the process of joining these other sectors by becoming a market-oriented industry. The rate of cost increases should be held down by a significant number of providers competing with one another for the right to sell healthcare benefits to consumers. The role of public policy is to ensure that the market works efficiently. This requires the following. First, some entity must provide quality measurements of healthcare providers. Second, consumers must have information on a consistent set of benefits, quality, and prices so that they can compare plans and providers and make informed decisions on healthcare coverage. Finally, competition must be enforced through antitrust legislation. The market approach has emerged only in the last several years, so states are just now entering a period in which they will be experimenting with how to promote competition and how to regulate the industry.

Quality and Consumer Information

Although states will continue their traditional role of inspecting health facilities and licensing providers, they are also starting to rely on other approaches to ensuring quality. They are participating, usually through the Medicaid program, in national initiatives by other purchasers and providers to develop a common data system to compare the quality of care delivered by managed care entities. The most common is the Health Plan Employee Data and Information Set, which contains nine indicators of quality; seven of these indicators are process oriented rather than output oriented. Moreover, because more care is being provided in ambulatory settings, there is increasing interest among states in measuring the quality of care delivered by practitioners. New York has released surgeon- and hospital-specific mortality rates for certain cardiac procedures. Significant improvements in mortality outcomes have already resulted from the public dissemination of this information.

States have been collecting healthcare data since the 1970s and early 1980s. As of 1996, more than 40 states have established, or are developing, data collection programs. Currently, approximately 14 states are collecting data on a statewide basis. In addition, many states require managed care organizations to provide information on quality. The challenge is to make the data and quality measures relevant to the provider decisions that need to be made by individuals, employers, and governments. The information is necessary not only to monitor the emerging market, but also to assist consumers with major healthcare decisions.

Antitrust Enforcement

Antitrust enforcement in the United States takes place at both the federal and the state levels. The federal government enforces antitrust provisions under the Sherman Act of 1890, the Clayton Act of 1914, and the Federal Trade Commission Act of 1914. Over the past 15 years, there have been a number of federal challenges, primarily related to the more than 400 hospital mergers. However, the impact of these challenges on the overall structure of the healthcare industry has been very small.

All states, except Pennsylvania and Vermont, have some type of antitrust laws that are generally enforced through their attorney general's office. Many states have also adopted immunity laws, which they were allowed to adopt under the authority of the 1943 Supreme Court decision in *Parker v. Brown* (Butler 1996). States can only adopt such laws, however, if the immune entities are under active state supervision. The applicability of antitrust laws is complicated by the nature of the changes that are taking place in the healthcare industry. This industry is being integrated both vertically, with physician hospital organizations, as well as horizontally, with physician networks. In a number of rural areas, state governments have often actually encouraged provider collaboration to maintain low costs and comprehensive benefit packages.

It is also true that there can be cost advantages for hospitals to share equipment and information. The problem is that some of these beneficial changes may not take place in states because of antitrust concerns. More than 20 states have enacted immunity laws to address this issue. The breadth and degree of active supervision required in these state immunity laws, however, differs, and therefore few providers have requested exemptions. Over the past several years, state antitrust officials have filed approximately 15 healthcare antitrust actions. Similar to the federal government, the impact of these cases has been marginal at best.

The short-term challenge for states is to determine where immunity is needed and, if it is needed, what kind of supervision is necessary. The healthcare industry is undergoing rapid change through mergers and acquisitions, so the issue of antitrust enforcement will become much more important in the future. In some geographic regions, such as the Minneapolis–St. Paul area, the market is already dominated by two major providers. If providers begin to take advantage of their market power and begin to lower quality or increase prices, states will need to become much more aggressive in enforcing antitrust laws.

Conclusion

The 1980s and even the early 1990s were periods of state activism on healthcare reform. Not only did a few states enact comprehensive re-form, but a large number of states initiated incremental changes. Most states, either through Medicaid or their own programs, also increased access for low-income people. As the nation moved toward the latter half of the 1990s, however, the state climate changed dramatically. The pre-vailing mood is now one that stresses austerity, efficiency, and monitoring the emerging healthcare market.

At the federal level, deficit reduction will be a political requirement over the next several years. This will mean little expansion in healthcare eligibility benefits and perhaps even some reductions as the emphasis, particularly in Medicaid, moves toward enacting efficiency changes and possibly even some limits on the rate of growth. A similar austerity climate will dominate states over the next several years as they reduce the rate of growth in total state spending, initiate few new programs, and limit program expansions. Reducing taxes and simplifying and streamlining regulations will dominate state activity. There will be few dollars for expansions in healthcare benefits, even assuming savings from

Section 1115 waivers. The budget savings from value purchasing will go back to state treasuries, not to expanding access. Consistent with the theme of austerity, states will continue to look for additional efficiencies through consolidating, restructuring, downsizing, and refocusing state healthcare agencies. The emphasis will be more on outputs than inputs, and the focus will be on the customers of healthcare.

The challenge over the next few years will likely be for states to begin to monitor and experiment with various policies to ensure that the healthcare market works to the benefit of consumers. This means overseeing the quality of providers as well as ensuring that consumers have sufficient cost and other information so that they can make informed decisions. Antitrust enforcement will become increasingly important as more mergers take place in the healthcare industry.

Having states focus on both increasing efficiency in state programs and making the market work is necessary given the voters' skepticism regarding eligibility expansions for low-income people. If states are able to attain the goals of providing efficient healthcare services and ensuring that the market works, they will help establish a stable and efficient healthcare industry.

After this period of consolidation and increasing efficiency, states may again choose to focus on increasing access. Yet states will continue to face two obstacles in attaining the goal of significant reductions in the number of uninsured people. The first problem is the substitution of state-financed healthcare coverage for low-income people for employer-sponsored coverage. Increasingly, there is evidence that low-income people with incomes between 100 and 300 percent of the poverty level have access to employer-sponsored healthcare, but will not purchase it if they are eligible for Medicaid. To some extent, this is a structural problem with the employer-based model. The second problem, which is major, is that the nation has a two-tiered healthcare system under which the federal government retains jurisdiction over self-insured plans through ERISA and state governments regulate the individual and small group markets. Given this, it is doubtful that either the federal government or states will be able to make major improvements to the existing healthcare system over the next several years.

Acknowledgments

The author thanks Randy Desonia, Jeff Harris, Jennifer Baxendell, Tess Moore, and Karen Glass of the National Governors' Association staff for their valuable contributions.

References

Advisory Commission on Intergovernmental Relations. 1993. *Characteristics of Federal Grants-In-Aid Programs to State and Local Governments: Grants Funded FY 1993.* Washington, DC: The Commission.

The Alpha Center. 1996. *State Initiatives in Health Care Reform.* Washington, DC: The Center.

Bureau of the Census. 1996. "Health Insurance Coverage: 1995." *Current Population Reports.* Washington, DC: U.S. Department of Commerce.

Butler, P. A. 1996. *Implications of Health Care Competition for Cost, Choice, Quality, and Innovation: The Role of Antitrust Policy.* Washington, DC: National Governors' Association.

Congressional Budget Office. 1996. *U.S. Congress, The Economic and Budget Outlook, Fiscal Years 1997–2006: A Preliminary Report.* Washington, DC: U.S. Government Printing Office.

Corporate Health Care Coalition. 1995. *ERISA Preemption: The Key to Market Innovation in Health Care Reform.* Washington, DC: The Coalition.

Curtis, R., and A. Page. 1996. *Improving Health Care Coverage for Low-Income Children and Pregnant Women: Optimizing Medicaid and Employer-Financed Coverage Relations.* Washington, DC: The Institute for Health Policy Solutions.

Dubay, L., and G. Kenney. 1995. *Revisiting the Issues: The Effects of Medicaid Expansions on Insurance Coverage of Children.* Washington, DC: The Urban Institute.

Kaiser Commission on the Future of Medicaid. 1996. *Medicaid Expenditures and Beneficiaries: National and State Profiles and Trends 1984–1994.* Washington, DC: The Commission.

Maralit, M., T. M. Orloff, and R. A. Desonia. Forthcoming. *State Health Agency Restructuring: A Fifty State Survey.* Washington, DC: National Governors' Association.

National Association of State Budget Officers. 1996. *1995 State Expenditure Report.* Washington, DC: The Association.

National Governors' Association. 1996. *State Medicaid Coverage of Pregnant Women and Children.* Washington, DC: The Association.

National Governors' Association and National Association of State Budget Officers. 1996. *The Fiscal Survey of the States, November 1996.* Washington, DC: National Governors' Association and National Association of State Budget Officers.

Weissman, J. 1996. "Uncompensated Hospital Care: Will It Be There If We Need It?" *Journal of the American Medical Association* 276 (10): 823–28.

V

The Search for Solutions II: Considerations for Comprehensive Reforms

18

Where Will Americans Obtain Their Health Insurance? The Job Link Revisited

Alain C. Enthoven

Consumer Choice Health Plan

My first intervention in the universal health insurance policy world took place in 1977 when I served as a consultant to U.S. Department of Health and Human Services Secretary Joseph Califano on the subject of health insurance. In his 1976 campaign, Jimmy Carter promised universal, compulsory, comprehensive, mandatory health insurance. I went to work for Secretary Califano to design an approach that might stand a chance of passing into law and that would not violate American cultural preferences for pluralism, individual choice and responsibility, and decentralized decision making. I spent 1977 developing what I called the Consumer Choice Health Plan (CCHP) that was a national health insurance proposal based on regulated competition in the private sector (Enthoven 1978). Briefly, in this plan the government would act as sponsor (i.e., system manager), contracting with the health plans over coverage and terms of participation, benefit standards, risk adjustment, enrollment processes, etc., and the government would pay defined contributions set at 60 percent of the average premium in each actuarial category, not dissimilar to the Federal Employees' Health Benefits Program (FEHBP). The competing health plans would set their own premiums with no government price controls or caps. Part of the government's contributions would be paid for by the abolition of the tax exclusion for employer-paid health benefits. The system would be driven by informed cost-conscious consumer choice. Coverage would be completely independent of employment. In the case of employed people, employers would participate in managing the enrollment and premium collection processes in the same way that federal agencies participate in the FEHBP on behalf of their employees.

The competitors in this system would have included prepaid group practices, individual practice associations (IPAs), health maintenance plans (the term then for primary care gatekeeper-based IPAs such as SAFECO and US Healthcare), and preferred provider insurance, which existed only in concept and under several names at that time (e.g., health alliances, variable cost insurance). Traditional fee-for-service indemnity coverage could also compete; however, because of its evident inability to manage costs, its prospects for survival in a competitive market would not be good.

In the current political frame of reference, this plan would be viewed as a far-left scheme, though not nearly as far left as the Clinton and Garamendi plans because, at that time, my intent was to create a workable market at the individual level, not to supplant it with government regulation of premiums. But my plan was not seen as far left at the time. The reactions were interesting. Single-payor-minded liberals looked at me as if I were somewhere to the right of Atilla the Hun. I was assured in no uncertain terms that health maintenance organizations (HMOs) were a West Coast idea that could and would never happen on the East Coast. (As it turned out, "never" meant not for another few years. Massachusetts now has a substantially higher percentage of population in HMOs than California [Hoechst Marion Roussel, Inc. 1995].) The most interesting reaction came from John Sears, Ronald Reagan's campaign manager, who said it was an interesting idea and offered to help. Before I could accept this offer, in view of the permanent Democratic majority in the Congress, I needed to get some Democrats out in front first—which I attempted to do with modest success.

Critique of Employment-Based Health Insurance

My first *New England Journal of Medicine* article included a brief critique of the employment-based system. Soon after, I expanded on that theme in an article for *Harvard Business Review* (Enthoven 1979). The following are some excerpts from that article.

> In this system, employees and their families lose their health insurance when the bread winner loses his or her job while, at the same time, a Medicaid beneficiary can lose Medicaid eligibility by getting a job, even a poorly paid one. . . . Today's familiar system

of job-centered health insurance is one of the main barriers to economic competition in health services. It is thus a major contributor to health care cost inflation. It is incompatible with universal continuous coverage. And it is the cause of many nonproductive administrative burdens. . . . Today's job-centered system . . . is largely the product of a series of actions by the federal government in the 1940s and 1950s whose primary focus was on wage controls, labor relations, and taxes, and not on the structure of the health insurance industry. . . . Two important economic effects of these tax laws are to subsidize employee decisions to select more costly health care systems and to encourage employee pressure for more employer-paid health benefits. . . . An equally important unintended effect of the tax laws . . . is to limit the employee's health insurance options to the plan or plans offered by the employer. . . . Both [employers and unions] emphasize benefits specific to the employer or union, and not the use of this medical purchasing power to create a market of competing provider groups in the community. . . . People who change jobs are often forced to change health insurance plans, with gaps in coverage, new starts on annual deductibles, and possible exclusions or waiting periods for pre-existing medical conditions. If they belong to a closed panel plan . . . they are likely to be forced to change doctors when they change jobs, which means new starts on medical records and doctor-patient relationships.

In March 1977, of 47.5 million husband-wife families, about 27.2 million had two or more earners. . . . In fact, in 1976, about 30 million people under 65 had duplicate hospital insurance. That is wasteful, can produce excess insurance [collecting twice for the same bill] and creates a need for complex coordination of benefit rules. . . . Each employer negotiates his own package with his insurance company, with a special mix of benefits, coinsurance schedules, and provisions concerning cash flow and experience rating. Many of the variations are idiosyncratic and add little or nothing to consumer choice or better health care at less cost . . . the job-link adds greatly to the time and cost required to market a new health plan. . . . There is little to lose and much to gain by cutting today's link between jobs and health insurance. (pp. 149–51)

I noted that many of these problems would remain even if the system were supplemented by special coverage for those left out, such as President Nixon's proposed Comprehensive Health Insurance Act of 1974 or President Carter's Private Guaranteed Health Plan proposal.

A few bills inspired by my writings were introduced in Congress: Ullman, Durenberger, Gephardt-Stockman, Jones, and others. The thinking in regard to CCHP may have helped influence legislation opening up Medicare to HMO competition. But the proposal went almost nowhere as far as public policy was concerned, at least in the short run.

Lessons Learned I: Incrementalism

That experience naturally led to introspection, a search for lessons to be learned. Perhaps the first and most important lesson the experience taught me was that incrementalism is the first law of our democracy. We simply do not make drastic discontinuous changes in our society through legislation, in spite of what President Carter and other politicians said. Of course, this was by design. The founding fathers, in strong reaction to the heavy-handed unchecked rule of George III, designed a government with separation of powers: two houses of the legislature—one representing population, the other territory—and maximum checks and balances. Legislative proposals get sliced and diced and come out in small bite-sized changes that can pass these multiple filters. President Clinton's Health Security Act went nowhere even in a Congress controlled by Democrats. The Kassebaum-Kennedy bill passed after extensive negotiations, but, contrary to what the president and congressional leaders said, it made small incremental changes. We do not and cannot carry out public policy the way it is done in European parliamentary systems. We have to work with incremental change that begins with where we are and that includes the employment-based system.

Incrementalism is not welcome news for health system reformers because the parts of the healthcare financing and delivery system interact with each other. It has often been said that "if you push down here (e.g., inpatient), it pops up there (e.g., outpatient)." In particular, as I explain below, to make health insurance available to Americans that are not in employment groups, it is necessary both to make the coverage available through pooled purchasing arrangements and to reduce the burden of adverse selection in the voluntary individual market by creating vouchers, individual mandates, or some policy to get the healthy to buy and maintain insurance coverage. A large step toward universal coverage will require several coordinated interventions.

Lessons Learned II: Americans Distrust Government

As I studied health policy, I became increasingly pessimistic about the ability of government to manage the healthcare system. I was not optimistic to begin with. I spent the 1960s serving in the Kennedy and Johnson administrations as point man for the Secretary of Defense in charge of bringing cost effectiveness to the U.S. Department of Defense, a quixotic task for a young man. The main things I learned at the Department of Defense were that the ideal weapon system is built in 435 congressional districts and it doesn't work (so that they will have to keep the plant open to "retrofit" it). I also learned that there is no political constituency or support for cost effectiveness or value for money in government. In healthcare, government was clearly the tool of well-focused and -financed provider interests. Medicare and Medicaid were founded on the "Guild Free Choice" model (Weller 1984). Medicare may not be the original "Provider Protection Act," but it did become the largest. These are models of virtually complete nonaccountability for providers. They illustrate that our government is incapable of acting as an effective purchaser, whether it is toilet seats for the Pentagon or coronary artery bypass grafts for Medicare.

Of course, I was not the only one to reach this conclusion, nor are these views confined to the far right. In the introduction to the *National Performance Review*, Vice President Al Gore wrote

> waste is not the only problem. The federal government is not simply broke; it is broken. Ineffective regulation of the financial industry brought us the savings and loan debacle. . . . It is almost as if federal programs were *designed* not to work. In truth, few are "designed" at all. . . . In Washington's highly politicized world, the greatest risk is not that a program will perform poorly, but that a scandal will erupt. Scandals are front page news, while routine failure is ignored. (Gore 1993)

And of course, as noted above, there is a reason for this. It is the way the founding fathers designed it. James Madison succeeded in making "ambition counteract ambition."

This is not to say that the record of government in healthcare is all bad. Medicare and Medicaid have served necessary purposes, though they were badly designed from the point of view of incentives. They should have been designed on the FEHBP model. I have frequently cited the FEHBP as an example of a good program because of its multiple choice, openness to managed care, and employee premium-price consciousness. The FEHBP started out well with a formula that produced approximately a defined contribution. But over time, it became increasingly dysfunctional as increasing numbers of health plans fell into the premium zone where the government's limit on contributions of 75 percent applied, so that a $1.00 in premium reduction became a $0.25 reduction to the employee making the choice—seriously interfering with price elasticity of demand. And government seems incapable of correcting this. The inability to modify the formula illustrates the rigidity characteristic of government. Moreover, mischievous proposals have been introduced in Congress, for example, to take away the power of the Office of Personnel Management to regulate benefit packages—a little thing that could destroy the program.

I have also previously cited the health benefits program of the California Public Employees' Retirement System (CalPERS) as a good example. As does the FEHBP, the CalPERS operates under a broad mandate, free of legislative micromanagement. The CalPERS offers a wide range of choice; has greatly facilitated market entry by managed care; has been a leader in quality accountability, benefit standardization, etc.; and does the job for a remarkably low administrative cost. But, unfortunately, it too suffers from a state employer contribution policy that leaves most employees' premium cost unconscious in choice of plan. The state has proposed a defined contribution, which unfortunately conflicts with union beliefs. So the issue is at an impasse.

I also note the Health Insurance Plan of California, a pooled purchasing arrangement for small employers in the private sector. The management of the plan has done an excellent job in devising strategies that work despite defective legislation. Among their innovations are risk-adjusted premiums, a "super directory" of providers participating in various health plans (see below), and improved information for consumers, including focus groups that find out what type of information consumers want most. The original legislation left the plan vulnerable to adverse selection. I believe that is the way the opponents wanted it.

There is an interesting question as to what separates these "good" programs from the type of bad program Vice President Gore wrote about. A key characteristic of FEHBP, CalPERS, and the Health Insurance Plan of California is that they operate under broad statutes, with authority to do the right thing, and with comparative freedom from legislative micromanagement. This is a topic worthy of more research.

Building on the Employment-Based System

So where do we go from there? In 1989, Kronick and I proposed an employment-based approach with what we called a "public sponsor" to aggregate and manage buying power to create managed competition for small employers and individuals, and an employer mandate (Enthoven and Kronick 1989). That approach attracted polite interest from the Bush administration until Chief of Staff John Sununu decreed, "If the American people want healthcare, they'll vote for Democrats. So we won't talk about it." Unfortunately, in view of the Clinton debacle, they did, and they didn't. And it also attracted the public support of presidential candidate Paul Tsongas.

Then, in collaboration with the Jackson Hole Group, I developed the idea of the Health Insurance Purchasing Cooperative (HIPC) for the small employment group market (e.g., employment groups up to 50 or 100) (Ellwood, Enthoven, and Etheredge 1992). The HIPC has the potential to ameliorate many of the problems of the employment-based system that are so severe in the small-group market. Risks and administrative costs can be spread widely. Employees in small groups can be offered the full range of managed care plans serving their area of residence. Employees changing from one employer to another within the HIPC can keep their own plan and doctors. The market is driven by consumer choice, not by employer choice. The HIPC can take over the administration of Comprehensive Omnibus Budget Reconciliation Act (COBRA) continuity, relieving the employer of the burden of administration and of adverse selection. The employee leaving one employer could still participate in annual multiple choice of plans, thus preserving competition. I envisaged the HIPC as a base on which access-to-coverage extensions could be built. For example, there could be a rule that once people were covered through an HIPC, they could maintain continuous coverage for as long as they paid the premiums. The threshold for membership might be reduced to firms of even two employees. Rules might be devised to permit individuals to join in a way that would not create a large burden of adverse selection, especially if combined with other policies (see below).

As mentioned above, there is an HIPC in California, the Health Insurance Plan of California. Managed by an agency of the state government, it now covers over 130,000 people in over 5,000 employment groups, ranging from 2 to 50 employees, through approximately 23 participating managed care plans (HMOs and preferred provider organizations).

The HIPC was the centerpiece of the Managed Competition Acts of 1992 and 1993, the former introduced and sponsored by the Conservative Democratic Forum in the House with 70 cosponsors, and the latter introduced under bipartisan sponsorship in both houses of Congress. In the 1993 legislation, states would have been charged with creating HIPCs, with all group insurance bought and sold through them for groups up to 100. The tax exclusion for health insurance would be available to employees in small groups only if the coverage were bought through the HIPC. This is logical because the tax exclusion of employer-paid health insurance acts as a powerful incentive to pool risks in employment groups. Because small groups are too small to spread risks or to achieve economies of scale in administration, it makes sense to use the tax exclusion to motivate them to join larger pools.

If large employers were to continue the trend toward offering employees a wider choice of managed care plans, we could move toward a situation in which few people would have to change health plans when they changed their jobs while keeping the same residence.

The debate over the HIPCs and the experience with them exposed three problem areas. First, many in Congress, including Democrats, feared that the HIPCs would become bureaucratic and unresponsive and that they represented an excessive concentration of state power. Therefore, support grew for the idea that the HIPCs should be voluntary, even competing. One trouble with voluntary HIPCs is the danger of adverse selection: The high-risk groups are eager to pool with low-risk groups, and the good risks want to stay out. So the voluntary HIPC could be killed in a spiral of adverse selection similar to what happens in the market for individual coverage. Health Insurance Purchasing Cooperatives that compete would be tempted to compete on risk selection. HIPC proponents thought through several methods to combat this, some of which were applied in the voluntary HIPC in California.

Health insurance is the pooling of risk, and, if given a choice, the good risks do not want to be pooled with the bad. So some form of incentive or compulsion is needed. This is, of course, the argument for the government as single payor. In our private voluntary system, there is pooling through employment groups primarily because of the important tax break for employer-paid health insurance.

The California HIPC is voluntary, and so far it has not been destroyed by adverse selection. There are four reasons for this. First, HIPC premiums are rated by ten-year age bands, so the young are not expected to subsidize the old. But of course that has a cost; it forces the elderly to pay more. Second, HMOs were eager to participate because they saw the HIPCs as a good way to penetrate the hard-to-reach small-group market, so the HIPC took advantage of this and only selected the lowest priced HMOs. Third, the HIPC required participating carriers to grant the HIPC most-favored-nation status: That is, health plans that contract with the HIPC must agree not to offer outside the HIPC in the small-group market a similar or richer benefit package at a lower price for persons of the same age, family size, or geographic region category (Enthoven and Singer 1996). And fourth, California insurance laws limit the range of premiums that insurers can charge outside the HIPC based on health status. That limits the ability of insurers to pick off the low-risk groups. There is a delicate ecology of incentives. So far, what has been done in California has worked. This is not to say how it would work if there were competing HIPCs. To guard against adverse selection, there needs to be a fairly strong incentive to pool insurance risks.

The second problem area in the debate over the HIPCs is the problem of slow growth. The California HIPC has been in place approximately three years, and it is adding covered people at the rate of approximately 5,000 per month, which is far too slow to make a dent in the problem of uninsurance in the small-group market in the foreseeable future. One proposed explanation for the slow growth is the HIPC's poor relationship with brokers. Another is that the HIPC lacks the resources to market the program effectively.

These problems relate to the issue of whether the HIPCs must be nonprofits. The nonprofit school argues that they should be driven by public benefit objectives rather than for-profit objectives. For-profit incentives might motivate undesirable risk-selecting behavior. On the other hand, nonprofit HMOs simply did not grow fast enough to meet the market need. And the present state of strong price competition now present in California and elsewhere could not have been reached without the dynamism of the for-profits (Enthoven and Singer 1996). The same may be true with respect to the HIPCs.

The third problem area is governance. I have already reviewed the characteristic failings of government that impair its ability to serve as an HIPC. The trouble with this is that government is overly influenced by well-focused, well-financed provider interests. But it is hard to find an alternative that is "less worse." What is needed is strong demand-side advocacy, tempered by social responsibility (i.e., the HIPC boards need to be motivated by a desire to get the maximum value for their small-employer members, while not excluding high-risk groups). One apparently attractive idea would be to have board members elected by the participating small employers. But that has problems. Would the typical small business take the time and trouble to learn the issues and to vote wisely? Or would special interest groups be able to elect their candidates? Would they become like school boards? Who would serve? Could conflicts of interest be prevented? Who better to serve on the board than a knowledgeable doctor, hospital administrator, and insurance agent? We end up with something that looks like poorly accountable government. I am currently searching for ideas on how to constitute the HIPC.

The HIPC in California is a state agency. In my view, it has been well run. But I worry what will happen when it becomes larger and more politically salient. (Pursuant to the founding legislation, which was a political compromise, a Request for Proposals has been issued to see if any nonprofit organization would take over the HIPC. It is not certain what the outcome will be.)

The CalPERS is a successful HIPC for the public sector. Its board is partly ex-officio (state treasurer, controller, etc.,) and partly elected by employees, and it strongly supports the interests of employees.

Employers Do a Better Job than Government Monopolies

Given that some public employers have been among the most enlightened sponsors of managed competition, I have concluded that the employment-based system, for all its defects and shortcomings, is less worse than a government-monopoly-controlled system as proposed by President Clinton or by other single-payor advocates.[1] Employers are not monopolies. They are interested in the health and satisfaction of their employees as well as the cost of care. They have to compete for employees. They do make mistakes. They stayed with open-ended fee-for-service for far too long. But eventually they have to change to meet market forces. We need to find ways to make the benefits of the employment-based system available to more Americans.

In recent years employers have been innovating in positive ways, public employers among them. First, they have phased in managed competition, which is mainly a multiple choice of managed care plans, employee responsibility for premium differences, some amount of benefit standardization, and comparative information on quality and satisfaction. The HIPC in California is leading the way with risk-adjusted premiums (with the help of a grant from the Robert Wood Johnson Foundation) and with the creation of a "super directory" linking doctors, medical groups, and health plans to make it easy for people to look up their favorite doctors, identify the health plans they contract with, and pick the low-priced plan among them, which they might as well do as the benefits are standardized. Employers are pooling in various ways. For example, the Buyers' Health Care Action Group in Minneapolis–St. Paul has put forward an innovative plan to create competition at the delivery system level, complete with risk adjustment and quality measurement. The Pacific Business Group on Health is pooling to negotiate with

HMOs to standardize benefits and contract for quality improvement. They and other groups are pressing the quality agenda. They emphasize measurement and continuous improvement. Major purchasers, private and public, are supporting FAcct, the Foundation for Accountability, which is working to advance the state of the art of population- and disease-specific outcome-based quality measures.[2]

A promising innovation is that many employers are purchasing healthcare information services for their employees so as to give them a good and independent source of medical information, to help them become better-informed consumers, and to be sure that they are not wholly dependent on their health plan for information about treatment options. PEPSICO is a good example. In their demands for quality measures, employers are asking for measures that apply to a health plan's entire population, not just their own employees. Basically, they are conferring a substantial benefit on the entire community.

A Program to Extend the Benefits of Employment-Based Coverage to Nearly All Americans

The following is a rough outline of an agenda for extending the benefits of employment-based coverage to most Americans who are not currently covered. It may disappoint the single-payor advocates and others who want wall-to-wall, one-class, universal coverage. But the experiences of 1993–94 taught us that universal coverage is not in the cards. What I propose is incremental, moderate, and will not do violence to American cultural preferences that favor decentralized decision making and that oppose further centralization of power in government.

First, healthcare costs should be reduced through managed care and managed competition. This is working now in California. In real terms, HMO premiums now contracted for in 1997 will be approximately 15 percent below 1994 levels (Enthoven and Singer 1996). Cost reduction is necessary to make coverage affordable to more families and to the taxpayers who are expected to subsidize those who need it (and others as well).

Second, the availability of affordable coverage should be expanded at stable rates by public policies designed to build the HIPCs for small employment groups in all states. The problem of slow growth should be solved by tax incentives or some other means. The problem of governance should be dealt with by trial and error. A variety of approaches should be tried. The need is to expand pooled purchasing arrangements for small groups with deliberate speed.

Third, the availability of coverage should be expanded further by encouraging such policies as indefinite guaranteed renewal in HIPCs. Also, we should experiment with inter-HIPC portability and then experiment with reaching out to individuals. This raises the specter of adverse selection in the voluntary individual market.

Fourth, the present tax subsidy should be converted from the present exclusion of employer-paid health benefits from employee taxable income into a refundable tax credit usable only for purchase of health insurance meeting certain standards. The present tax revenue loss would permit a credit of approximately $500 per person (i.e., $100 billion for 200 million Americans not covered by government programs). The substitution of the tax credit for the exclusion is supported widely by economists across the ideological spectrum, and it is favorable from the point of view of efficiency and incentives and from the point of view of equity and target efficiency. (Currently, many upper-income people receive a strong incentive to buy coverage, but would buy coverage without it.) It would make this large drain on the federal budget finite and controllable. Also, this would be a start on a universal voucher. From the present point of view, it could be an effective way of ameliorating the problem of adverse selection in the individual market because it would give healthy people an incentive to buy coverage.

But there is a serious, potential problem with the tax credit approach (i.e., depooling). As noted above, the present tax exclusion contains a powerful incentive to obtain one's coverage through the employment group. The credit might leave people free to buy coverage where they like; therefore, good risks form the good-risk pool and bad risks end up in the bad-risk pool, in effect, recreating and generalizing all the problems we have in the individual market now. So the credit would have to be linked to its use through some type of large pool that could spread risks widely and achieve economies of scale in administration and that was not selected primarily or substantially on the basis of medical risks.

The credit for exclusion, of course, implies a substantial amount of income redistribution. Perhaps it could be offset by a reduction in the marginal income tax rates of upper-income families. The financial effect on such families would not be large. But the revenues are needed to pay for the credits. There should be some offsetting savings in reduced need for public programs as coverage expands. (Credits not taken up should be paid to local public direct care systems that take care of the uninsured or to a fund for compensating hospitals for uncompensated care.) The redistribution that does take place does not raise anyone's marginal tax rate.

This type of approach will become increasingly important if more and more workers become temporary, part-time, self-employed contractors or otherwise without employer-paid benefits, as is increasingly the trend, or as employers keep dropping coverage. (Indeed, this is the approach that ought to be followed for pensions.)

Fifth, the Managed Competition Act was justly subject to the criticism over its proposal to subsidize coverage for people between 100 and 200 percent of the poverty level, based on a sliding scale with income, implying a very high marginal income tax rate such as 35 percent. When combined with income taxes, payroll taxes, Earned Income Tax Credit phase-out, and phase-out of other benefits, this would lead to a prohibitive marginal tax rate on reported income and a powerful reporting or working disincentive. With the universal tax credit, the benefit reduction rate would not have to be so high. If health cost reduction brought family coverage down from $5,000 to $4,000 (in today's prices, which seems entirely feasible in view of California's experience) if the universal voucher were $2,000 for a family of four, then perhaps a $2,000 subsidy for the near poor would be phased out over $15,000 of income, for a benefit reduction rate of 13.3 percent. Therefore, the next step might be to revisit the sliding-scale subsidies in the Cooper and Chafee bills as a way of providing coverage for the near poor.

Sixth, if the above does not get the job done, the next step to consider might be an "individual-employer" mandate: In lieu of an increase in the minimum wage, a law should be passed that requires employers and employees to segregate 50 cents an hour of the total compensation package and put it into an employee account to be usable only for the purchase of qualified health insurance coverage. If the employee does not use it, the money would be paid to the local government as a contribution to the safety net. Thus, it would be a "free rider" tax. This should be much less objectionable to employers than the open-ended mandate in the Clinton proposal. It would not have the political appeal of a proposal to "make the employer pay for it," but it would have the advantage of honesty. Fifty cents an hour would be approximately $1,000 per year for a fully employed person. Combine that with a $500 tax credit and one has a powerful incentive to buy coverage. Employers would be required to offer or broker coverage, though not necessarily "pay for it," other than the 50 cents per hour. Small employers could do this by joining a HIPC.

Some will object that such a mandate is a tax. Of course, it is a tax. It is a tax on people who generate a negative externally (i.e., who act irresponsibly and take a free ride on the safety net). Others will object that this is a tax on those least able to pay. I point out that the "credit for exclusion" trade already redistributes a substantial amount of income. It would redistribute even more if it were supplemented by additional vouchers for the poor.

Seventh, combined with the finite mandate should be special programs for special populations such as college and university students, a group with many uninsured. Stanford University has mandated coverage for its students—either through a policy purchased through the university or by proof of coverage through parents. Government could offer special incentives for managed care companies to develop special-purpose products if the market does not, and to colleges and universities to mandate and market some coverage.

Finally, there always will be a requirement for publicly supported direct care systems to act as a safety net. There will always be people whose lifestyles or conditions do not fit well with signing up for a health plan and paying premiums. As it is today and has been traditionally in the past, this is a good role for academic health centers. The burden on government to support the public direct care system could be made much smaller by the policies I have outlined here.

Notes

1. The Clinton plan was a "single payer in Jackson Hole clothing." See Enthoven and Singer (1994).
2. Foundation for Accountability, 220 NW Second Avenue, Suite 725, Portland, OR 97209.

References

Ellwood, P. M., A. C. Enthoven, and L. Etheredge. 1992. "The Jackson Hole Initiatives for a Twenty-First Century American Health Care System." *Health Economics* 1 (3): 149–68.

Enthoven, A. C. 1978. "Consumer Health Plan." *New England Journal of Medicine* 298 (12) and (13): 650–58 and 709–20.

———. 1979. "Consumer-Centered vs. Job-Centered Health Insurance." *Harvard Business Review* 57 (1): 141–52.

Enthoven, A. C., and R. Kronick. 1989. "A Consumer-Choice Health Plan for the 1990s." *New England Journal of Medicine* 320 (1) and (2): 29–37, 94–101.

Enthoven, A. C., and S. J. Singer. 1994. "A Single Payer in Jackson Hole Clothing." *Health Affairs.* 12 (1) (Special Issue) 81–95.

———. 1996. "Managed Competition and California's Health Care Economy." *Health Affairs* 15 (1): 39–57.

Gore, A. 1993. "Creating a Government that Works Better and Costs Less." In *The Report of the National Performance Review.* New York: Plume, Penguin.

Hoechst Marion Roussel, Inc. 1995. *Managed Care Digest.* Indianapolis, IN: Hoechst Marion Roussel, Inc.

Weller, C. D. 1984. "'Free Choice' as a Restraint of Trade in American Health Care Delivery and Insurance." *Iowa Law Review* 69 (5): 1351–91.

19

Employer-Based Health Insurance: R.I.P.

Uwe E. Reinhardt

Introduction

As other chapters in this volume report, the number of Americans caught at any time without any health insurance whatsoever has been growing steadily over the past decade. The best current conjecture is that the number is likely to grow steadily in the coming decade.

At this time approximately 40 million Americans report to be without health insurance, among them are approximately 10 million children. Less well known is the fact that just as many Americans appear to be "underinsured," although the definition of that category is necessarily subjective. To be underinsured means that gaps in coverage leave an insured family exposed to a significant risk of losing a large fraction of its income to illness. In fact, as Moon (1996, 11) has shown, underinsurance afflicts even millions of elderly Americans with Medicare coverage. According to Moon's estimates, close to seven million elderly Americans with incomes at 125 percent of the poverty level or below currently must devote an average of between 27 to 33 percent of their meager incomes on out-of-pocket spending for healthcare, including insurance premiums for Part B of Medicare and Medigap policies.

This lack of insurance coverage is a uniquely American phenomenon. In no other country in the industrialized world can illness visit nearly as much economic hardship on individual families as it can in the United States. In no other industrialized country are there millions of uninsured citizens who literally turn into healthcare beggars when serious illness strikes (Fragin 1997). Unpaid medical bills are a major source of personal bankruptcy in the United States and appear to vary, across states, with the percentage of uninsured families (see Bleakley 1996). Given the comprehensive, universal health insurance coverage in other nations, that phenomenon would have to be a rare occurrence there. Finally, in no other country is there the hand wringing and finger pointing among sectors of the healthcare industry over who does and does not carry a "fair" share of the economic burden that is posed by the nation's uninsured. That issue simply cannot arise in other countries.

The phenomenon of the uninsured and underinsured, of course, would not be considered a social problem in the first place if Americans deemed it acceptable to ration healthcare strictly by price and ability to pay, as are many other ordinary goods and services. However, survey after survey suggests that, like citizens in other industrialized countries, the American public tends to view healthcare as a social good that should be made available to all who need it, without regard to the recipient's ability to pay for that care (see, for example, Taylor and Reinhardt 1991). Rare would be the politician or corporate executive who would have the temerity to propose openly that, say, preventive healthcare services for American children should be rationed by the ability and willingness of their parents to pay for such care, even though tacitly this country has countenanced that very regimen for decades.

Given this widespread *professed* sentiment for the socialization of the cost of healthcare, it can be asked, and it should be asked, why the structure of the American health system does not reflect that sentiment, why the problem of the uninsured has been so chronic in the American healthcare system. The answer is that the majority of American families have been adequately and often quite generously covered by employment-based private health insurance coverage, and that elderly Americans and millions of low-income, younger Americans have been covered by Medicare, Medicaid, and other government programs. Finally, the uninsured, most of whom are healthy most of the time, so far have been able to receive critically needed healthcare on a charity basis, although that approach does cast them into the undignified role of healthcare beggars just at a time when efforts should be made by society to shore up a person's dignity.

As a national health insurance system, this mosaic always has had several shortcomings that are becoming more pronounced at this time. First, the system perennially exposes American families to the financial risk of illness, because job-based insurance is lost with the job. Second, the system is extraordinarily expensive in terms of the slice of the gross national product that the rest of society must cede to the providers of healthcare. Third, both the employment-based health insurance system and the informal insurance system represented by charity care show signs of erosion, which may expose many more million American families in the future to financial ruin through illness.

At this time, policymakers face a fundamental question: Should public policy be used to shore up the eroding employment-based system and the informal system of charity care—either through mandates, tax preferences, or targeted public subsidies—or should these two systems be left to wither on the vine, so to speak, while public policy concentrates on their gradual replacement with alternative and possibly superior models of health insurance. This chapter argues for the second approach on the grounds that the many drawbacks of the employment-based health insurance system outweigh its many accomplishments. Chief among these drawbacks is that the job-based system is inherently fickle and, thus, inadvertently cruel. A second major drawback is that the system relies for its existence on an inefficient and regressive tax preference. Third, the job-based system traditionally has been one of the major cost drivers in American healthcare. Although currently employers do appear to have better control over the cost of the system, there is no guarantee that they will be able to do so in the future. On the contrary, there is evidence that they may not be able to do so (Thorpe 1997).

This chapter is organized as follows: The second section immediately following offers the thesis that the plight of the uninsured is tolerated by Americans not because Americans are unusually callous toward the poor, but in part because the American health system has priced kindness out of the nation's soul. The third section then turns to the factors that have caused the price of kindness to escalate so much in the United States. I argue that government is a culprit in this process, but that it is by no means the only culprit and probably not even the chief one. That honor goes to the private, employer-based health insurance system. The merits and shortcomings of that system are explored at some length in the fourth section, mainly to make the case that we ought not to deplore the gradual erosion of employer-provided health insurance and should instead explore alternatives that are more defensible on both ethical and economic grounds. By the same token, it is not clear that we should mourn the gradual collapse of the informal, rickety insurance system that the nation's hospitals have offered critically ill, low-income, uninsured Americans by means of charity care whose cost is shifted to paying patients. That informal, catastrophic insurance system is merely a bandaid over this festering social problem and thereby has shielded the conscience of policymakers from the problem. That bandaid may be ripped off by the tide of health reform that is now sweeping the country. In the final section of the chapter I suggest one of many alternative policy responses to that contingency and to the possible demise of employer-based health insurance.

Pricing Kindness out of a Nation's Soul

In a modern society, the basic human needs of its less fortunate members cannot be met solely by kind acts that are rendered, one on one, by the donor to the recipient. For the most part, the donors must purchase kind acts from the commercial sector, either through the offices of privately funded and administered not-for-profit organizations or, more commonly, through the offices of government. There is solid empirical evidence that the fundamental law of demand applies here as it does for anything else people demand: The potential donors' demand for charitable acts that are to be bestowed on less fortunate members of society is related inversely to the cost of these kind acts to the donor (Schwartz 1970; Clotfelter 1983; Slemrod 1988). That is precisely why legislators the world over seek to encourage the financing of charitable acts by making such donations tax deductible to the donors.

Figure 19.1 illustrates this phenomenon graphically. Modeled in the figure are two hypothetical countries that are assumed to be alike in every relevant respect but one. By assumption, the demand for kind acts in the two countries is identical, but at any volume of kind acts that the more fortunate citizens would purchase for their less fortunate fellow citizens, the supply price of kind acts in country "A" is much higher than that in country "B." If a survey research team sought to plumb the nation's soul by probing public attitudes toward charity in the two countries, the teams might not detect any discernible cross-national difference in the distributive ethic that respondents in the two countries would like to see imposed on their respective health systems—that is, in fact, what one tends to find in such surveys (Taylor and Reinhardt 1991). On the other hand, research teams that observed the number of kind acts actually purchased in the two countries and bestowed on the poor would discern a sizable difference in charitable activity. On that criterion, the citizens of country "B" would appear much kinder and gentler than would the citizens of country "A," as would be inferred by the different kind act utilization rates on the horizontal axis of Figure 19.1. There is no paradox here, for between professed noble sentiments and actual noble acts stands a powerful intervening variable: the price

Figure 19.1 The Demand for and Supply of Kind Acts, Country "A"
and Country "B"

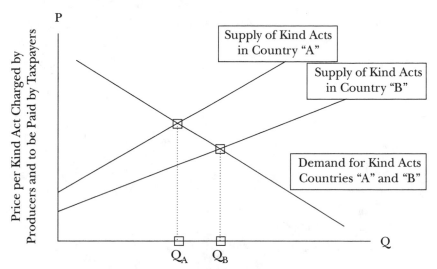

Number of Kind Acts Taxpayers Wish to Purchase
on Behalf of Less Fortunate Fellow Citizens and
Number of Kind Acts Producers of These Acts Will Supply

of noble acts. That price can create a deep gulf between what we say and
what we do.

Can anyone doubt that the United States approximates country "A"
in Figure 19.1 and the rest of the industrialized world country "B"? If
so, Figures 19.2 and 19.3 might put these doubts to rest. Figure 19.2
indicates the most recent, available, comparable data on per capita
health spending in selected countries of the Organisation for Economic
Co-operation and Development (OECD). To be sure, differences in per
capita income alone can explain close to 80 percent of the cross-national
differences in per capita health spending. But in 1993 the United States
spent more than $1,000 on healthcare per capita than can be explained
by its higher per capita income. That higher spending occurred in spite
of the fact that the population of the United States is much younger
than are the populations of most other countries in the OECD. Only
approximately 12.5 percent of the American population was over the
age of 65 in 1993. The comparable numbers for Europe fall between
14 and 16 percent, a percentage the United States will attain only after

Figure 19.2 Per Capita Health Spending and per Capita Gross
Domestic Product, 1993 (U.S. Dollars, PPA Adjusted)

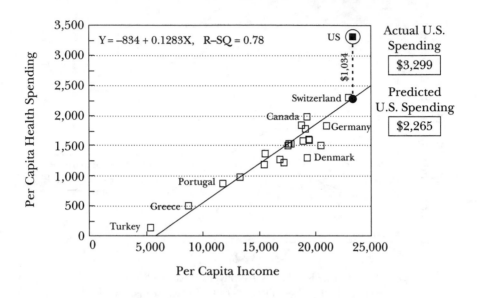

Source: Data furnished by Organisation for Economic Co-operation and Development.

the year 2015 when the baby boom generation retires (see Figure 19.3).
It is known that the higher health spending in the United States does
not result in superior measurable health status indicators. Indeed, on
measures such as infant mortality the United States actually fares rather
poorly (Schieber, Pouillier, and Greenwald 1994). This circumstance
raises the question as to what *real* benefits Americans actually buy with
their higher *monetary* outlays on healthcare.

A recent, large research project undertaken by McKinsey & Co.,
under the tutelage of an advisory board of highly distinguished academic economists and clinicians, sought to discover the sources of these
cross-national differences in real per capita health spending. The team
explored health spending in 1990 in the United States, the United King-
dom, and [then] West Germany. After all relevant adjustments that could
be made, the team concluded that, in 1990, German patients actually
used $390 more of real medical inputs (physician visits, hospital days,
pharmaceutical products, and so on) per capita than did Americans,
a finding the team interpreted as lower productivity in Germany. On

Figure 19.3 Percentage of Population over Age 65, 1993

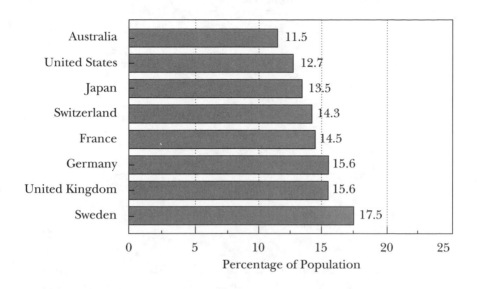

Source: Organisation for Economic Co-operation and Development (1996).

the other hand, Americans were found to spend $360 more per capita on "administrative costs" than did Germans. Americans also spent $257 more per capita on "other inputs." These two items alone wiped out any cost advantage Americans registered relative to the Germans because of the more sparing use Americans make of real medical inputs. These cost differences, it must be noted, were calculated by assigning to the real medical inputs used in the two countries the identical money prices. In fact, Americans paid the providers of these real inputs an average of 40 percent more money per unit of real resources than did the Germans. Overall, Americans spent approximately $1,000 more per capita on healthcare than did the Germans in that year.

Figure 19.4, taken directly from the report, illustrates these remarkable findings graphically. These data are perfectly compatible with the hypothesis embodied in Figure 19.1, as are a number of other cross-national studies on the use of real resources per capita that found other nationals to use more *real* healthcare resources per capita than do Americans, although they transferred less money per real resource to providers and spent, according to some studies, less on administrative costs (Fuchs and Hahn 1990; Pauly 1995; Welch et al. 1996).

Figure 19.4 Sources of Difference in Healthcare Spending (U.S.
            Dollars per Capita, 1990, PPP)

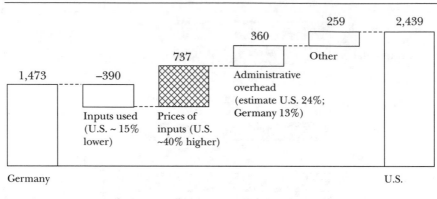

Source: McKinsey & Co. 1996.

If one accepts the hypothesis that it is not necessarily callousness
among the American people that leads them to tolerate considerable
social pathos in the midst of an otherwise superb healthcare delivery
system, the question arises as to why the cost of healthcare is so high
in the United States. The commonplace explanation, recited time and
again in the debate on American health policy, is that government is the
chief culprit, that government has driven up both the money prices of
health services and their use rates. That facile explanation, however, is
at best a half truth. A closer look at history and the data suggests that the
private sector has been just as much a cost driver in American healthcare
and may even have been the chief culprit. It has been so by virtue of
this country's unwieldy employer-based health insurance system, which,
throughout the post–World War II period and until the early 1990s,
had set for the entire American health system the extraordinarily high
standards for healthcare prices that government had no choice but to
follow. In the process, although surely inadvertently, the employer-based
health insurance system has been instrumental in pricing kindness out
of America's soul.

Because that proposition is controversial, it is explicated more fully
in the next two sections.

Government as a Cost Driver in Healthcare

When the Medicare and Medicaid programs were legislated in the mid-
1960s, after decades of legislative struggle, these two programs were

initially thought of as mere appendages to the general, private health system. As such, they were expected to adapt themselves to the standards set by the private sector. To thoughtful persons it must have been clear from the outset, however, that the two programs would quickly take on a life of their own, mainly by virtue of their sheer size. For many medical interventions used mainly by elderly people (e.g., cataract surgery, hip replacements, heart surgery), Medicare quickly became the single most important buyer.

While prices and spending under Medicaid for the poor and disabled were controlled by varying mechanisms and to varying degrees of success by the states, the federal Medicare program experienced very rapid cost growth during its early years. That cost growth, however, was not a completely unanticipated consequence. It was the price that Congress and the designers of the Medicare program had to pay to gain the acquiescence of the politically powerful providers of healthcare who had reason to fear the monopsony (single-buyer) market power that usually is created with tax-financed, government-run health insurance programs. That compromise with providers in 1965 put a stiff price on kind acts in America for the ensuing two decades. Remnants of that compromise linger to this day, mainly in Medicare's payment for skilled nursing facilities and especially for home care, where noble sentiments turn out to be particularly expensive at this time.

The payment system that was put in place in 1965 was inherently inflationary. Every hospital in America was to be reimbursed by Medicare, retrospectively and individually, for the full cost that hospitals reported to have incurred in the care of the Medicare beneficiaries. For investor-owned hospitals, this arrangement became a pure cost-plus pricing scheme, with a generous guaranteed profit margin under which such a hospital literally could not lose. Every physician, on the other hand, was to be paid their "usual, customary and reasonable" fee for each codified service on a list of some 7,000 distinct items. A particular physician's "usual" fee for a particular service was the median of the frequency distribution of the fees that this particular physician had billed in the previous year for that particular service. It was one of two price ceilings that Medicare imposed on physicians in the following year, although the physician was free to charge more and thereby push up their "usual fee" standard for the following year. A particular physician's "usual fee" for a particular service was judged "reasonable" if it did not exceed the 75th percentile of the frequency distribution of the fees for that particular service charged by all physicians in the physician's market area. This unwieldy payment system, of course, forced every item on every bill submitted by every individual physician to a particular patient through two price-ceiling filters: first, the filter to determine whether the actual fee billed was equal to or less than that physician's usual fee and, second, the filter to determine whether that physician's usual (median) fee for that service was "reasonable" (did not exceed the 75th percentile of fees in the area during the previous year). The entire system was administered through more than 130 private insurance carriers coordinated in their efforts by a rather small staff of federal Medicare bureaucrats. Not surprisingly, each carrier soon developed its own rules for claims processing, including their own definition of many codes. Variations in coding practice made it difficult to compare physician fees across regions.

It would tax the imagination to think of a payment system that would be more unwieldy, more impenetrable to analysis and control, and more inherently inflationary than the system that was imposed in 1965 on the noble gesture called "Medicare." No one should have been surprised that the cost of such a system would soon be out of control. But it was also not surprising that, even as in 1970, Congress began a long drawn out, valiant struggle to rein in this inflationary system. By the mid-1970s, the standard of "reasonableness" for physician fees was put under a ceiling that was determined by a national medical practice cost index. At the same time, extensive research was funded by Medicare to shift the payment of hospitals from the uncontrollable, retrospective basis to a prospective one, and research was also begun to develop a common, national relative value scale on which Medicare could base a common fees schedule for physicians.

By the mid-1980s the shift to prospective payment of hospitals was fully under way. It was completed by 1987. That highly innovative compensation method—a system of flat fees for each of some 5,000 diagnostically related groups of cases—has since been copied elsewhere in the world. Furthermore, by the early 1990s, Medicare had placed physicians on a uniform fee schedule that was based on carefully re-searched relative costs for at least the physician component of costs. That fee schedule, too, now serves not only Medicare, but is also widely used by private insurance carriers in the United States in their negotiations with physicians.

Figures 19.5 and 19.6 illustrate the fruits of Medicare's cost-containment methods. These figures show that, during the period from 1980 to about 1992, real per capita spending by Medicare actually increased much *less* rapidly than did spending per capita in the private sector. Indeed, Medicare's main problem in the 1980s was the rampant price inflation in healthcare that was tolerated by private insurance carriers.

Figure 19.5 Trends in per Enrollee Expenditures for Medicare and Private Health Insurance and Gross Domestic Product per Capita, 1980–93

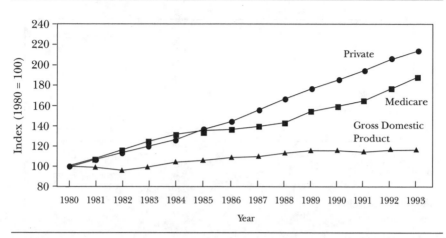

Source: Physician Payment Review Commission analysis of information compiled from the Health Care Financing Administraiton and the Congressional Budget Office.
Note: Values are adjusted for inflation and are expressed in 1980 dollars.

So effective had Medicare become in controlling its costs that private insurance carriers and business executives wailed loudly about a "cost shift" from Medicare into their budgets—that Medicare was not shouldering its "fair share" of hospital costs (Schramm 1994). Even as late as the mid-1990s, the fees paid physicians by Medicare were only approximately 65 percent of the average comparable fees paid physicians by private insurance carriers (Physician Payment Review Commission 1996). Similarly, while Medicare tried to rein in the vast excess capacity of the hospital sector by paying hospitals less than the full cost of hospital care, that excess capacity was maintained easily with the aid of the enormous profit margins private insurance carriers were content to pay hospitals throughout the 1980s and, it would appear, to this day (see Figure 19.6).

It has been only since about 1993 that the private sector, by then truly desperate over the high double-digit increase in private health insurance premiums, has set to work in earnest on cost control. In that endeavor, private employers were helped greatly by the general economic recession of 1988–92 and the fear of job loss triggered by corporate reengineering and downsizing. That fear enabled private employers to shift their employees from their hitherto open-ended,

Figure 19.6 Hospital Payment Cost Ratios, 1980–93, Medicare, Medicaid, and Private Payors

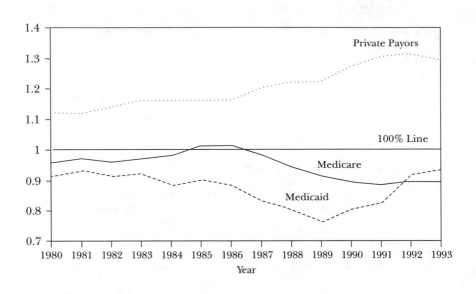

Source: Prospective Payment Assessment Commission (1995, Table 1-8).

free-choice indemnity insurance policies into health plans that limit the insured's choice of healthcare provider at time of illness. Once employees were willing to acquiesce in that limitation, it was possible for health insurance plans to contract selectively with doctors and hospitals. Selective contracting, in turn, meant effectively that a particular hospital or physician could literally be "fired" from a health plan, either because that provider did not grant the plan adequate discounts from regular fees or because that provider's statistical practice profile was deemed too service intensive and therefore too expensive. That shift of market power from the supply to the demand side, of course, can easily be diluted and reversed by the current trend among health plans to widen the network of providers with whom they contract and to offer enrollees so-called "point-of-service" riders that permit easy access to providers outside the health plan's contracted network. That weakening in market power manifests itself in the recent increases, once again, in employer-paid health insurance premiums (Thorpe 1997).

The turmoil surrounding the health reform debate during 1992–94 and the political stand-off between the Clinton administration and

Congress since 1994 has left the Medicare program unattended except through whatever regulatory cost control measures Medicare was already authorized to pursue. Left adrift, the program by now has fallen behind the private sector in its ability to control the growth of its overall spending and will stay behind for a few years to come. There is no reason to assume, however, that this state of inaction will remain permanent. On the contrary, it is possible that government in the future will be able to enlist the power of the managed care industry far more effectively—and with greater attention to the requirements of true *managed competition* among health plans—than private employers have been able to do so far.

In short, the often stated maxim that throughout the past decades government has been the chief culprit behind the rising cost of health-care is not supported by the data, unless one wishes to argue that much money could have been saved simply by rationing the nation's poor and elderly out of health services altogether—by leaving them to their own fate and budgets. It is easier to make the case that, for all the many positive contributions private employers have made to American medicine and to the well-being of their employees, private employers actually have been the chief cost drivers in the American health system, at least until very recently.

In fact, it can be argued that the positive contributions that private employers have made to American medicine have been facilitated mainly by the massive, virtually uncontrolled flows of funds private employers have been content to channel to the American health system, dragging in its wake the Medicare and Medicaid programs. As can be inferred from their annual reports, raising fees to keep up with private sector fees and refraining from other forms, cost controls have always been an *explicit* policy guide for the Prospective Payment Assessment Commission and the Physician Payment Review Commission that jointly advise Congress on the payment of healthcare providers under Medicare.

Employer-Based Health Insurance: Merits and Shortcomings

Approximately 65 percent of Americans under age 65 obtain health insurance coverage through employer health plans as workers, dependents, or retirees (*Medical Benefits* 1996). However, total payments by all private health insurance, including individually purchased policies, currently account for only approximately one-third of all national health spending in the United States (Levit, Lazenby, and Sivarajan 1996). The rest is paid by various government programs (approximately 43 percent) and with out-of-pocket spending by patients at the time healthcare is received.

The engagement of private employers in the financing of healthcare is not uniquely American. On the contrary, most countries find it expedient to siphon off the contributions for their social insurance systems at the nexus of the payroll, mainly because compliance at that nexus is very high. The role of private employers in those systems, however, is relatively passive. Aside from programming the requisite codes into their payroll accounting routines and periodically sending checks to the health insurance funds, private employers tend to have representatives on the governing boards of these funds. As a general rule, however, they do not intrude into the employee's choice among insurance funds—to the extent that employees have that choice—let alone into the active management of their employees' healthcare and health. Such activities would be considered inappropriate intrusions into the employees' private lives. This form of intrusion is the very staple of employer-based health insurance in the United States, where employee benefit managers and their outside consultants see it as their mandate to help manage their employees' private lives. Curiously, American employees have always tolerated this intrusion into their lives, even at the risk of losing their privacy (Schultz 1994).

It is doubtful that anyone setting out to design a nation's health insurance system from scratch would ever stumble on the idea of delegating to private employers the task of procuring health insurance outright for their employees and, with it, the task of managing outright the employees' healthcare and even their health. The practice has its origin in World War II, in a classic maneuver by private business firms to evade the price and wage controls then imposed on that sector by government. Presumably these controls were based on the ethical premise that, if millions of American draftees were asked literally to walk into live gun fire in exchange for only meager, government-set wages, it was only fair that the folks who made the ammunition not be allowed to profit unduly from the resulting shortage of labor at home. In an attempt to walk around these wage controls, private employers then seized on the idea of bidding for scarce labor with newly established fringe benefits, which, curiously, were not considered by the law to be under the wage caps. To this dubious evasion of war-time wage controls go the roots of employment-based health insurance in the United States.

In subsequent years, this particular form of healthcare financing grew by leaps and bounds, mainly because employers and organized labor had extracted from the government a much cherished tax loophole that gave employers powerful leverage in the market for health insurance. Although employers could treat the procurement of health insurance for employees as a normal, tax-deductible payroll expense, these outlays were not added to the taxable income of employees. On grounds that could never be defended with an appeal to either fairness or economics and that literally defy logic, self-employed Americans or those purchasing health insurance on their own were never accorded this complete tax shelter.

Employer-Based Health Insurance and Social Equity

Those who favor the socialization of the financial burden of illness, spreading responsibility over larger groups—the present author included—must acknowledge the salutary contribution private employers have made toward that goal. Typically, employers procure health insurance for their employees by means of group policies whose premiums are "experience rated" or "priced actuarially fairly" *for the entire firm,* which means that they reflect the *total* expected cost of procuring healthcare for all of the firm's employees. As argued below, economists believe that the great bulk of these premiums are shifted backwards to the employees in the form of lower take-home pay. However, usually only the *average* premium per employee is shifted backwards to the individual paycheck. Relatively more sickly employees performing the same job as relatively healthier employees do not receive commensurately lower take-home pay—at least not yet. It follows that from the perspective of individual employees the typical group health insurance policy procured by American employers is "community rated" within the firm. Because the arrangement forces a redistribution of income from relatively healthy to relatively sick employees, one may view them as miniature socialized health insurance systems.

Although advocates of socialized health insurance should applaud this salutary effect of employer-based health insurance, the premiums it implicitly imposes on individual employees must be judged regressive, because they are akin to a fixed head tax on each employee, regardless of the individual employee's income. Low-wage employees therefore contribute a much higher *fraction* of their gross wages to their employer's socialized health insurance system than do high-income employees. By contrast, the social insurance systems in continental Europe, Asia, and Latin America tend to levy premiums as a constant percentage of the individual employee's gross wages.

The regressivity of the American approach is amplified further by the dubious tax preference granted employer-provided health insurance. In absolute dollars, the tax shelter bestows much greater benefits on high-income employees facing high marginal tax rates than it does on low-income employees facing low marginal tax rates (Butler 1995). Oddly enough, this built-in regressivity of the tax preference never seems to have troubled the leaders of organized labor, nor the usually progressive champions of labor in academia, in the media, and in politics.

The employer-based health insurance system, American style, also has an inherent tendency to foster discrimination in the labor market against the chronically ill. The lower the number of employees in a firm, the more problematic will be the implicit community rating of health insurance contributions over the small "community" within the firm, because the more visible will be the cost push that a very sick employee— for example, one with AIDS or cancer—can exert on the employer's average insurance premiums. Indeed, the delicate managerial issues raised by that circumstance could explain in part the reluctance among small enterprises to offer their employees health insurance. It probably is a contributor to the overall number of uninsured in this country.

Employer-Based Health Insurance and the Problem of Not Having Insurance

From the viewpoint of the family, probably the most serious drawback of employer-based health insurance is that the protection is tied to one particular job and is lost with that job. That turns out to be a major reason for the lack of insurance among chronically ill Americans who may be unemployed because they are ill. Short of their spending down to outright poverty, when they might become eligible for Medicaid, these chronically ill persons are literally left on their own in the United States. The very thought would be anathema to other nations.

Although legislation that was shepherded through Congress in 1996 by Senators Kassebaum and Kennedy makes employer-provided group health insurance more portable between jobs and during self-employment or unemployment, the premiums charged under the mandated guaranteed issue of insurance can be "actuarially fairly" priced, which therefore moves insurance out of the reach of families beset by serious existing medical conditions. Quite aside from the perennial insecurity that such a dire prospect visits on every employed person who currently has insurance, the prospect naturally contributes to immobility in the labor market through "job lock," that is, staying in a job solely for the benefit of having health insurance. That job lock would not be present under fully portable health insurance. One econometric study has shown, for example, that far from reducing overall employment in the private sector, the introduction of fully portable national health insurance in Canada during the 1970s actually appears to have *increased* overall employment levels in Canada, presumably (according to the authors), through the greater labor mobility that the policy created (Gruber and Hanratty 1995).

The lack of portability that is inherent in the American employer-based health insurance system is so severe a flaw that probably no other country would ever contemplate copying that approach. Indeed, it is hard to imagine that any American policy analyst would ever contemplate it for the United States, were that system not already in place. The flaw was visited on the United States by sheer historical accident. It is one for which American families pay dearly in terms of perennial anxiety and, from time to time, in terms of real physical hardship. It is a truly ugly facet of our employment-based health system.

Employer-Based Health Insurance and the Problem of Underinsurance

During the first two to three decades following World War II, the American economy reigned unchallenged in the world. In that secure environment, many American employers and their workers had persuaded themselves that private companies could provide American families with reliable social insurance, under employer-sponsored "defined-benefit" plans that cover both pensions and healthcare. Retiree health benefits were often promised during negotiations over total compensation as a substitute for cash wages.

Consequently, millions of retired workers now look to their former employers as a complement to the Medicare program, which, in spite of its enormous outlays, nevertheless covers less than half of the average annual healthcare cost of the elderly (Health Care Financing Administration 1995). Although Medicaid and other public sources pay for approximately another 18 percent, approximately 37 percent of total health spending by the elderly is covered by private sources. Among these private sources are out-of-pocket payments by beneficiaries themselves, private insurance purchase directly by the elderly themselves, and, for many of the elderly, supplemental insurance coverage provided by their erstwhile employer. As noted, this entire arrangement sill leaves many low-income elderly exposed to very high burdens of out-of-pocket health spending (Moon 1996).

To the extent that private business firms will find themselves unable in the future to own up to the expensive promises that they have made to their employees, their possible withdrawal of that support could contribute significantly to the problem of underinsurance in America and to genuine social pathos. Given the pressure on corporations to produce increased earnings in a globally competitive market, that prospect is very real. It is made all the more likely by Statement No. 106 of the Financial Accounting Standards Board (FASB) that, effective in 1992, forced employers at long last to account honestly for these promises in their financial reports to shareholders.

Until the early 1990s, private employers did not have to recognize on their income statements or on their balance sheets the liability that is incurred in a given year when workers are promised future health benefits in retirement. This huge gap in the Generally Accepted Accounting Principles that govern business accounting in the United States, literally allowed corporations to pay their workers partially with funny money. For decades, the managers of these private corporations kept the ever mounting liability that was incurred in this way perfectly secret from their shareholders and from the investing community. Naturally, they also did not then, and even do not now, have set-aside funds for the future day when these promises will have to be honored. Only in 1992, when FASB-106 forced private employers to recognize on their income statements the expense of these promises *when they are made*, and to show the associated cumulative liability openly on their balance sheets, did the world learn of the staggering mortgages past management had written stealthily, year after year, on the future cash flows and net worth of their enterprises.

General Motors furnishes a dramatic illustration of this stealth approach to health insurance. Between 1991 and 1992, in one year, the net worth of General Motors shrank by $21 billion, from $27 billion to approximately $6 billion, as that firm was finally forced by FASB-106 to report to shareholders the cumulative pre-tax tax liability of $33 billion that it had incurred through promised retiree health benefits (General Motors 1992). More ominously, in the footnotes of its annual report the firm announced that, while being forced to put this liability on the balance sheet, General Motors' compliance with that new rule did not amount to an acknowledgment on the firm's part of any *legal* liability actually to own up to the promises it had made earlier to its current and former workers (General Motors 1993). To appreciate the temptation that future managers of General Motors will face to welsh on these promises, one need only imagine how many automobiles the company would have to sell to cover a pre-tax liability of $33 billion. Although General Motors' predicament in this respect is dramatic, many other companies with large, aging work forces face similarly burdensome and hitherto unacknowledged liabilities for promised retiree health benefits.

It is remarkable that Americans have been content for so long to anchor an important part of their families' financial security in particular firms whose financial strength is contingent on the managerial acumen of a handful of future managers, whose very existence can be threatened by the vagaries of the dynamic global market, whose management can change its ethical precepts over time with changing circumstances, and who can at any time marshall the legal prowess to break promises made to employees decades earlier. In no other industrialized nation is the economic security of citizens during retirement that closely tied to the economic fortunes of a particular business enterprise and to the personal integrity of the few managers who control that enterprise. Workers should worry how long this brittle, private social security system can survive in the global market economy of the late twentieth and the early twenty-first centuries. Sooner or later, the public sector may well have to step into the breach to assume some of the mortgages that were recklessly and stealthily written years ago by private employers.

Employer-Paid Health Insurance and Healthcare Costs

The ultimate incidence of the cost of employer-provided health insurance is not well understood outside the economics profession. It may be one reason why labor and its champions always have so staunchly defended that peculiar form of healthcare financing and, in particular, the inefficient and regressive tax preference on which it rests.

Although the private organizations for whom employees work may write checks to cover taxes and other costs (including the cost of fringe benefits bestowed on employees), the organizations themselves ultimately cannot absorb any costs, because they are not human beings. They are merely legal constructs surrounded by three groups of human beings: the organization's clientele, its employees, and its owners. Few people seem to ponder from whom business actually recovers outlays that it makes voluntarily or is forced to make on behalf of its employees. For example, many otherwise intelligent commentators seem sincerely to believe that "fat-cat corporations" do not bear their fair share of the nation's tax burden. Anyone who sincerely believes that "fat-cat corporations" should pay higher taxes probably also believes that the premiums for health insurance purchased by employers for their employees are absorbed by "the company" and probably believes in many other comforting fairy tales of this sort.

How an organization recoups its costs from its clients, employees, or owners depends on these groups' relative sensitivity to such cost shifts (Krueger and Reinhardt 1994). The suppliers of equity capital have numerous alternatives worldwide to deploy their funds and therefore are able to resist attempted backward shifts of the cost of fringe benefits into lower returns to capital. Similarly, in a highly price-competitive global market, the demand for the output produced by American employers typically tends to be relatively price sensitive. Empirical research suggests, however, that the supply of labor to the labor market tends to be relatively insensitive to take-home wages and salaries (Gruber and Krueger 1991). Not surprisingly, then, empirical research on the ultimate incidence of employer-paid fringe benefits strongly suggests that, in the longer run, most or all of the premium for employer-financed health insurance is, indeed, shifted backward to the employees in the form of lower take-home pay (Krueger and Reinhardt 1994). This means that these premiums should be viewed as merely one part of total labor compensation, which is the "price" of labor that is determined jointly by employers and employees in the labor market. As the Congressional Budget Office (1992) has observed on this point:

> Although employers initially pay a significant portion of employer-provided health insurance, in the long run employers shift most of the cost to workers in the form of lower wages or less generous nonmedical benefits.

Ignorance among the rank and file of the ultimate incidence of employer-paid health insurance premiums may well explain the traditionally high tolerance among workers for premium increases in the private sector—increases that reached the high double digits in the later 1980s and far outranked increases in per enrollee spending under the public health insurance programs. Management and the leaders of unions probably did understand that the bulk of those premiums eventually would be shifted backwards to employees in the form of lower wages (see, for example, a remark by Douglas Fraser [1989], past president of the United Auto Workers in the *New York Times*). The rank and file, on the other hand, appear sincerely to have believed that this cost was borne by someone else—by the "company." Either party to the deal therefore deemed healthcare cost control to be the other party's problem. The result was an expensive *pas de deux* that came to an end—or at least a temporary halt—only when the huge bite that these premiums took out of the employees' take-home pay became simply too large to ignore, even by the rank and file.

In the meantime, however, this expensive *pas de deux* undoubtedly helped drive up the cost not only of employer-based health insurance, but of all government-run health insurance programs as well—in the manner suggested above. The rising cost of government programs, in turn, made policymakers and the general public ever more reluctant to embrace further expansions of government-financed insurance for the uninsured—even for children! Through this dynamic employer-based health insurance in the United States, it has helped price kindness out of America's otherwise kind soul, however unwittingly (Reinhardt 1993a).

Employer-based health insurance, of course, helped drive up not only the money prices paid for particular health services in the United States. It also is the source of much of the high administrative overhead that makes American healthcare so expensive—an added cost burden made clearly visible, for example, in the cross-national study by McKinsey & Co. (see Figure 19.4). It is the employer-based insurance system that channels the financing of healthcare into a myriad of capillaries, each with its own rules, forms, and claims-processing bureaucracy that engulfs insurers, providers, and patients alike in a paper war that should belong to an earlier age. As President Bush observed in his health reform proposal presented in 1992, hospitals and physicians were billing the bulk of their claims under Medicare electronically. At the same time, the bulk of private insurance claims were still on paper and remain on paper to this day (White House 1992).

The Future of Employer-Based Health Insurance

There is mounting evidence, some of it reported in other chapters of this volume, that employment-based health insurance coverage has declined in recent years and will be likely to erode further in the future (*Medical Benefits* 1996). Many employers no longer cover certain benefits for dependents; others are phasing out retiree health benefits. And many small business firms do not offer their employees health insurance at all.

A major policy issue at this time is whether the government should shore up the employment-based system, with further tax breaks or targeted subsidies, or whether it should ready the nation for an alternative approach to health insurance, not necessarily a government-run system on the model of Medicare or Medicaid. To think about that question, readers may find it helpful to construct for themselves a traditional "T account," entering on its credit side all of the advantages offered by employer-based health insurance, entering on the debit side all of its shortcomings, and then mentally drawing a balance for the account. In this author's view, that net balance comes up a debit.

On the credit side of the ledger, one must enter the fact that the employer-based health insurance system in this country has provided the bulk of American families with adequate health insurance—most of the time. Until about the early 1990s, that coverage typically had been generous to a fault. It covered all imaginary contingencies, with few questions asked.

On the credit side also one could enter the energy and imagination that the employee-benefit managers in the private sector, and their many consultants, have brought to their task over the decades. That effort has not been to minimize the employer's debits to the payroll account. Typically, employee-benefit managers have sought to enhance the welfare of employees and their families, even if only as long as the employee worked for the firm.

For the most recent period, in particular, one must give these employee-benefit managers credit for their success in breaking the back, at long last, of the premium inflation that employers suffered during much of the 1980s. Although so far the bulk of private employers still remain relatively unsophisticated buyers of healthcare, who offer their employees only a single health plan (48 percent), two plans (23 percent), or three (12 percent), some of the larger employers have recently made major contributions to solving the twin problem of cost and quality in American healthcare (Etheredge, Jones, and Lewin 1996). They have unleashed upon these problems the energy and the ingenuity that resides in both the public and the private sectors of the economy, but that only the private sector can mobilize swiftly, flexibly, and single mindedly. Many useful insights and innovations are likely to spring from these efforts, among them valuable insights on what will not work. One must give private employers credit for these efforts. In principle, one would like them to continue on that path, for if they continue to be successful in their efforts at cost control, private employers may help make affordable again the kindness that these same employers had helped price out of American health policy during the 1970s and 1980s.

Together, these several credits of employment-based health insurance, and other credits that readers may think of, do add up to something of an accomplishment. But the debits of the system deserve far more attention than they have traditionally received. First among these debits is the fragility of employer-based health insurance. The system operates strictly on the "out-of-sight, out-of-mind" principle. All of the efforts that are bestowed by employee-benefit managers on an employee cease the minute that employee is dropped from the firm's payroll. Whatever protection families enjoy beyond that point comes to them courtesy of special government legislation.

A second major drawback of the employer-based system is that it probably can exist only by virtue of an inherently inefficient and highly regressive tax preference. It is this tax preference, rather than a particular genius for purchasing insurance, that has given employers a completely unwarranted comparative advantage in the procurement of health insurance and, with it, a completely unwarranted control over the private lives of their employees. (The resulting lack of personal privacy is a third major drawback [Schultz 1994].) That this tax preference has not traditionally been available to self-employed and unemployed Americans will forever remain a moral stain on the American health system.

A third major shortcoming of the current employer-based system is that it insulates employees from the true cost of healthcare in this country and from knowledge of who actually bears that cost. Usually the thought is that only government programs provide that insulation. They do. But the employer-based system does so as well. Economists are convinced that employees do bear most of the premiums in the form of lower take-home pay. Yet rare and probably nonexistent is the employer who forthrightly tells employees "but for the $400 a month I paid for your and your family's health insurance coverage, your paycheck would be considerably higher."

Finally, as Etheredge, Jones, and Lewin (1996, 93) have pointed out, the search by employers for improved cost and quality control in healthcare is "mostly driven by socially amoral economic forces." It is precisely their ability to engage socially amoral economic forces, and not a special genius for innovation, that allows private employers now to be so innovative in healthcare. Their experiments in health insurance can proceed like tests in a laboratory without safety precautions, or with precautions only for the employees within the laboratory. At any moment, private employers need not and usually do not worry about the welfare of anyone not in their employ at that time (retired workers possibly excepted). Private employers can pursue their cost-containment strategies without any concern over the effect that the price discounts they extract from hospitals and doctors might ultimately have on the informal catastrophic health insurance system that doctors and hospitals traditionally have maintained for the uninsured—particularly for the uninsured and chronically ill. Private employers enjoy the luxury of being able to experiment boldly in healthcare on the assumption that government will sweep up the social pathos such experimentation might inadvertently beget. Employing the ingenuity of private employers in this way may be a productive social policy as long as the government is able and willing to function as that shovel brigade. If not, some unfortunate Americans are likely to be in for a very rough time in the years ahead.

On balance, it can be asked whether a system with so many inherent flaws merits shoring up through public policy—its numerous virtues notwithstanding—or whether it had not best be left to its own slow demise. Some thoughts on that option conclude the present chapter.

Alternatives to Employment-Based Health Insurance

If universal health insurance coverage is a national goal, then a health insurance system seeking to own up to that goal must make it mandatory that every resident in the United States have adequate insurance coverage. The requirement of "adequate coverage" does not imply first-dollar coverage for, except perhaps, the very poorest families. In principle, that coverage should be broad enough to preclude a person literally having to beg for healthcare at the time illness strikes. It should also preclude the practice of healthcare "mooching" practiced by some younger Americans who could, in principle, afford adequate health insurance coverage, but who prefer to use their funds for other goods and services when they are healthy, secure in the knowledge that a kindly nation will give them critically needed care—even expensive care—when they are sick.

Such an insurance system should also be fully vested in the individual and fully portable between jobs and during self-employment and unemployment.

A third desideratum is that such an insurance system should be based on whatever subsidies are needed by low-income families and an honest tax-and-transfer mechanism that holds this transfer up for public accountability. To have integrity, this mechanism should come equipped with an accounting system that can highlight the cost of the system per client served.

Fourth, such an insurance system should not insulate people from knowledge about the cost of healthcare in this country, even in cases where a person does not fully bear that cost with their own resources. At the least, people should know how much they directly and indirectly pay for their own healthcare.

The American health insurance system has never owned up to these minimal requirements of a sensible health insurance system and, as noted, the employer-based system has been one of several reasons for this shortcoming.

Health insurance proposals abound that would meet some or all of the desiderata spelled out above (Danzon et al. 1991; Pauly and Goodman 1995; Butler 1991). Some of them are being proposed in this volume (see, for example, Pauly in this volume). Early in the first Clinton administration, I proposed an alternative to the president's concept. The president's plan was based on a government-mandated reinforcement of employer-based health insurance (Reinhardt 1993b). The alternative that I proposed was one based on a mandate on people having adequate health insurance coverage. Employers would at most help their employees own up to that mandate, if employers wished to do so. A sketch of the plan is as follows.

Under the plan, every individual would have been mandated, subject to penalties, to have health insurance coverage for a basic package of health benefits that would have to be determined by the political process. Initially, that package would not have to be very generous, but it would be adequate to protect even low-income families from unmanageable financial hardship due to illness. Taxpayers would have to demonstrate their insurance status by clipping a copy of their policy to their tax form. In the absence of such a policy, they would be required to include in their tax payment a separate check equal to x percent of their taxable income, specifically for health insurance, with an upper limit on the absolute amount. Persons not filing income taxes would have to be captured elsewhere—ultimately when they contact the health system, but preferably through contact with the relevant state authority (e.g., the state health department).

All of the earmarked taxes collected by the government from individuals would be pooled at the federal level in a health insurance fail-safe fund. That fund could be supplemented through various excise taxes (e.g., taxes on alcohol and tobacco) and, most importantly, through tax funds flowing into it from the gradual abolition of the tax preference now accorded employer-provided health insurance. The ultimate goal would have been to abolish that tax preference altogether. The added billions of taxes from ending this preference alone would have been enough to provide adequate financing for universal health insurance.

The federal government would be a mere collector of the fail-safe funds, but it would not use them to administer a new, huge federal health insurance program, such as Medicare. Instead, these funds would be devolved to the states, on the basis of a capitation payment that would be roughly the same across regions. Each state would issue its uninsured a voucher large enough to offer the uninsured a choice of several health maintenance organizations or other health plans willing to offer enrollees the basic benefit package against the monetary value of the voucher. In some states, this stipulation would have required additional funding of the voucher from state sources. In the plan presented in 1993, the states would have had the option of offering their uninsured, for their voucher, entry into the federal Medicare program or the state's Medicaid program; but that feature would not be necessary for the operation of the plan.

In the absence of sanctions, the fail-safe component of the health insurance system outlined above would, of course, have been subject to adverse risk selection. For example, business firms with relatively older or sicker or lower-wage employees probably would prefer to dump the latter into the federal fail-safe system, while firms with younger or healthier or better paid workers would prefer their own private coverage. Similarly, healthy people would tend to favor actuarially fairly priced private insurance; chronically ill persons would gravitate toward the fail-safe system, driving up its average cost. If such choices were feasible on an annual basis, the system could be stabilized over time.

Here, as in other health insurance proposals that rely on competition among private health plans, there would have to be a risk adjustment mechanism available to compensate individual health plans for adverse risk selection. That problem is not inherent solely in the fail-safe plan proposed here. It is inherent in any system in which private health insurers compete, on price, for enrollees.

A complete specification of the fail-safe plan would go beyond the intended compass for this chapter, indeed, I am not wedded to this particular approach. As noted, there exist many alternatives to the current employer-based insurance system, all of them based on an individual mandate, rather than on a mandate on employers to cement in place the existing system.

It would be predicted, of course, that the elimination of the tax preference for employer-provided health insurance, with the availability of the fail-safe system, actually would hasten the erosion of the current employer-based system. The thrust of this chapter, and its main objective, has been to suggest that this development should not be deplored as an unintended consequence. The existing employer-based health insurance system is propped up artificially by an inefficient and highly inequitable tax preference without which that system would not have developed in the first place. In the longer run, after a potentially somewhat rocky transition, the demise of that system probably would be for the national good.

References

Bleakley, F. R. 1996. "Personal-Bankruptcy Filings are Soaring: High Debt, Downsizing and Medical Woes are Cited for Four-Month Record." *The Wall Street Journal* (8 May): A2.

Butler, S. M. 1991. "A Tax Reform Strategy to Deal With the Uninsured." *Journal of the American Medical Association* 265 (19): 2541–44.

———. 1995. "A Policymaker's Guide to the Health Care Crisis. Part I: The Debate over Reform." *Heritage Talking Points.* Washington, DC: The Heritage Foundation.

Clotfelter, C. T. 1983. "Tax Evasion and Tax Rates: An Analysis of Individual Returns." *Review of Economics and Statistics* (August): 363–73.

Congressional Budget Office. 1992. *Economic Implications of Rising Health Care Costs.* Washington, DC: U.S. Government Printing Office.

Danzon, P., P. Feldstein, J. Hoff, and M. V. Pauly. 1991. "A Plan for 'Responsible National Health Insurance'." *Health Affairs* (Spring): 5–25.

Etheredge, L., S. B. Jones, and L. Lewin. 1996. "What is Driving Health System Change?" *Health Affairs* 15 (4): 93–101.

Fragin, S. 1997. "Uninsured: The Health Care Crisis Report." *New Woman* (May): 127–33 and 168–70.

Fraser, D. 1989. Quoted in "A National Health Policy Debate." *Dartmouth Medical School Alumni Magazine* (Summer): 30.

Fuchs, V. R. and J. S. Hahn. 1990. "How Does Canada Do It? A Comparison of Expenditures for Physicians' Services in the United States and Canada." *New England Journal of Medicine* 323 (13): 884–90.

General Motors. 1992. *Annual Report 1992.*

———. 1993. *Annual Report 1993.*

Gruber, J., and M. Hanratty. 1995. "The Labor Market Effects of Introducing National Health Insurance." *Journal of Business and Economic Statistics* (April): 163–74.

Gruber, J., and A. Krueger. 1991. Incidence of Mandated Employer-Provided Insurance: Lessons from Workers' Compensation Insurance." In *Tax Policy and the Economy*, edited by D. Bradford, 111–44. Cambridge, MA: MIT Press.

Health Care Financing Administration. 1995. *Medicare: A Profile.* Washington, DC: U.S. Department of Health and Human Services.

Krueger, A. B., and U. E. Reinhardt. 1994. "The Economics of Employers versus Individual Mandates." *Health Affairs* 13 (2): 34–53.

Levit, K. R., H. C. Lazenby, and L. Sivarajan. 1996. "Health Spending in 1994: Slowest in Decades." *Health Affairs* 15 (2): 130–44.

McKinsey & Co. 1996. *Health Care Productivity.* McKinsey & Co.

Medical Benefits 1996. "Recent Trends in Employer Health Insurance Coverage and Benefits." *Medical Benefits* 13 (19): 1.

Moon, M. 1996. *Medicare Now and in the Future*, 2nd ed. Washington, DC: The Urban Institute.

Organisation for Economic Co-Operation and Development. 1996. *Policy Implications of Aging Populations.* Unpublished document, Organisation for Economic Co-Operation and Development, Paris.

Pauly, M. V. 1995. "U.S. Health Care Costs: The Untold True Story." *Health Affairs* 14 (3): 152–59.

Pauly, M. V., and J. C. Goodman. 1995. "Tax Credits for Health Insurance and Medical Savings Accounts." *Health Affairs* (Spring): 125–39.

Prospective Payment Assessment Commission. 1995. *Medicare and the American Health System.* Report to Congress. Washington, DC: The Commission.

———. 1996. *Annual Report to Congress.* Washington, DC: The Commission.

Reinhardt, U. E. 1993a. "An 'All-American' Health Reform Proposal. *Journal of American Health Policy* (May/June): 11–17.

———. 1993. "Reorganizing the Financial Flows in American Health Care." *Health Affairs* (Suppl.): 173–93.

Schieber, G. J., J.-P. Pouillier, and L. M. Greenwald. 1994. "Health System Performance in OECD Countries." *Health Affairs* 13 (4): 100–12.

Schramm, C. J. 1994. "What Price Controls Wrought." *The Wall Street Journal* (24 May): A16.

Schultz, E. E. 1994. "Medical Data Gathered by Firms Can Prove Less Than Confidential." *The Wall Street Journal* (18 May): A1 and A5.

Schwartz, R. A. 1970. "Personal Philanthropic Contributions." *Journal of Political Economy* 78: 1264–91.

Slemrod, J. 1988. *Are Estimated Tax Elasticities Really Just Tax Evasion Elasticities? The Case of Charitable Contributions.* NBER Working Paper No. 2733. Washington, DC: National Bureau of Economic Research.

Taylor, H., and W. E. Reinhardt. 1991. "Does the System Fit?" *Health Management Quarterly* 13 (3): 2–10.

Thorpe, K. 1997. *Changes in the Growth in Health Care Spending: Implications for Consumers.* Executive Summary. National Coalition on Health Care.

Welch, W. P., D. Verrilli, S. J. Katz, and E. Latimer. 1996. "A Detailed Comparison of Physician Services for the Elderly in the United States and Canada." *Journal of the American Medical Association* 275 (18): 1410–16.

White House. 1992. *The President's Comprehensive Health Reform Program.* Washington, DC: U.S. Government Printing Office.

20

Trading Cost, Quality, and Coverage of the Uninsured: What Will We Demand and What Will We Supply?

Mark V. Pauly

Introduction

Whatever happened to the healthcare crisis? If you are the average American, not poor but not too rich, not young but not too old, and if you pay attention to the things that really matter to you—whether your wages are growing, whether you have more money to spend on the things you really like, whether your family stays healthy and happy—you might be prompted to ask that question. To be sure, if you read too many East Coast newspapers, you still might be a little concerned—the newspapers will have exposés of what a few health maintenance organizations (HMOs) are not telling a few of their members, and you know that the plan you choose (which so far has not given you much trouble but then you have not been very sick) might not let you use some hospitals. But, all in all, you note that things are pretty good—the quality of care and your satisfaction, which always were high, are staying high, and the premiums you pay and your employer's complaints about what he is paying are, for once, getting no worse, and maybe even getting a little better.

The story would, however, be quite different if you asked one of the 40-million-odd uninsured Americans if they are seeing a disappearing

A version of this chapter was presented as The Eleventh Annual William Campbell Felch Lecture for the American Society of Internal Medicine, Chicago, October 10, 1996.

problem. The number of uninsured has increased by approximately 40 percent since 1985, more rapidly in periods of recession, less rapidly in the intervening periods of positive but feeble economic growth. Even now, as the overall unemployment rate sinks to an eight-year low, the number of uninsured apparently continues to creep up (Sheils and Alecxih 1996). Moreover, there is evidence that the availability of care to uninsured people is shrinking and is under attack by the pressure on providers coming from the growth of managed care plans.

To what extent does this less-emphasized development diminish both our appreciation for and our enjoyment of the slowdown in private sector spending growth? Is the second change, perhaps, also responsible for the first? Is it theoretically possible, practically feasible, and politically desirable to avoid a negative correlation between the welfare of the privately insured and that of others? I believe that the answers to all of these questions are affirmative, but not easy and surely not automatic. In what follows I offer some prediction of where things might be going, what changes are needed, and what actions will impede desirable changes. I also argue strongly that the problem is not one of market failure, but of government failure. The chapter closes with a new variant on a proposal that meets the challenges set out.

What Competitive Markets Will and Will Not Do

To avoid the twin dangers of overselling and underselling private sector healthcare reform, one should note the social tasks that competitive markets can perform. Markets are good at three things: (1) ensuring that costs are minimized for whatever quantity and quality of output is produced; (2) producing the mix and variety of products, by type and quality, that people prefer; and (3) getting valued products to people willing and able to pay the most for them.

There are, however, two roles in which competitive markets cannot be cast: (1) *No Robin Hoods.* Markets will distribute goods based on the distribution of purchasing power; they will not redistribute to or cross subsidize lower income people. (2) *No Bailouts.* Some people will make choices that, after the fact, will expose them to risk unless they have already bought insurance. Absent previously purchased insurance, competitive markets will not make transfers from winners to losers.

How Healthcare Used to Be: Myth and Reality

Some critics of market competition hold it up against an idealized version of past arrangements, held in the golden glow of memory. In this happy lost time, doctors and hospitals treated all patients regardless of their ability to pay, and kindly insurance plans spread the cost of doing this evenly over everyone in the community.

The facts were rather different. Some poor people were helped, but many were not. Uninsured low-income people have always had 25–33 percent fewer doctor contacts and hospital days than the insured. At one time, the Blue plans often charged community rates, but at that time the share of the population with any insurance was below 50 percent. By the time that share had risen above 80 percent, most large employers had become self-insured, and most of the remainder (except in a few eastern states) were experience rated to some extent. Individual insurance was also largely risk rated. So the "good old days" were far from good.

The truth is, however, that there are clues (not proof) that things have been getting worse lately. Although the national average percentage of hospital revenues devoted to charity care of the poor has yet to fall, there is some evidence, primarily from California, that the combination of the growing market share for HMOs and highly competitive hospital markets does lead to a decline in bad debt and charity care (Gruber 1994). Furthermore, although small-group insurance has always been medically underwritten to some extent, there are numerous assertions that underwriting is now stricter and more aggressive than it used to be (Jones, Cohodes, and Scheil 1994).

It is not just the increase in the numbers of the uninsured that is striking and worrisome. There are two other changes that affect this minority, one well known and the other less so. The well-known change is that the uninsured will have a harder time getting care when they do not pay for it. It is a true and praiseworthy American tradition that we have relied on private organizations, especially nonprofit firms, to adjust around the edges when government fails to help some as much as others would want. These organizations have used two spigots to draw the resources they need for charitable work. One is in the form of philanthropic donations—cash, volunteer work, and lifelong dedication by religious organizations—to help those who need help. The other spigot operates through the selling of *other products* for more than they cost and using the profits to cover the cost of charitable activities. Raising $15.43 from a bake sale and earning $15,430,000 in net income from care provided to commercially insured patients, from an accounting perspective, look the same except for the exponent; of course, the consumers of cupcakes may be more aware of the intended use of their overpayment than the consumers of insured hospital days.

The problem, of course, is that one spigot may be going dry. Managed care plans in many markets have attained sufficient size and power that they can demand to pay providers' prices that are closer to their costs, and threaten to take their business elsewhere if providers resist. This has meant some limitation, compared with an earlier period, on the ability of not-for-profit providers to overprice services sold to some customers so as to underprice services sold to (or required by) the uninsured. The most sophisticated study of this phenomenon, using information from California, finds that two things must be present for behavior to change: There must be managed care penetration, and there must be competition among multiple hospitals in local market areas. Interestingly, this study found that, despite the Comprehensive Omnibus Budget Reconciliation Act, the impact of greater competition on provision of charity care was limited to the emergency room. In local markets where HMOs grew in importance and hospitals competed, there was a reduction in emergency room bad debt and charity care (Gruber 1994).

Even when the uninsured are treated, and even before the advent of managed care, they get less treatment on average than the insured. Test frequency, costly procedures, and good outcomes are all lower for the uninsured when matched against apparently equally ill insured persons. We know the uninsured, even at present, are twice as likely to be hospitalized for "avoidable" conditions such as asthma; they have a higher risk of death once hospitalized; and, at the other end of the spectrum, they postpone or fail to receive needed care at higher rates than the insured; and they are less likely to obtain preventive care. This bad state would presumably be made worse if the amount of charity and bad debt care were further reduced, and it is likely that the loss of access might have some serious negative impacts on health. These effects are likely to be much worse for approximately half of the uninsured, those with incomes below 150 percent of the poverty level, than for the growing proportion of those with incomes above the poverty level.

Of course, no one has done a randomized trial to measure the effect of the absence of insurance on healthcare use or health, selecting a sample of people and assigning one group to insurance and the other to a situation of no insurance. The differences in outcomes in existing studies could still be due to subtle initial differences in severity (possibly themselves related to earlier patient behavior in the absence of insurance). But the circumstantial evidence lines up with common sense.

The less obvious change is that the absence of insurance is becoming more of a disease of lower-middle-class housewives and children than of either poor or nonpoor workers. The broadening of Medicaid coverage in the early 1990s actually decreased the proportion of poor people who are uninsured (Brown 1996). The proportion of workers with coverage has stayed fairly constant. A growth in the number of low-income households in the same period was still enough to keep the number of poor uninsured from falling, but the growth of the uninsured since 1990 has been disproportionately among people whose incomes are less than four times the poverty level, but still above the poverty level, and who are dependents of workers (Sheils and Alecxih 1996).

These, then, are the current facts as we know them. But where is it all leading? Specifically, if things keep going as they have been, will (or when will) the medical care industry have to change so as to deal with this environmental shift? It seems fair to say, for reasons discussed below, that the numbers and growth of the uninsured are at present largely invisible to the average American. However, if the growth in numbers continues, and if the uninsured are denied care, their problems will become more salient just when the financing and delivery system is moving in the direction of making the problem worse. When will the time bomb explode and, when it does, who will hear it and be affected by it?

An Invidious Distinction

The following addresses the question of what policy analysts noneuphoniously call the "provider point of view." In theory, and with some confirmation in practice, there are three different types of providers with different expected responses to this changing scene. One set roughly corresponds to "most hospitals," the other set probably corresponds to "most physicians," and the third set corresponds to "most providers of outpatient tests and other things physicians order but do not produce themselves."

Most private hospitals in the United States are legally not-for-profit corporations. The number of for-profit or investor-owned hospitals ebbs and flows, but so far has actually stayed a relatively small proportion overall, though such hospitals are becoming more numerous in some cities and suburbs. Some particular corporate chains have expanded (at the moment Columbia/HCA), whereas others have stopped expanding or have begun contracting out; overall the proportion of beds in "proprietary" hospitals has not increased over the long term (Gray, in this volume).

One might think that not-for-profit firms are guaranteed to behave differently than for-profit firms. The evidence on the behavior of not-for-profit and for-profit hospitals is controversial and, in many ways, conflicting. There is, however, one consistent and strong finding: For-profit hospitals tend to locate in places where there are fewer low-income or uninsured people than do not-for-profit hospitals (Norton and Staiger 1994). Somewhat less certain, but still a reasonably firm conclusion, is this: When for-profits and not-for-profits are located in places where there are few poor people, they tend to behave in much the same fashion with regard to cost, quality (insofar as we can measure it), such bad debt and charity care as they do provide, and most other things. The for-profits tend to charge higher prices to private insurers, thus reducing those insurers' profits and/or raising the costs of insurance benefits to local employers (Gray 1986). The real difference between for-profits and not-for-profits then is not so much in the day-to-day behavior as it is in the environments in which they are located.

The only relevant comparison group for the not-for-profit hospitals in areas with many uninsured people are government-owned hospitals. The latter provide more charity care and incur lower reported costs; in both cases the subsidies from taxpayers for charity care and capital probably account for the differences. The fragmentary evidence suggests that, when either private not-for-profit or public hospitals have some power to set prices above costs for paying customers, they do so to some extent but then use some of the would-be profits to provide more charity and bad debt care. It is not a one-for-one substitution; not all of the market power turns into charity, because some goes for medical education, some for technology, and some for a rainy day. It therefore follows that not all of the consequences of reduced market power will fall on charity care or that these consequences will be immediately apparent.

Indeed, it is even possible that hospitals will try to keep up with their charity care burden as long as they can, raising prices to the remaining nonmanaged care customers, and then merge or exit before they have to cut back, especially on the more crucial inpatient side. But whatever the not-for-profit hospital's choice over possible short-run responses, the long-run response is clear: Even after it cuts back to the bare minimum amount of charity care, if (as is typical) the not-for-profit is in a neighborhood with a disproportionate share of uninsured people, it will not be able to survive as an independent entity—nor will it be very attractive as a merger partner, unless it has either a good name or a distinguished medical staff.

Consider, first, a simplified story in which all hospitals in a town have an equal chance of attracting uninsured people, poor and not so poor. The laws on emergency care, and the inevitable credit problems with all care, mean that some of their clients will not pay enough to cover the full cost of the services they receive. Will inability to cover the cost of this minimum required level of charity care in the face of price-competitive insurance plans drive these hospitals out of business?

In this simple case the answer is no. If all hospitals provide the same (positive) level of charity care, and if insurers wish to purchase hospital care for their members, the price for that purchased care will have to cover the cost of the care plus the cost of hospital-provided charity care. No hospital can legally cut below the minimum, and, unless insurers can find a way to get by with no hospital care, they will have to pay this price.

Outcomes are quite different, however, in the more realistic case in which uninsured people are not uniformly distributed across hospitals. Competitive health insurance plans will reduce the ability of hospitals to charge prices to paying customers that exceed prices charged by other hospitals; hospitals with a heavy charity care or bad debt load may therefore find it impossible to provide the care that they cannot avoid while still covering their costs.

These firms will then cease to exist. The nonpaying patients who used these hospitals will go to other hospitals (although inconvenience may deter some). It is not the presence of uninsured people but rather their uneven distribution that causes the major problems. The final equilibrium, if there is one, will have the following characteristics:

- there will be fewer hospitals in places where the uninsured are numerous;
- the uninsured will be distributed more evenly than at present over the remaining hospitals;
- competitive hospitals will tend to provide only uninsured care that is required by law or unavoidable because they sell on credit; or
- hospitals that retain market advantage in terms of location (relative to paying customers), quality, or reputation will have a reduced ability to care for the uninsured and may still provide more than the minimum amount, but may also attract larger numbers of uninsured if they do so.

For those who care about the uninsured, there is good news and bad news. The good news is that some cross-subsidized care will remain, both because it is required by law and because some bad debt is unavoidable, and it may even be provided in a more evenly distributed fashion at better hospitals. The bad news is that it will be in shorter supply and delivered in a smaller number of less-convenient hospitals than at present.

The effect of the changes on self-employed physicians (those in private practice, either solo or group, who still manage the bulk of the medical services provided in the United States) is explored below. What economists predict as a response to the growth in competitive managed care depends on assumptions about their objectives. The simplest story is to assume that physicians are like other people who provide their services or efforts in exchange for money. Whereas there doubtless are exceptions for special cases and special circumstances, their primary motivation in rendering services is to obtain income, enough to cover both the costs of resources they must pay for and to compensate them for their work.

Physicians now face three types of customers. Some patients have insurance that tells the doctor: "This is how much we will pay for your services for our insured; take it (and provide services) or leave it." Except for the small 15 percent balance billing margin, now used by fewer and fewer physicians, this is how Medicare and Medicaid usually work, and a number of managed care plans do the same thing in terms of an offer, though the form of that offer is sometimes a complex combination of capitation, fee-for-service, and withholds. Other patients have insurance that reimburses them but still permits the physician to set his own price— conditional, of course, on the patient's willingness to pay that price and stay with that doctor. This subset of full-paying customers is shrinking in many places, but it still exists. Finally, there are the uninsured: people who will have to rely only on what they can pay out of pocket, and, most often, that may not be very much.

Suppose the first of the changes discussed occurs: Managed care plans (and probably Medicare too) pay less than before, less than what was charged in the "price-setting" market and perhaps less than is needed to keep up with inflation. Will this lower private income affect charity care? Economic theory says the physician really has only two choices when it comes to uninsured customers: either continue to accept them or accept fewer customers. Physicians' incomes will be reduced by the spread of managed care, but that will not necessarily cause charity care to fall because the profit-motivated doctor does not have to collect more from paying customers to make charity care feasible. Moreover, the strategy of "cost shifting" to whomever is left paying full charges that not-for-profit hospitals may pursue (up to a point) should not be available to the physician, because this physician would already have been charging the price-setting customers the profit-maximizing price (which would largely have been paid by their insurers). That is, because the physician is permitted to earn and retain profits or net income, and presumably prefers more such net income to less, the physician would not have been subject to the same desire to restrain prices as would the not-for-profit community hospital. (Also, physicians, even physician corporations, are usually not beholden to local businessmen who sit on their boards of directors.)

So compared to what hospitals face, there is good news and bad news with regard to physicians. The good news is that managed care plans should not expect physicians to accommodate lower prices by charging other people more, and so this may make insurers less likely to cut physician fees. The bad news is that if managed care plans still cut fees, then a physician's only recourse is to accept a lower net income, and that lower net income itself may reduce willingness to treat uninsured or poorly insured patients who cannot pay charges in full. Because a given percentage reduction in price paid by patients who have switched to managed care generally takes a bigger percentage bite out of not-for-profit hospitals' surplus than out of physicians' net incomes, we might expect the physicians to cut back care to the uninsured somewhat less than what hospitals would be financially compelled to do. On the other hand, because patients who switched to HMOs are now financially less interesting than they were when they paid full fees, a physician may decide to attract more paying customers—but to do this fees may have to be cut, or more of those who cannot pay fees in full but can pay something may have to be accepted.

Paradoxically, for physician services, the spread of price-cutting managed care may actually help uninsured lower-middle-income people. If they can afford to pay something, they may find doctors more willing to take them. At least this is what economists would say.

Physicians in private practice are, in most states, not under the same legal obligation as hospitals to treat emergency cases, though they doubtless feel a moral obligation to the uninsured. But, as with the rest of us, this moral obligation has limits and becomes more difficult to discharge when those limits are further collapsed by income cuts from other sources.

The most certain punch line here seems to be that the advent of a larger number of uninsured patients coupled with lower payments from managed care will make physicians truly miserable: They will face lower incomes, and they will face more people who need their services without being able or willing to pay the fees. For fee-paying consumers, there *may* be an offsetting greater willingness to accept them if they can pay something, but there are no guarantees.

The most serious bottleneck in delivering care to the uninsured is probably not the reluctance of not-for-profit hospitals or physician professionals to render care.[1] Instead, it is the unwillingness of firms that produce outpatient services and products to provide these often essential items without receiving revenue in return, specifically clinical labs, outpatient diagnostic centers, pharmacies, and suppliers of other similar complementary goods. Many of these firms are for-profit entities, and even those owned by physicians or hospitals are often so distant from the patient that they are operated in a for-profit fashion.

Here again there is bad news and good news. The bad news is that even when physicians seek to provide needed care to uninsured people, the difficulty of getting these providers of complementary medical resources to go along is serious indeed; most uninsured will often find arranging for these services the most difficult hurdle to overcome. One piece of good news is that as the numbers of uninsured increase, this hurdle will not get any higher for each uninsured person. The other piece of good news is that these firms should not cut their uncompensated care further when HMOs cut into their process, because they would not have been providing more than the bare minimum of such care anyway. These for-profit firms will be reluctant to provide care to nonpayors, whether there is one or a million such persons or whether insured customers pay a lot or a little, because they have not promised to accept either a charitable or professional responsibility toward the insured. They take the simple, but not illogical, view that if society wants services provided to people who do not pay, then society rather than the people who choose to own their stock should be the ones who pay. Increases in the number of uninsured or declines in revenues will not change this view, either for the better or the worse.

How Far Will It Go and How Long Can It Go On?

Virtually everyone agrees that the high and growing number of uninsured is a problem. Virtually no one agrees on what should be done about it. Even more ominously, many people currently agree that it is not worth doing something about. This author has argued elsewhere that the latter was at the heart of the failure of Clinton health reform (Pauly 1996c). The plan's most valuable accomplishment would have been the achievement of universal insurance coverage. And yet there was virtually no discussion of morality, compassion, or even more mundane but crucial issues such as how much good the uninsured would get from different levels and types of insurance coverage. Instead (simplifying only slightly), the administration's main argument for health reform was contained in the small space between two contending slogans pitched at the insured middle class: "Healthcare that is always there," and "Health insurance for you as good as members of Congress get." According to the inside story told by Johnson and Broder (1996), there are political operatives who still believe the effort would have been successful if the second motto had been used rather than the first.

Why was there no appeal to justice? The answer is that insiders thought justice would not sell because middle-class taxpayers believed that even without universal coverage everyone would get some type of healthcare somehow, and that beyond that they did not much care. Tautologically, but truly, the problem was just not bad enough, and there was no cheap way to solve it.

In rehashing the failure of the great healthcare crusade, the question abould be addressed: If the problem of the uninsured continues to worsen, how bad does it have to get before there is some action, and what is that action likely to be?

High numbers of uninsured either impose costs on others or make them feel guilty. To respond positively, it would help if taxpayers had growing real incomes and fewer public obligations. I believe (and hope) that economic growth will be healthy enough to increase our willingness to be taxed to help others, but I do not believe that public budgets will create much breathing room for additional spending on the uninsured. Quite the contrary. The inexorable burdens of paying interest on the national debt, coupled with virtually certain increases in payroll and general revenue taxes to pay for pensions and healthcare for the elderly, are likely to sop up (and then some) any substantial excess willingness of taxpayers to be taxed for the purpose of subsidizing large contributions to adult uninsureds. Money that ought to go to improve the lot of the uninsured will instead go to help middle-income Medicare beneficiaries.

Although the situation for the uninsured may not get as bad as one's worst fears, it will get worse. What then? There are two possibilities. The first is that not-for-profit firms, no longer able to use would-be monopoly profits to help the poor, turn (or return) to the traditional source of funds for their charitable activities: philanthropic donations. In addition to philanthropic foundations, this means businesses, consumers, and perhaps even individuals willing to volunteer or work for less than market wages to help the sick poor.

One thing we may expect (or hope) will change will be an increase in the willingness of people in the community to make philanthropic donations to not-for-profit hospitals to help cover the cost of care for the sick poor. In this sense, such hospitals will find it worthwhile to return to their origins and their original reason for being and tap the community willingness to make explicit transfers to the poor (Pauly 1996b).

One may fear that years of government and private cross-subsidies may have caused the philanthropic urge to atrophy. It will doubtless be difficult to replace entirely the lost cross-subsidy. But the fundamental notion is that the amount of subsidization of care for the poor that ought to occur is the amount that people in the community are willing to make available, either through voluntary charity or through elected governments. If they are stingy, there is no analytic basis for claiming that "we" want greater subsidies to the poor.

Of course, free rider and information problems may make the voluntary charity solution imperfect and doubtless will trigger the discussion of larger explicit government support through expanded Medicaid or some similar program. The alternative to private philanthropy is for government to step in and step up its support of care for the sick poor. Suspend for the moment your disbelief about political feasibility. Generally the best institution in society to make transfers, either from the rich to the poor or from the healthy to the unhealthy, is government. And generally, economists say, the fairest and most efficient way to make such transfers is for government to use explicit transfers and taxes as the means. Roundabout approaches, such as "community benefits" obligations laid on private firms or subsidies to private charities generally are less efficient in that some of the money never reaches its intended destination. Moreover, and here I personally feel strongly about this, the great advantage of explicit taxes and transfers is their political transparency: In a democracy the citizens have the right to know how much charity they are being asked to do, how much they are paying for it, and where it goes.

By now sad reality may set in. What is to prevent the bad outcome in which citizens are unwilling to give philanthropic donations and are unwilling to support higher taxes that are needed to make greater public transfers? I would regard it as a very sad situation indeed, but, from an analytical viewpoint, that selfish verdict would have to be accepted.

There is an important point here. The worsening of the lot of the uninsured under market competition, if it occurs and is not offset by government, would not be an example of market failure. Rather, it would be an example of serious "government failure" (at least in the sense of citizens collectively making a bad decision), an example of political failure, and perhaps of moral failure. Markets would be doing what they do best. It would be government that would be failing to do what it should do. Market competition will have abolished a type of charity that citizens, when faced with the challenge to pay for it explicitly and consciously, determined to be not worth its cost. If one believes that democratic government works well, one would have to conclude that formerly we were more charitable than we really wanted to be. If one thinks that we should be more charitable, one will need to get government to work differently.

The last version of a "failure" argument would be one that proposed that all, or most, citizens really *do* want to be taxed more to help the poor and the ill, but sometimes "our" government, due to defective political institutions, fails to reflect this desire. But then one would have to explain why our political choice system fails.

Limits on Equity

It is obvious that the level of intensity, volume, and quality of care desired by upper-middle-income people would set a standard of cost per capita that, if applied to the uninsured, would be too expensive for taxpayers to pay. This is a hard, but unavoidable, conclusion: In some way, the care that can be provided to and financed for the poor must contain some limits on beneficial but very costly care—not because taxpayers do not have the money, but because they are not willing to give it up for improvements in quality or access that, although beneficial, are not valuable enough to them. If so, something we can call "quality" will differ for those with enough income to spend or enough fear to assuage, compared with what will be available to the erstwhile uninsured and underinsured. (Of course, quality already differs.) Can we, as a society, cope with the institutional arrangement of two-class insurance when we explicitly choose that arrangement? How do we avoid self-contradiction, what is the best design we can offer, and where do we get the money for the "adequate class" insurance for the currently uninsured?

What to Do in Theory

There are three (and only three) ways to solve the problem of the uninsured:

- Hold down or reduce the price of insured medical care, compared with the alternatives that uninsured people face, so that insurance will become more feasible and more attractive.
- Provide subsidies to induce (and make possible) the purchase of insured medical care.
- Mandate the purchase of insured medical care.

As already suggested, as long as people place a positive value on medical care, they will be interested in ways of achieving access to it. They will choose among alternative ways with an eye to both the price and the "outcome" of those ways. For people at almost all income levels, it is not an option to expect to pay out of pocket for all care in all illnesses. The possibility is real for a very large medical expense, relative to one's current income or what one could expect to earn in a lifetime; both the desire to have access to the care and the desire to avoid financial risk (random cuts from income to be spent on other things) suggest that the self-insured, pay-for-it-all strategy is an option only for a tiny minority of corporate executives and U.S. senators.

So for almost everyone the choice is between buying insurance that covers at least high-cost illnesses, if not more, or going without insurance and hoping for free or reduced-price care. As already noted above, the previously high rate of growth in private insurance premiums for insurance of given coverage (higher than the rate of growth in Medicare costs per beneficiary for most of the 1980s and early 1990s), has for the past three years or so fallen dramatically. The total private premium for a given level of coverage is still growing, probably in the last year at a rate slightly in excess of the economywide inflation rate, but it is growing much less rapidly than its long-term real trend.

The alternative to private insurance is to be uninsured and to use the emergency room, charity care, and public clinics as the source of care. One could look at this "system" as a kind of free insurance plan for which we are all eligible in principle. It is not a very good insurance plan, but it certainly is cheap. More important, the better it gets, relative to the *net benefit* from private insurance, the more attractive it becomes. There is some good evidence to suggest, for example, that both the expansion of Medicaid benefits in the late 1980s and the availability of guaranteed access to hospitals for the uninsured in some states in the same period contributed to a drop in private insurance purchasing by families at the low end of the income distribution (Rask 1991; Cutler and Gruber 1996). Because employer contributions to *family* coverage dropped, as a proportion of premiums, more than employer contributions to *worker-only* coverage, this type of theory may explain as well why coverage for dependents dropped.

This discussion implies that policies that would raise private insurance premiums would be likely to cause the problem of the uninsured to become worse again. It also implies, regrettably, that providing easier access to free care to people who could afford to buy private insurance may induce them to drop themselves (or, say, their enviably healthy high school graduate dependents) into the ranks of the uninsured.

Subsidies provide another possible influence on insurance purchases. We now provide substantial subsidies for private insurance, almost $100 billion worth. This subsidy takes the form of a "tax expenditure" in which the compensation paid to employees in the form of a portion of health insurance premiums, rather than as cash, are free of federal income and payroll taxes and many state and local taxes (Pauly 1996a). The problem with this subsidy is that most of it goes to higher-income workers who probably would have bought insurance anyway, and little of it goes to the lower-middle-income workers. In addition, because it is open-ended, it provides an incentive to buy more generous benefits than are appropriate. In effect, we have a sizable subsidy to undeserving upper-middle-class people who then buy more insurance than they need.

The policy message would appear to be an obvious one: Subsidies need to be redirected. The theory on this is virtually impeccable; redistributing subsidies to lower-income people while curtailing them for the rest of us would improve both efficiency and equity. The only fear that some have is that removal of subsidies to employment-based group insurance might cause some increased risk segmentation; but the impact is likely to be small and easily dealt with by other, more targeted means. However, despite the overwhelming case, the political process is resistant. The following returns to the question of why this is so and what we might do about it.

So Who Pays?

The most fundamental problem in planning or forecasting future treatment of the problem of the uninsured is one of the oldest of all problems: money. If we are to deal appropriately with the still-growing ranks of the uninsured, we need to determine (and get our fellow citizens to agree) who will pay for what.

The uninsured are increasingly less accurately classified as "the poor": They are middle class, and they are often dependents of workers. The traditional patchwork solution for the uninsured poor—the tax-supported public hospital—is increasingly unsuited to the characteristics of the current uninsured population. In particular, the low amenity levels and the "rationing-by-time cost" that have traditionally characterized public hospitals and clinics do not fit either the needs or the desires of a largely working middle-class population. The separate delivery system of the sick poor will not be accepted by this population.

Instead, the best vehicle for financing and delivering services to the currently uninsured is through the structure of a formal insurance plan, but one that is both inexpensive and subsidized to make it attractive to this population. In some cases, and in some states, an expanded Medicaid managed care plan with heavy provider price discounting comes close. Advocates of TennCare (or of what the Oregon plan may (someday) come to be), believe that these arrangements might fit this need, although critics of the specifics of those plans beg to differ. However, an expanded, fully state-organized and state-supported Medicaid-type program is probably not the way to go for the long term. One reason is that the heavy price concessions that have made these plans financially feasible to some extent for the state probably cannot be supported over the long run by hospitals and physicians whose revenues are shrinking. Moreover, it makes more sense to group the lower-middle-class uninsured with other middle-class people seeking a frugal but tolerable plan than it does to link them to the poor.

One way to think about how to open up such options would be for the government to first perform an appropriate role of gathering information. A bidding process might work here, but one that itself works in reverse. Instead of proposing a product and asking for the lowest prices, the entity arranging the bids would propose a price (premium per member per month) and ask health plans to "bid" on the services, access, and networks they would offer for that amount of money. The idea would be to use a bidding type arrangement to elicit descriptions of what the best $4,000 plan for a family, the best $3,000 plan, etc., would look like. The process would differ from conventional bidding in that the organizer of the scheme would not anoint one of the offerings as the winner. Rather, consumers could choose among the options, because people with different tastes may have different definitions of what is best.

This scheme cannot do the impossible and provide a really cheap and really great plan that has so far been overlooked or hidden by managed care firms. The result of posting options will be rather to inform both the potential enrollees and the taxpayers who might subsidize them of the best options, the "frontier plans," among which they might choose. To close the loop in a voluntary fashion, however, it is quite clear that larger and better subsidies than those that now exist will need to be offered to the lower-middle-income populations that represent the source of most of today's uninsured and most of the growth in the uninsured.

How to Pay

The general outlines of an efficient and equitable scheme to answer the question of what to do about the uninsured have already been offered in several different settings and under a variety of assumptions (Pauly et al. 1991; Pauly and Goodman 1995). The plan uses refundable tax credits to pay the subsidy and largely finances it by eliminating the current tax subsidy to employer-paid health insurance for the upper-middle-class.

Previous writings explore some of the reasons why Americans do not seem to be concerned enough about the fate of the uninsured to do something serious about it (Pauly 1996c). There probably is no possible scheme that can be guaranteed to motivate taxpayers to pay more or to offset an incorrect perception that everything is under control. To some extent, it may be necessary to allow the number of uninsured to rise further, to drive a few decent hospitals out of business, and to cause more of a ruckus for this question to become politically salient in a way that is more genuine than the Clinton health plan and that will generate more than a modest expansion in children's coverage. Nevertheless, the following offers some new thoughts on a slightly modified and repackaged version of the tax credit approach, which could be used either for coverage for children or for coverage for all of the uninsured.

There is a major technical problem in constructing a subsidy plan for the currently uninsured. Taxpayers, even kind and benevolent ones, will not be eager to waste their money subsidizing many who need no help so as to help a few who do (Danzon 1984). The problem is that there is no obvious way to channel subsidies only to the uninsured. Although the majority of the uninsured are lower-middle-income, the majority of lower-middle-income families are insured. If we pay a subsidy only to those who are currently uninsured (e.g., as the Vaccine for Children program does on a small scale), we are in effect encouraging people to become uninsured. But if we pay a subsidy to all lower-middle-income people, we are subsidizing many who do not need help. Although perfection cannot be expected, a scheme is needed that discriminates in some fashion to select those who most need help.

Here is a way to begin to solve this problem. Interestingly, it was first proposed years ago in the Gephardt-Stockman bill, so potentially it has bipartisan respect.[2] The currently insured overwhelmingly receive their insurance through employment, and that insurance now receives a large subsidy. Even though the value of the tax exclusion is lower for lower-middle-income workers than for those with higher incomes, it is still positive and, to the extent that it avoids the payroll tax at a

15 percent rate, is not negligible if it exists at all. Only the insured obtain this subsidy, and it depends solely on obtaining coverage that meets the minimum standard. One way to avoid piling subsidies on top of subsidies—to direct new subsidies primarily to the uninsured—is to offer a tax credit of a certain dollar amount toward health insurance for all lower income people (probably adjusted for family size), but also to require any employment exclusion tax subsidy to be deducted from this credit. Thus, if the credit was $2,000 and an insured family currently saved $1,000 on income and payroll taxes because of the exclusion, its net credit would be $1,000. For a currently uninsured family the credit would be the full $2,000. At any income level, a family could decline the subsidy.

Formally, this scheme is equivalent to the "surrender your tax exclusion for a credit" proposal John Goodman and I made (Pauly and Goodman 1995); the insured family in effect gives up its $1,000 exclusion for a $2,000 subsidy. But by repackaging the credit as the *net* credit, it looks different. In this scheme, no one is forced to give up anything; you cannot be worse off. You never really give up anything; at worst, you receive a zero additional net credit because your tax exclusion was worth more than the maximum credit to which you are entitled. Most importantly, this scheme automatically gives a larger new net subsidy to those who are uninsured than to those who are currently insured. It surely has a lower net tax cost than just giving a $2,000 credit to every lower-middle-income family, while leaving the treatment of employer-paid premiums intact.

But it will cost something. We know where we must get the additional financing. As there is no hidden pot of gold that the Internal Revenue Service has identified, we will need to go to the upper-middle-income population that is the source of taxable wealth in the United States. How much will we need from them, and how will we get them to part with it?

What to Do?

How much such a scheme will cost obviously depends on the value of credit provided to people at different income levels, and the answer to that question is a political answer: How much quality and how much assurance of coverage do we want to buy? Given the current state of knowledge, we might parse out this questions as follows: (1) Consider the poor and the near poor (say up to 125 percent of the poverty *level*).

We want to give them a credit large enough to pay in full for a reasonable but frugal insurance plan. (2) Consider people who are lower-middle-income, say from 125 percent to approximately 250 percent of the poverty level. (The median income is approximately 250 percent of the poverty level.) They would be offered a credit worth approximately two-thirds the cost of the frugal policy. For Medicare Part B, a subsidy of approximately 50–75 percent of the premium is enough to get virtually everyone to buy in, so such a share is a reasonable guess as to what will get most of the uninsured to participate. There will always be some holdouts, and how much more we want to spend rounding them up is a question for taxpayers. (3) For the richer remainder of the population, only a small token credit should be offered—say approximately $750 per family. About 15 percent of the uninsured have incomes above 400 percent of the poverty level, though it is unclear whether we really should feel sorry for them. But with such a credit they will at least have $750 to spend on a catastrophic policy—and the great bulk of people at this income level already get tax subsidies worth much more than $750. There will be very low additional cost, and at least the remaining high-income "daredevils" will now have $750 worth of coverage.

Even for those lower income families for whom the credit is closer to their current tax subsidy, there may be some budgetary offsets. Consider a hypothetical citizen in a 33 percent tax bracket buying a $6,000 policy with a $2,000 valued tax exclusion who is offered a $2,000 credit. One might think he should be indifferent, but there is a difference. To get the $2,000 exclusion, he would have to spend at least $6,000 on a policy, but to get the $2,000 credit he would not need to buy as expensive a policy.[3] He may therefore accept the credit, cut back the insurance plan to one that costs, say $5,000, and save $1,000 on insurance premiums as well. However, if he gains from substituting a credit for the exclusion when the amount is balanced, someone with, say a $2,200 exclusion, may also be willing to exchange it for the $2,000 credit—saving a net $800 and making the U.S. Treasury $200 richer.

To get defensible (though not necessarily correct) estimates of the budgetary cost of a scheme modeled along these lines, one would have to specify exactly the subsidies for each coverage one has in mind and then turn it over to the expensive process of running a microsimulation model. In lieu of the time and expense to do this, it's reasonable to conclude with a tautology: If the problems of the uninsured get bad enough, and bother the rest of us enough, there will be potential political support for at least a small credit and hopefully eventually for a larger one.

What Will It Take?

Asking economists to forecast politics sounds like compounding imprecision, and no claims to accuracy or foresight are made by this author. Nevertheless, if the problem of the uninsured continues to worsen in terms of sheer numbers and continues to veer in the direction of children and nonworking spouses, the level of political concern will rise. Better information on how much of an impact loss of insurance coverage has on the uninsured middle class will also help; taxpayers can too easily dismiss the current data as applying only to the poor. A concerted effort to design something sensible and to outline starkly the need for it might be effective.

What would be undesirable is a continuation of our current post-Clinton-plan strategy of ineffective piecemeal reform, in which politicians try to provide apparent benefits of little actual value at zero government budgetary cost. Without universal coverage, using federal mandates on coverage or premium structure is likely either to make no difference or to raise costs for employment-based benefits enough to discourage almost as much additional coverage as it encourages.

Real reform will cost real money, but it will solve real problems. Some wrenching social decisions—how much quality is enough, how much do we care about our fellow citizens, how much residual uninsurance are we willing to tolerate?—need to be posed and addressed. The strategy of ignoring the problem or looking for solutions costless to the government budget but therefore either ineffective or harmful to private budgets needs to be avoided. I believe it is possible to put together an effective strategy that the middle class will decide that it can afford. Things can get better before they get much worse.

Notes

1. I am indebted to Giles Bole for this point.
2. It was devised by John Hoff.
3. One of the issues in designing a tax credit policy is whether the minimum policy whose purchase makes one eligible for the credit needs to cost more than the credit and, if so, how much more.

References

Brown, E. R. 1996. "Trends in Health Insurance Coverage in California." *Health Affairs* 15: 118–30.

Cutler, D., and J. Gruber. 1996. "Does Public Insurance Crowd Out Private Insurance?" *Quarterly Journal of Economics* 11: 391–430.

Danzon, P., with F. Sloan. 1984. "Covering the Uninsured: How Much Would it Cost?" Leonard Davis Institute of Health Economics. Policy Decision Paper No. 9, Philadelphia, PA.

Gray, B. H., ed. 1986. *For-profit Enterprise in Health Care.* Institute of Medicine, Washington, DC: National Academy Press.

Gruber, J. 1994. "The Effectiveness of Competitive Pressure on Charity: Hospital Response to Price Shopping in California." *Journal of Health Economics* 13: 183–213.

Johnson, H., and D. Broder. 1996. *The System: The American Way of Politics at the Breaking Point.* Boston, MA: Little, Brown.

Jones, S., D. Cohodes, and B. Scheil. 1994. "The Risks of Ignoring Insurance Risk Management." *Health Affairs* 13: 108–22.

Norton, E., and D. Staiger. 1994. "How Hospital Ownership Affects Access to Care for the Uninsured." *Rand Journal of Economics* 25: 171–85.

Pauly, M. 1996a. "An Efficient and Equitable Approach to Health Reform." Paper delivered at the Galen Institute, Washington, DC.

———. 1996b. "Health Systems Ownership: Can Regulation Preserve Community Benefits?" *Frontiers of Health Services Management* 12 (3): 3–34.

———. 1996c. "The Fall and Rise of Health Reform." Dialogue, pp. 7–14 in *Looking Back, Looking Forward "Staying Power in Issues of Health Care Reform."* Institute of Medicine. Washington, DC, NAP.

Pauly, M., and J. Goodman. 1995. "Tax Credits for Health Insurance and Medical Savings Accounts." *Health Affairs* 14 (1): 125–39.

Pauly, M., P. Danzon, J. Hoff, and P. Feldstein. 1991. "A Plan for Responsible National Health Insurance." *Health Affairs* 10 (1): 5–25.

Rask, K. 1991. "Public Insurance Programs: The Impact of Uncompensated Care Reimbursement Funds and Medicaid." Ph.D. diss., Health Care Systems Department, University of Pennsylvania.

Sheils, J., and L. Alecxih. 1996. *Recent Trends in Employer Health Insurance Coverage and Benefits.* Washington, DC: The Lewin Group, Inc.

21

Seeking More Efficient Healthcare Subsidies

Robert B. Helms

The issue of universal coverage for medical care is not a new one. It has been a central part of the health policy debate for most of this century and has been discussed seriously at the national level several times during the past 50 years. What is new about the argument today is the effect of the changing healthcare market, especially the effect of economic competition on the ability of healthcare providers and institutions to provide care. What, if anything, can those of us who have pointed to the lack of competition in the past as a source of inefficiency say about the provision of healthcare to the uninsured now that we seem to have a little more competition? If there are going to be public subsidies to help the uninsured, are there any principles that can guide us about how to provide these subsidies?

There are some principles that we can follow, but these principles will not satisfy everyone. There is no magic pot at the end of a rainbow that will allow us to painlessly expand the ability of a significant portion of the population to increase their consumption of society's scarce resources. The possibility of improving healthcare use will have to come from improvements in the economic performance of the healthcare sector. Improving the economic performance of any industry is never easy, but it can be achieved if public policies are based on economic realities rather than sidetracked by wishful thinking or the pleadings of special interests.

Political rhetoric in health policy debates about universal coverage traditionally have been filled with criteria that have little to do with improving economic performance, criteria such as maximizing political advantage for one or more politicians, improving the health status of one or more segments of the population, or improving the financial condition of some set of healthcare providers. To obtain real improvement in the economic performance of the health sector, we will have to base our policies on the broader concept of economic efficiency.

Using the concept of economic efficiency as a guide to policy could get one into a lot of theoretical trouble. For those not bred and born in this theoretical briar patch, the following explains what efficient economic markets mean to economists and why at least some of us believe that policies that attempt to establish efficiency-promoting incentives can improve the economic well-being of all of us. Economic efficiency is a broader concept than just reducing costs or eliminating waste. As the final users of goods and services, consumers play an important role in determining the amount and characteristics (including quality) of the output of an industry. Industry producers take this information, usually conveyed through market prices, and produce the amounts and types of products and services desired by consumers in the least costly manner. To minimize their costs of production, they must use available technology and information to combine the resources they choose to use in the most efficient manner. In other words, an economically efficient industry will produce the products and services that consumers want and will produce them at the lowest possible cost, given the state of technology and the prices of all possible resources. And in a changing world, the efficient industry will continually adjust to changes in consumer desires and changes in the relative costs of resources, although this adjustment to change will never be instantaneous.

As a guide to public policy, and especially in healthcare, two broad criticisms are often made about this concept of economic efficiency. Both criticisms are related to two of the assumptions that are made in formal models of economic efficiency, the assumptions of perfect (zero-cost) information and perfect competition. Needless to say, neither condition is met in the real world. Information is costly to produce so that neither consumers making choices in the market (say among health plans or physicians) nor producers who organize resources (for example, substituting nursing for physicians' services or outpatient for inpatient care) have complete information about the total costs and characteristics of all choices.

Markets also fall short of economic efficiency because of two types of monopoly power, both of which have played important roles in the history of medical markets. First, producers can restrict output and charge higher prices and thereby increase their own profits when they can exclude or intimidate (actual or potential) rivals. Or buyers of goods or services can reduce their cost of production (pay lower wages) if they can exclude or intimidate rival purchasers of these resources (this condition is called monopsony). Monopoly power can derive from legislation that excludes potential competitors from markets or professional intimidation that restricts the competitive behavior of market rivals.

So if economic efficiency is so difficult to achieve in medical markets, is it of any use as a practical guide to health policy, or as an attempt to seek a better way to subsidize healthcare for those we would like to help? There are two basic reasons why economic efficiency is a useful guide. One, the concept of economic efficiency helps identify a set of policies that can improve the efficiency of the market, that is, use available resources and technologies to satisfy consumer wants. Policies that systematically eliminate market restrictions that inhibit competition or help to reduce the cost of producing useful information should improve the efficiency of medical markets, even if they do not achieve some theoretical perfect state. Those who develop health policy have heated arguments about which policies will actually move the country in this direction, but my list would include tax policies to eliminate unintended subsidies for employer-sponsored health insurance, the elimination of state laws that reduce competition (e.g., professional licensing laws, restrictions on advertising, so-called preferred provider laws, state certificate-of-need laws), strong antitrust policies to prevent market dominance and restraints of trade, and the elimination of the emerging set of anticompetitive federal and state mandates on health insurers and managed care firms. I do not believe that a market dominated by any one of the current fads in health policy, managed care, old-fashioned fee-for-service, or consumer choice under medical savings accounts, would necessarily bring about an efficient outcome. For that reason the preference is for policies that eliminate known inhibiting factors in the market so that competition between providers and consumers making informed choices become the driving forces behind market change.

The second justification for using economic efficiency as a guide to policy is that the alternatives are much worse. History is full of examples of kings, elected politicians, central planners, and dictators (some of whom claimed to be benevolent) who have claimed that they knew how to improve the well-being of people. Some may have increased their own personal wealth, but there is little evidence that any of them have consistently improved the wealth of their nations and left their people better off than they would have been with free and open markets.

This propensity to argue for one simple solution is common among healthcare providers, healthcare policy professionals, and even some health economists. In fact, few are completely innocent of this desire to promote an oversimplified policy prescription. None has the knowledge or foresight to predict where an efficient healthcare sector would end up. The best health economists can do is to recommend eliminating those factors known to inhibit competition and consumer choice and hope that healthcare markets will perform more like other efficient markets.

It might be possible to develop a formal model specifying the conditions necessary to reach an efficient level of public subsidies. But it would be extremely abstract and involve personal values and unbiased market prices that can be conceptualized but would be impossible to obtain. Instead, more useful would be the development of some practical principles that might be used to move the country toward a more efficient healthcare system. The goal of these principles would be to complement other reform initiatives rather than exacerbate the distorting incentives that are currently the source of excessive use of healthcare services and the inequitable access to public subsidies.

The following sections outline four principles that might lead in the direction of more efficient public subsidies that are designed to provide healthcare to people currently uninsured. In the discussion of each principle I present some of the economic and political trade-offs that should be considered.

Do Not Increase Taxes or Budget Deficits

First is the killer constraint: We cannot have more of something such as healthcare for the uninsured without having less of something else. Nevertheless, it still leaves some options. There is little popular support for raising taxes or running even higher budget deficits to expand healthcare coverage, which means that we have to look for cuts in other budget expenditures if we are going to spend more public funds on healthcare.

However, before considering ways to expand coverage, it is important to know what it might cost. Using 1993 data on utilization rates of both the insured and the uninsured, Long and Marquis (1994) estimate that it would cost $19.9 billion to close the "access gap" for the uninsured. Using the same 1993 data, they also estimate the total cost of healthcare for the uninsured to be $60.5 billion. This estimate might climb even higher if we account for some increase in medical prices and the greater number of uninsured. Although Long and Marquis emphasize the smallness of this cost relative to total resource cost, it is large enough to illustrate that providing some adequate insurance to the uninsured is not a trivial political issue (the provision of this health insurance cannot be accomplished by a rider on some convenient piece of legislation).[1] In today's political and budget climate, with the emphasis on reducing government expenditures, a move to increase expenditures of even this relatively small size is not a trivial matter.

Therefore, if we cannot increase the government deficit or raise taxes, what options are left? Here are four options:

1. *Cut other government expenditures.* All nonelected policy analysts have a long list of expenditures outside their field of expertise that could be reduced to make room for more expenditures within their field. But even if all the health policy analysts in the nation could agree on such a list, developing it would not be a productive exercise. People in the health policy field have a responsibility to look for healthcare budget savings and then let the politicians decide between health and nonhealth budget cuts. However, with healthcare expenditures amounting to 12.3 percent of the gross domestic product in FY 1993, 19 percent of the federal budget in FY 1996, and, on average, 7 percent of state budgets in 1992, there are some possibilities.

2. *Reduce the level of benefits within existing programs.* Again, all health policy analysts have their own list of covered benefits they would like included in government programs that are often based on political reasons rather than any strong medical rationale. My list includes a large fraction of disability benefits (a program that appears subject to great abuse because it is so difficult to restrict the program only to the deserving disabled), some of the health expenditures for veterans (there are more efficient ways to help veterans), and some of what is now included as overhead for National Institutes of Health research grants. Reaching any agreement about what to cut, however, is likely to be unproductive until we have better information about medical outcomes and cost effectiveness upon which to make recommendations.

3. *Reduce government payment rates for health services.* This is the option of direct price controls that seems to be favored by the majority of health policy analysts and some health economists who (unlike this author) have lost, or never had, faith in the healthcare market. Government controls are a bad idea. If undertaken effectively, they have the advantage of obtaining immediate reductions in expenditures. But sooner or later, these controls

create their own set of problems as program managers face consumers and providers with strong incentives not to play by the rules. This is not a policy that will move the healthcare system in the direction of economic efficiency.

4. *Improve the efficiency of government healthcare programs by changing the incentives of consumers and providers.* This approach holds the greatest promise of simultaneously extending coverage to the uninsured and seeking to improve the economic efficiency of the healthcare system. But it will not be easy. Managed care in Medicare and Medicaid has some potential to reduce low-valued use of healthcare facilities and services. The problem is that public programs using managed care are now basing their payment policies on private sector fee-for-service prices rather than exerting an independent push toward efficiency. Managed care in the private sector is being pushed by employers, which results in some gains in efficiency, but not nearly as much as would occur if consumers had stronger incentives to seek out more cost-effective providers, regardless of how they are organized. A change in tax policy will be necessary to encourage consumers in the private sector to exert a stronger influence on the market. The more efficient the private sector becomes, the greater will be the benefit to public programs that use the same healthcare providers. Meanwhile, as Dowd, Feldman, and Christianson (1996) show, Medicare is not doing a good job of promoting efficient managed care because of its crude method of setting capitation rates based on average county fee-for-service costs. Reforming Medicare's payment methodology for managed care plans and purchasing practices would help, but the biggest roadblock to change is the lack of incentives of Medicare enrollees to seek out cost-effective providers. There needs to be a more balanced approach using more cost sharing or deductibles or some type of defined contribution plan to give consumers stronger incentives to seek value.[2] Competition from managed care and stronger consumer incentives should also improve the efficiency of the fee-for-service sector.

Give Consumers a Stronger Role in Seeking Cost-Effective Medical Care

I recently completed a review of the literature on the effects of tax policy on the demand for health insurance and medical care (Helms

1996). This review led me to two conclusions. First, there is strong evidence from Feldstein's (1981) and others' research that the exclusion of health insurance from taxation substantially increased the demand for employment-based health insurance, and that this tax-induced increase in insurance played a strong role in increasing both the use and the cost of medical services. Second, the highly technical nature of this literature has not helped create a more widespread appreciation of the role of tax policy in medical markets. These have been relatively large tax subsidies for the purchase of employment-based health insurance for more than 50 years. The result of these subsidies has been to transfer income to higher-income working people, increase the cost of healthcare to all people (those with and without insurance), and to make it more difficult for people to purchase cost-effective insurance.

If tax policy has had these effects, it seems logical that this country cannot expect to achieve more efficient healthcare markets without substantially changing tax policy. Economically efficient competition in healthcare markets will require stronger incentives for consumers to seek cost-effective care. The current movement toward more managed care may help create more competitive markets, but the system will not achieve the full potential of competition unless consumers also have stronger incentives to seek out cost-effective care from cost-effective providers. Providers will have little incentive to change their competitive behavior unless they get a strong message from consumers.

Encouraging consumers to be more involved is not just a matter for the private sector. It will also be necessary to reform public health programs, especially Medicare, so that consumers exert a stronger influence on the demand side. The most effective way to improve consumer incentives would be to provide subsidies in the form of a defined contribution. Not only would this give recipients incentives to spend their subsidy wisely, but it would make it easier for Congress to determine what it wants to allocate for health subsidies and to be more explicit about adjusting these subsidies by income, geography, as a reward for military service, or whatever criteria it would deem worthy.

Public Subsidies Should Be Explicit

Europeans often use the term "transparent policies" to describe the objective of making it easily apparent who benefits and who pays for a given policy. In the United States we use a host of terms such as cross-subsidies, cost shifting, and hidden costs to complain about policies that are anything but "transparent." Health policy analysts generally agree that our tax system boosts the demand for and the cost of healthcare for all people (including the uninsured), that Medicare and Medicaid payment policies force providers to at least try to shift costs onto other payers,[3] and that policy proposals to increase coverage such as mandated employer coverage or guaranteed issue may impose hidden costs on employees. Of course, the objective of making public subsidies explicit faces strong political opposition. If one describes the art of politics as convincing voters that they can be provided something for nothing, then the last thing a politician wants to see is an attempt to make the costs of public programs explicit. Yet if subsidies are made explicit, the advantage is that we are able to better evaluate the costs and benefits of public programs. It also has the advantage of not distorting other health market prices so that, at least in principle, all healthcare markets would be under stronger pressure to improve their economic efficiency.

A corollary principle is to make explicit any attempts at income redistribution among income classes, populations, or areas of the nation. Again, this goes against the political grain because the predominant incentive for politicians is to redistribute income to middle-income taxpayers for which the political payoff is greatest. When the regressive effects of tax subsidies for employment-based health insurance and payroll tax financing for Medicare are considered, a plausible case can be made that there is a net transfer from low-income people to middle- and high-income people from the total of health and tax policies (McClellan and Skinner 1997).

Despite rhetoric to the contrary, the Medicaid program is not a model for redistribution from the wealthier to the poorer states. In 1993 the eight states with the largest Medicaid programs received 49 percent of the federal dollars, with New York leading the way. Even though wealthier states pay higher federal taxes than do poorer states, they are encouraged by the 50 percent minimum federal matching rate to expand their use of optional benefits. Even with federal matching rates above 50 percent, poorer states (mostly southern) choose not to expand their Medicaid programs. The result is smaller federal subsidies to most of the nation's poor people than may be apparent if one looks only at the higher federal matching rates for low-income states. If the redistributive effects of health programs are made explicit, it might help to identify any political games being played with health policies and raise the demand for a distribution formula based more on some measure of medical benefits and less on politics.

Minimize the "Woodwork Effect"

The "woodwork effect" is the term used by policy and budget analysts at the U.S. Department of Health and Human Services to describe the effects of ill-defined eligibility and coverage regulations that allow people to "come out of the woodwork." The result is program enrollment and costs that far exceed the original expectations for the program. The woodwork effect is a common feature of all federal health programs with Medicaid, Supplemental Security Income disability, and veterans' benefits supplying some of the most notable examples. The unpredictable increases in costs occur despite the efforts of Health Care Financing Administration bureaucrats and an army of government auditors. Again, they are a predictable result of politics—members of Congress wish to appear to be the ones who provide benefits rather than the ones who deny benefits. The bureaucrats are then left with the dirty work of drawing the line between those who are entitled to benefits and those who are not. For most bureaucrats (political and career) charged with running these programs, there are more rewards for expansive definitions of eligibility and coverage than for being tightfisted. The result is budget expenditures that continually increase above the previously predicted baselines and a growing mistrust of government among taxpayers and voters. This situation helps feed the popular mistrust toward those pleading for any small increase in public subsidies for the uninsured, for children, or for any so-called worthy cause.

There may be no practical way to eliminate the woodwork effect, especially if we continue to have open-ended entitlement programs. This effect could only be minimized by some combination of fixed annual congressional appropriations, vouchers, per capita program caps, or some form of block grants. To make such programs effective in controlling costs, they must be designed in such a way so as to entice consumers not to overuse the system. The alternative is to continue to rely on price controls and direct utilization controls that seldom work because both patients and providers have strong incentives to use more resources.

Conclusion

Schroeder (1996) recently asked in the *New England Journal of Medicine* if the uninsured will "always be with us." The answer to this question is, yes, some of them will always be with us, but we could greatly reduce their number if we pursued health reforms designed to improve economic efficiency. It is conceivable that by eliminating the present tax exclusion for employment-based health insurance and turning Medicare into a defined contribution plan, it would be possible to enlist the cooperation of both consumers and providers and thereby increase the degree of effective competition in medical markets. Lower healthcare costs and more efficient forms of insurance would make coverage of the uninsured more feasible.

However, there is currently no sign of the political will to make these large changes that would move us toward more efficient healthcare markets and more efficient public subsidies. The nature of our political system is that Congress is more likely to follow the "squeaky wheel gets the grease" principle. Congress is far more likely to respond to loud cries for help from organized sets of providers rather than taking the steps to fundamentally reform healthcare policy. Congress will be increasingly preoccupied with Medicare as the cost of that program continues to grow. This will make all other aspects of healthcare policy (Medicaid, the uninsured, the veterans, the Indian Health Service, the National Institutes of Health, military medicine, etc.) more difficult to deal with.

Those of us contributing to this volume, as well as the larger community of health policy analysts, know enough about what is wrong with the healthcare system to design a more efficient set of policies, including a more efficient set of healthcare subsidies for the poor and medically needy. However, given the preoccupation with other issues, it is likely that we will never be asked to do so.

Notes

1. The Long and Marquis procedure may likely underestimate the total cost that would have to be incurred to include coverage in the federal or state budgets. Multiplying 40 million uninsured by the average annual cost of private sector insurance ($2,900) yields a crude estimate of $116 billion as the cost of covering the uninsured through insurance. To obtain the net cost to governments, we would have to subtract the value of care presently received by the uninsured. That number is not available, but past experience teaches us that a new federal program would have a difficult time restricting itself to paying only the net costs. The displacement of private insurance coverage by recent expansions of Medicaid eligibility illustrates this effect (see Cutler and Gruber 1996).
2. The elderly already pay a relatively high proportion of their health expenditures as out-of-pocket expenditures. But much of these aggregate out-of-pocket expenditures are for health services not covered by Medicare, so they exert the behavior-modifying change in consumer behavior primarily

on the noncovered services. Hospital and physician services that are covered are often shielded from the effects of statutory deductibles and copayments by supplemental insurance policies. Vouchers and other policies could also increase the incentives for consumers to choose cost-efficient care, but we have not exhausted the potential in fee-for-service Medicare for cost sharing to promote more efficient consumer choice.

3. Attempting to shift costs is not the same as actually doing it. For a careful analysis of cost-shifting issues, see Morrisey (1994).

References

Cutler, D. M., and J. Gruber. 1996. "Does Public Insurance Crowd Out Private Insurance?" *Quarterly Journal of Economics* 111: 391–430.

Dowd, B., R. Feldman, and J. Christianson. 1996. *Competitive Pricing for Medicare.* Washington, DC: The AEI Press.

Feldstein, M. 1981. *Hospital Costs and Health Insurance.* Cambridge, MA: Harvard University Press.

Helms, R. B. 1996. "The Tax Treatment of Health Insurance: Early History and Evidence." Paper delivered at the Galen Institute conference, 25 March.

Long, S. H., and M. S. Marquis. 1994. "The Uninsured 'Access Gap' and the Cost of Universal Coverage." *Health Affairs* 13 (2): 211–20.

McClellan, M., and J. Skinner. 1997. *The Incidence of Medicare.* Cambridge, MA: National Bureau of Economic Research, Working Paper 6013, April.

Morrisey, M. A. 1994. *Cost Shifting in Health Care: Separating Evidence from Rhetoric.* Washington, DC: The AEI Press.

Schroeder, S. A. 1996. "The Medically Uninsured—Will They Always Be With Us?" *New England Journal of Medicine* 334 (17): 1130–33.

22

The Case for Universal Health Insurance Coverage

Thomas Rice

Many reasons have been given to justify the need for universal health insurance coverage in the United States, including:

- obviating the need to provide a vast network of healthcare facilities for those who get sick but cannot afford coverage;

- giving government more clout in its dealing with providers who historically have been able to shift costs from one payor to another; and

- improving the health, and as a result, the productivity of the population.

Although reasons such as these are indeed important, they pale in comparison with what I would argue is the primary reason for which we should provide health insurance coverage to everyone: Universal coverage is consistent with prevailing notions of social justice.

Even though social justice is not an issue foreign to U.S. policy, other reasons have been more central in the debate over universal coverage. Why might this be the case? Some of the blame goes to the power of economic thinking in formulating social policy. Although some economists have given considerable thought to the area of social justice, these issues play little part in the traditional microeconomic model. Rather than concerning itself with how people come into possession of their initial stock of wealth, economic theory devotes nearly all of its attention to how people allocate the resources *over which they have already been assigned property rights* (Young 1994).

Under the traditional model, competition is used to ensure that resources are used efficiently. Where people obtain these resources is not typically considered because economic tools provide no basis for determining what is the appropriate initial allocation. Rather, such issues fall under the purview of distributive justice and moral philosophy. Individual economists might advocate that resources be redistributed (typically through cash grants rather than in-kind services), but this is based on their own opinions, not the tools of the trade.

Whether the United States should rely on market forces in the delivery of healthcare services is an issue subject to much debate—but this is not our subject here. The problem that is considered in this chapter is that market forces do little if anything to ameliorate the problems of those who have been endowed with few resources (in fact, they might make it worse). If competition is not the answer for helping those who are left behind, then the answer must obviously lie in some way with government involvement. The specific application considered here is whether the U.S. government should enact universal health insurance coverage.

This chapter is divided into two main sections, one theoretical and the other applied. The first section, which is devoted to theory, argues that our reliance on utilitarian philosophy has resulted in a mind set in which we look toward market forces—inappropriately as it turns out—for answers to social questions. Alternative philosophies, such as those advocated by John Rawls, Amartya Sen, and others, provide a more appropriate means of dealing with the problems of the disadvantaged. The second section of this chapter then applies this conceptual background to the issue of universal health insurance coverage.

Utilitarianism versus Alternative Philosophies

Utilitarianism is the belief that social welfare is simply the sum or aggregate of all individuals' welfare. Utility is a personal psychological perception, and, to the economist, is based on the goods possessed by a person.

Early utilitarians believed that these utilities could not only be quantified, but could also be added across individuals. Modern economics rebelled against such a concept, relying instead on the notion of "ordinal" rather than "cardinal" utility. Under ordinal utilitarianism, individuals must be able to choose only which bundle of goods they prefer to any other, rather than quantify how much utility is derived from each.

Modern economic theory is based on the concept of ordinal utilitarianism. Arrow, a strong advocate of the use of ordinal utility in evaluating social welfare, has stated that

> The implicit ethical basis of economic policy judgment is some version of utilitarianism. At the same time, descriptive economics has relied heavily on a utilitarian psychology in explaining the choices made by consumers and other economic agents. The basic theorem of welfare economics—that under certain conditions the competitive economic system yields an outcome that is optimal or efficient . . . —depends on the identification of the utility structures that motivate the choices made by economic agents with the utility structures used in judging the optimality of the outcome of the competitive system. (Arrow 1983, 97)

This section explores two problems with the concept of ordinal utilitarianism employed by modern economics, each of which has important implications in making the case for universal health insurance coverage. The first issue concerns the lack of breadth of the concept; it ignores issues of social justice and fairness. The second concerns its lack of depth; utilitarianism is defined solely in terms of a single, goods-based, psychological metric, ignoring other potentially important conceptions of what drives individual and social welfare.

Social Justice and Fairness

Modern economics in general and utilitarianism in particular do not concern themselves with what is right or fair. Rather, the simple possession of goods brings utility to individuals and therefore to society, which is conceived as simply the aggregate of all individuals.

No concern is given to whether the overall distribution of wealth is *justified.* This is not to say that issues of income distribution are ignored. In fact, the people in a society may indeed be concerned about distributional issues and may choose to tax the rich to provide for the poor. But if that occurs, it is the result of social choice and not necessarily based on social justice.

To understand this distinction—which is a crucial one—it is useful to consider the difference between altruism versus equity. The former is based on preferences; for example, I want the poor to have more so I provide donations or vote to increase taxes. Thus, providing for the poor makes *me* better off because their welfare enters my utility function. In contrast, according to Wagstaff and van Doorslaer (1993, 8):

Social justice (or equity), on the other hand, is not a matter of preference. As [Anthony] Culyer puts it: " . . . the source of value for making judgements about equity lies outside, or is extrinsic to, preferences. . . . The whole point of making a judgement about justice is so to frame it that it is . . . a judgement made independently of interests of the individual making it." Social justice thus derives from a set of principles concerning what a person ought to have *as a right.*

As might be imagined, different philosophers (and economists) have reached different conclusions about what things people should have as a right. At one extreme, Nozick (1974) has proposed a libertarian philosophy in which the distribution of wealth is just if (1) the original assignment of wealth was arrived at fairly, and (2) the current distribution was arrived at through voluntary exchange. It is certainly a matter of opinion, however, as to whether the original distribution was arrived at in a just fashion; as a result, this philosophy has been aptly coined as one of "finders keepers" (Elster 1992; Stone 1996).

The most well known modern exposition of social justice and rights is the book by John Rawls (1971), *A Theory of Justice.* Rawls' theory, which he calls "justice as fairness," provides an alternative to utilitarian philosophy. To determine what is fair, he invokes a concept called the "original position" in which people choose the principles of a just society from a position where "no one knows his place in society, his class position or social status, nor does anyone know his fortune in the distribution of natural assets and abilities, his intelligence, strength, and the like" (Rawls 1971, 12).

In addition, one does not know the sort of society in which he or she will be placed; it may be a democracy or, alternatively, a dictatorship in which there is a small ruling class, with the rest of the population assigned to slavery. Rawls calls this lack of information about one's talents and standing a "veil of ignorance." His goal is to determine what system of justice that rational, self-oriented people would choose when placed in the original position. The other term that needs definition is "primary goods," which are defined as "rights and liberties, powers and opportunities, income and wealth" (Rawls 1971, 62).

Rawls posits that people in the original position would accept the proposition that primary goods "be distributed equally unless an unequal distribution of any, or all, of these values is to everyone's advantage. Injustice, then, is simply inequalities that are not to the benefit of care" (Rawls 1971, 62).

The punch line—the system of justice that Rawls believes would be adopted by a society whose members consider these issues under the veil of ignorance in the original position—is what he calls the "difference principle." Under the difference principle, society is better off only when it makes its least well-off people better off. In other words, society's resources should be devoted to increasing the primary goods possessed by the most disadvantaged people. The only time that resources will go to the group that does not occupy the bottom rung is when by doing so, benefits will trickle down to the most disadvantaged group.

This result—that in the original position people will adopt the above method of allocating primary goods—is called "maximin." In essence, people will choose to maximize the lot of those who have the minimum. Society is no better off if one person has more primary goods if those goods possessed by others do not increase. The only way to increase social welfare is to equalize the goods possessed, and then provide more to everyone.

Why would people, placed in the original position, come up with such a conception of justice? Rawls has a simple answer:

> Since it is not reasonable for [a person] to expect more than an equal share in the division of social goods, and since it is not rational for him to agree to less, the sensible thing for him to do is to acknowledge as the first principle of justice one requiring an equal distribution. Indeed, this principle is so obvious that we would expect it to occur to anyone immediately. (Rawls 1971, 150–51)

Although Rawls did not list health as one of the primary goods, some analysts have disagreed with this decision. According to Green (1976, 120), "Access to healthcare is not only a social primary good, but possibly one of the most important such goods [because] disease and ill health interfere with our happiness and undermine our self-confidence and self-respect." The types of services that would be included as part of a universal health plan would include such things as "basic preventive and therapeutic services."

Before moving on to a critique of the theory, it is important to make a note of its policy implications. Although the theory is abstract and cannot be applied directly to many problems, there is one overriding implication: Society should engage in far more redistribution than it does currently. This is because much if not most redistributive programs are not targeted solely at those who are worst off in society. In fact, one could argue that relatively little goes to this group. In this regard, Tullock (1979, 172) has written:

So far as I know there is absolutely no reason to believe that majority voting or any of the variants of democratic government transfer an "optimal" amount. Indeed, I would argue that they do very badly, since the bulk of the transfers they generate are transferred back and forth within the middle class; and, so far as I know, there are no arguments that would indicate that these transfers are desirable.

Though it is usually praised even by its critics, a number of objections have been leveled against Rawls' philosophy. Here is one of them because it has a direct bearing on the issue of universal health insurance coverage.

Just as utilitarianism is limited in its conception of how resources should be distributed, so, it can be argued, is Rawls' theory. In the theory, the only basis for redistribution is where a person stands in society with respect to his or her possession of primary goods. This viewpoint would appear to be rather limited:

- Under the theory, people are entitled to an equal share of resources irrespective of their work effort, motivation, etc. This is because what a person is born with is, according to Rawls, really just the result of a "natural lottery," which "is arbitrary from a moral perspective." As a result, he believes that "even the willingness to make an effort, to try, and so to be deserving in the ordinary sense is itself dependent on happy family and social circumstance" (Rawls 1971, 74). Thus, if a person exhibits a lack of motivation it is not clear that he should be endowed with less of a share of primary goods because, in essence, it really isn't the person's fault. Needless to say, relying on such criteria to carry out policy could result in a very large sacrifice of efficiency.

- Equalizing resources does not necessarily solve people's problems because they still might not be born with the wherewithal to use these resources in a manner that will be of benefit to them. In fact, some people might need more resources than others (e.g., the disabled).

One reason that *A Theory of Justice* was such an important book is that it allowed others, who may not have totally agreed with Rawls, to formulate their own bases for thinking about alternative conceptions of social welfare. Rawls poked a number of holes in the utilitarian philosophy; since then others have enlarged them.

It is often difficult for readers to understand why most philosophers do not believe that people should be granted full property rights over the resources that they have inherited or earned. Rawls (1971, 102) states that, "No one deserves his greater natural capacity nor merits a more favorable starting place in society," and, interestingly, most philosophers and even many economists agree. Arrow (1983, 98–99), in writing about Rawls' book, notes that under the theory:

> Even natural advantages, superiorities of intelligence or strength, do not in themselves create any claims to greater rewards. . . . Personally, I share fully with this value judgment. . . . But a contradictory position—that an individual is entitled to what he creates—is widely and unreflectively held; when teaching elementary economics, I have had considerable difficulty in persuading the students that this *productivity principle* is not completely self-evident.

The literature on moral philosophy is very clear that, in creating a fair society, something must be equalized. Sen (1992, 17) provides a reason:

> It may be useful to ask *why* it is that so many altogether different substantive theories of the ethics of social arrangements have the common feature of demanding equality of something—something important. It is, I believe, arguable that to have any kind of plausibility, ethical reasoning on social matters must involve elementary equal consideration for all at *some* level that is seen as critical. The absence of such equality would make a theory arbitrarily discriminating and hard to defend. A theory must accept—indeed demand—inequality in terms of many variables, but in defending those inequalities it would be hard to duck the need to relate them, ultimately, to equal consideration for all in some adequately substantial way.

Sen notes that even Nozick's libertarian philosophy does call for the equalization of something—libertarian rights.

Unfortunately, deciding that something ought to be equalized does not solve most of our problems—rather, it seems to raise more questions than it answers. The main problem, of course, is that it does not tell us *what* should be equalized. Before confronting this, it is important to distinguish between two similarly sounding, but quite different concepts: "equality" and "equity." The former implies equal shares of something, the latter a "fair" or "just" distribution, which may or may not result in equal shares.

The difference between the two terms can be seen by examining the two common forms of equity: horizontal equity and vertical equity.

Horizontal equity implies that similar people are treated the same with respect to some characteristic (the choice of which is a major issue in itself)—what is referred to here as equality. But vertical equity is much different; it is, according to Mooney (1996b, 99), "the unequal but equitable treatment of unequals." For example, we might, in the name of equity, establish a lower tax rate for the poor than for the rich.

The distinction between these terms is further illustrated by Stone (1996), who discusses how to divide up and distribute "a delicious bittersweet chocolate cake" among students in her public policy class. One way, of course, is to give equal slices to all, but that seemingly fair method may lead to protests that "equality" does not result in an "equitable" distribution. Some possible objections to equal slices noted by Stone, each of which results in a different distribution of cake, include:

- everyone in the university should get a slice, not just class members;
- higher-ranked persons deserve bigger slices (or more frosting);
- because males traditionally have had less access to homemade cake, each sex should get half the cake to divide among their members;
- those who were given smaller main courses should get more cake;
- people who can't appreciate the cake should get less (or none);
- *access* to the cake, not the cake itself, should be equalized by giving everyone a fork; competition for the cake would then ensue;
- the cake should be distributed by lottery; and
- the allocation should be decided on by voting.

It is not hard to come up with close analogies to each of these arguments when allocating scarce medical goods and services.

As noted above, to be persuasive in issues involving resource allocation, it is necessary to advocate the equalization of something. What is being equalized under utilitarianism? The answer is not as straightforward as it might seem because, as noted above, the concept embraces several different formulations. In general, though, utilitarianism is not about equalizing something so much as maximizing something else (Sen 1992). Under classical utilitarianism, the sum of all individuals' utility is being maximized. Under ordinal utilitarianism, society is best off when each individual succeeds in maximizing his own utility, although some income redistribution is likely to be necessary to maximize social welfare.

We are most concerned with ordinal utilitarianism because it forms the basis of modern economics. If one had to venture a guess as to what was being equalized under ordinal utilitarianism, one possibility is that each individual's interests are being treated equally; my utility counts as much as yours.[1] Another might be this: People have equal rights to produce and trade so as to maximize their utility. This is not to say that they have equal ability or opportunity to do so; rather, in a competitive market there are no explicit restrictions on participating in the marketplace. It is not hard to see why moral philosophers, in considering the vagaries of social advantage in the real world, would view this concept as wanting.

What, then, should be equalized? One line of thought, advocated by Dworkin (1981), is that "resources" should be equalized—a philosophy that would appear to be not terribly different from Rawls' equalization of primary goods.[2] Another, by Roemer (1995) and many others, is that "opportunity" should be equalized. The idea is that people should be responsible for their own actions once there is established a "level playing field."

To operationalize this, Roemer distinguishes between factors that are beyond a person's control versus within his or her control. He gives the following example. Suppose we want to compensate people when they contract lung cancer (so that they can afford their medical care). We first come up with a list of factors over which people have little control; examples he uses are age, ethnicity, gender, and occupation. We then look at smoking behavior within these subgroups. Suppose that the average 60-year-old male black steelworker has smoked for 30 years, and the average 60-year-old female white college professor has smoked 8 years. These figures provide a way to gauge the behaviors of others who fall into these subgroups. If we then have a black steelworker contracting lung cancer who smoked for 20 years, and a professor who smoked 15, the former would receive more compensation—because his behavior was more responsible *given the circumstances over which he had little or no control.*

A final candidate for equalization, advocated by Sen, is particularly relevant in the next section of this chapter when the theory is applied to universal health insurance coverage. This is the equalization of capabilities that "reflect a person's freedom to choose between alternative lives" (Sen 1992, 83). The idea here is to give people the wherewithal to be able to achieve the things they want. It is designed to focus not on resources themselves, but what resources can do for a person.

Equalizing capabilities is different from the other theories discussed above. It differs from Rawls' theory and from equalizing resources, because under those systems people are given physical resources but not necessarily the ability to use them to achieve what they want.

And it differs from equality of opportunity because giving someone the opportunity does not necessarily mean that they will be able to effectively use it to their own advantage. Equality of capabilities might mean that more resources would be given to a disabled person because such a person could need more so as to be capable of achieving their goals. Or it might mean actually giving unskilled laborers the skills to achieve more—rather than simply plying them with cash grants.

In summary, the utilitarian viewpoint does not consider matters of social justice and therefore provides an inadequate basis for confronting issues such as what sorts of goods people should be provided as a right—including, of course, health insurance. The work of Rawls and subsequent philosophers provides the conceptual underpinnings for making such a determination. Alternatives discussed included providing everyone with the same set of primary goods, equal resources, equal opportunities, and equal capabilities. The latter—equalizing capabilities— is especially appealing because it would allow people to meet their own goals.

Alternative Concepts of Utility

Economists do not typically inquire into why people derive utility from particular goods. Through its reliance on ordinal utilitarianism, modern theory is interested simply in which bundle of goods a person prefers; the preference need not be justified. An economic system that is best able to satisfy such preferences is then desirable because the preferences themselves are beyond questioning. Sen has deemed this a "welfarist" viewpoint—the only thing that matters in evaluating an economic system is how well it satisfies these preferences.

Several objections to this viewpoint can be raised:

- It essentially sanctions preferences that we might view as immoral; for example, equal favor is given to those preferences that may involve harming others as compared to those that we might find to be more lofty. In this regard, Sagoff (1986, 302) writes, "It cannot be argued that the satisfaction of preferences is a good thing in itself, for many preferences are sadistic, envious, racist, or unjust."

- It also sanctions preferences that might be, in some sense, faulty (e.g., behaviors that are self-destructive). One example is short-sightedness. Sagoff (1986, 304) writes, "Literary and empirical studies amply confirm what every mature adult discovers: happiness and well-being come from overcoming or outgrowing many of our desires more than from satisfying them."

- It focuses on goods rather than other values such as freedom. This leads to the seemingly faulty prediction that people would be equally happy with a particular bundle of goods that was assigned to them versus the same bundle of which they freely chose (Hahnel and Albert 1990).

It turns out that this conception of utility also does a poor job in predicting other aspects of people's behavior. One concerns why people even bother to vote. Given the infinitesimally small chance that your vote would decide an election, why go to all the effort? Another example is income taxes; why be honest when it is so easy to cheat and so hard to be caught? (Aaron 1994). As a final illustration, it is useful to summarize Margolis' (1982) discussion of people's contributions to charity.

Suppose that a public radio station embarks on a fundraising campaign and you decide to contribute $10 (but not $11); that is, you maximize your utility by spending $10 for this charity in the place of spending it on other goods and services you could purchase. But just as you are about to call in your pledge, the station announces that someone else has just given $10. Under the conventional economic model, this new information will make you forgo your contribution—the station is already $10 richer; you can now keep the $10 and be that much better off than before. Not contributing allows you to have your cake and eat it too.

If people really behaved this way, there would be no way public radio (or for that matter, almost any charity) could exist. Once a single large donor announced his or her intention, it would be nearly impossible to get anyone else to contribute. Everyone else would "free ride" onto this donation. The outcome would be economically inefficient because far less would be contributed to charity than is desired by the public.

Fortunately, something still drives people to contribute to charities. To explain paradoxes such as these, it is necessary to have a broader definition of utility. An example from Sen is recycling behavior as an example of commitment—a behavior that people engage in, even though it may not seem to be in their self-interest. Another formulation is from Margolis, who explains people's behavior by positing that they possess two distinct altruistic motivations. One, which he calls "goods altruism," is the one we normally conceive; people receive utility when other, less well-off people have more goods to consume. The other is "participation altruism," a very different concept. Under it, you get utility from the act of giving resources away (including your time) because it makes you feel good about yourself. This dual form of altruism, according to Margolis, can explain the paradoxes discussed above (why a person would vote, give to charity, not cheat on taxes, etc.).

More recently, Aaron (1994, 15–16) has provided a critique of utility theory, calling for "a new economics of human behavior." Although it is beyond the scope of this work to spell out the details, he believes that

> each person [has] more than one, possibly many, utility functions. In one or more of these sub-functions the arguments, as in standard theory, are particular goods and services. In others the arguments are intangible objectives such as adherence to duty, altruism, or spite, characteristics necessary for reputation or self-respect. Particular economic commodities may enter more than one function. In contrast to standard theory, however, the marginal utility of a given object may vary widely in different utility functions and may even have different signs.

Viewpoints such as these are heretical to adherents of ordinal utilitarianism, who believe that people's utility is derived largely if not solely from the goods that they possess. But if utility is derived in large measure from something else—say, being part of a community that provides for its members—then there is a strong basis to consider providing certain goods to those who do not have them. Health insurance, it will be argued, is one of these.

Implications for Universal Coverage

The preceding section attempted to demonstrate two key issues that have direct implications for the issue of universal health insurance coverage. First, there are certain things that people should have as a right; health insurance is one of them. And second, there are aspects of social welfare over and above the utility that people derive from the goods that they consume; good health is one of them. These are discussed in reverse order, below.

Focusing on Health, Not Utility

Under the conventional economic model, society strives to allow people to maximize their utility. Because utility is purely subjective, not directly measurable, and not comparable across different people, public intervention is typically not advised. Rather, people should choose to spend their resources in whatever manner they think will maximize their welfare.

But as argued above, there are various shortcomings with this viewpoint, one of which is that it is silent on a basic issue of social justice: People should not be penalized over things about which they have little or no control. It was argued that, for a theory to have any moral sway, something very important needs to be equalized. It was further argued that this "something" has to do with people's opportunities or, alternatively, their capabilities to achieve their life goals.

For decades, health economists have debated whether there is something "different" about healthcare.[3] Much of this literature has focused on informational problems—certainly an important issue, but not terribly convincing because there are major (although perhaps not quite as severe) information problems in other sectors of the economy. Other literature has focused on the fact that there are perhaps stronger positive externalities associated with healthcare—that is, people derive satisfaction knowing that other people are healthy. Arrow (1963, 954), for example, has stated, "The taste for improving the health of others appears to be stronger than for improving other aspects of their welfare." Although this provides a perhaps somewhat stronger case for health being special, one can still imagine other things—food, education, housing—that are equally compelling.

Rather, what would appear to be truly different about health concerns opportunities and capabilities: Good health provides people with the opportunity and capability to achieve other desired things. As Culyer (1993, 300) has written, "One reason for such beliefs may be to do with the important role [things like health] have in enabling people to fulfill their potential as persons. . . ." Such a viewpoint is consistent with the reason given by Thurow (1977, 93):

> Society's interest in the distribution of medical care springs, not from unspecified externalities that affect private-personal utility, but from our individual-societal preferences that "human rights" include *equal* "right" to health care.

The idea that there are other nonutility aspects of welfare that should be considered by society has been coined as the "extra-welfarist" approach. (Under a welfarist approach, only individual levels of utility matter to society.) In healthcare, these aspects have to do with either or both access to healthcare services and good health itself.[4] Some researchers, such as Aday, Andersen, and Fleming (1980, 26), have advocated that access to healthcare service is a key dimension of equity, whereby "The greatest 'equity' of access is said to exist when need, rather than structural or individual factors, determine who gains entry to the healthcare system." More recent work by Mooney and his colleagues (1991, 479) appears consistent with this viewpoint. They advocate "equal access for equal need," because this "provides individuals with the *opportunity* to use needed health services."

Other analysts, notably Culyer (1989), have advocated that health status rather than access to care be considered the key outcome[5] and the determinants of health as the key research issue.[6] If one considers health rather than utility as an outcome, the meaning of economic efficiency is very different than the one typically used in economics. Under this conception, Culyer (1993, 312) states that efficiency is achieved "by prioritizing the more 'urgent' and so distributing health between A and B that, at the margin, the cost of A's and B's additional health is equal to the social value attached to the health of each."

Under this type of allocation rule, we are interested not so much in what people demand as in how much of an improvement in health can be purchased with a given amount of money—a very nonwelfarist viewpoint. Both this view as well as the one centered on access to care seem to dictate health policy worldwide much more so than the conventional economic model. The view that centers on access as the key outcome is consistent with the fact that most government-sponsored healthcare programs seek to equalize people's ability to obtain needed medical care. The view that focuses on health itself as the key outcome forms the basis of the growing reliance on analyses of the cost-effectiveness of healthcare and on the relatively new focus on clinical outcomes and effectiveness in the field of health services research. Both views, however, are consistent with the notion that society as a whole gains when no one faces severe financial impediments to receiving needed care. They are also consistent with the notion that society would greatly benefit if everyone had health insurance coverage.

Health Insurance Coverage as a Right

If, as was just argued, societies believe that equal access to either healthcare services or equal access to good health is necessary in the name of social justice, then there is a clear-cut justification for universal health insurance. Recent research on views about equity in several developed nations, conducted by Wagstaff and van Doorslaer (1992) show that such programs are consistent with the prevailing ethical viewpoints in nearly all developed nations. They report that

> There appears to be broad agreement... among policy-makers in at least eight of the nine European countries [studied] that payment towards healthcare should be related to ability to pay rather than to use of medical facilities. Policy-makers in all nine European countries also appear to be committed to the notion that all citizens should have access to health care. In many countries this is taken further, it being made clear that access to and receipt of health care should depend on need, rather than ability to pay. (p. 363)

The case for universal coverage is compelling when one considers the alternative conceptions of social welfare that were discussed above. If, as Margolis and Aaron argue, people have more than one element in their utility, functions—in addition to regular "goods-based" utility, they also derive satisfaction from helping others—then they would derive utility from being part of a society that helped those who do not have access to healthcare or good health.

In this regard, Mooney (1996b, 100) writes that

> Individuals recognise that they are members of a society and that they get some form of utility or increased well-being from being in a society, being able to make a contribution to that society, and being an active participant in that society. The source of this form of utility seems much more to be non-individualistic or at least stemming from a recognition on part of the individual that he or she is a member of a society and that such membership does convey certain benefit but also perhaps certain responsibilities.

This attitude has been denoted by the term "communitarianism," where, as applied to health, there is a "desire on part of the members of that society to create a just health care service as part of a wider just society" (Mooney 1996a, 101).

In summary, the case for universal coverage is very strong. Universal coverage is consistent with prevailing notions of fairness; people should not be penalized for circumstances—such as their sociodemographic background or their current state of health—over which they may have little control. In addition, unlike other characteristics, good health is instrumental in allowing people to have the capabilities to achieve their personal goals. Consequently, financial barriers to obtaining healthcare

are doubly unfair because they not only result in poorer health, but because they also frustrate people's ability to attain the other things that they desire. Furthermore, most people would appear to be endowed with a communitarian spirit in which they draw pride in being part of a society in which the well-being of others is an important part of their own welfare. It is thus no surprise that nearly every developed nation is committed to providing healthcare to its population regardless of ability to pay. The United States has much to learn from these societies that have found it worth their while to provide universal health insurance coverage.

Acknowledgments

I express my appreciation to Gavin Mooney and Deborah Stone for providing comments on this material. All conclusions and errors, however, are my own.

Notes

1. Gavin Mooney, personal communication, 1997.
2. Dworkin devotes several pages to explaining the difference between his theory and Rawls'. One difference is that Dworkin claims that his theory is tailored to the individual, whereas Rawls focuses on one representative person in a social class. It would also appear that individuals are more responsible for their actions (how they spend their resources) under Dworkin than under Rawls.
3. See, for example, Pauly (1978) and Reinhardt (1978).
4. For a good discussion of pros and cons of equalizing health, use, or access, see Chapter 5 of Mooney (1994).
5. Some of Culyer's more recent writing has begun to move away from this position. He writes, "I now think that it more helpful in studies of distribution to focus on the need for health care than on the need for health . . . [Adam] Wagstaff and I have also come to a stipulative definition of need as 'the minimum resources required to exhaust an individual's capacity to benefit from health care' " (Culyer 1993, 318).
6. For a thorough model of the determinants of health, see Evans and Stoddart (1990).

References

Aaron, H. J. 1994. "Public Policy, Values, and Consciousness," *Journal of Economic Perspectives* 8: 3–21.

Aday, L., R. Andersen, and G. V. Fleming. 1980. *Health Care in the U.S.: Equitable to Whom?* Beverly Hills, CA: Sage Publications.

Arrow, K. J. 1963. "Uncertainty and the Welfare Economics of Medical Care." *American Economic Review* 53: 940–73.

———. 1983. "Some Ordinalist-Utilitarian Notes of Rawls's *Theory of Justice*." In *Social Choice and Justice: Collected Papers of Kenneth J. Arrow*. Cambridge, MA: The Belknap Press of Harvard University.

Culyer, A. J. 1989. "The Normative Economics of Health Care Finance and Provision." *Oxford Review of Economic Policy* 5: 34–58.

———. 1993. "Health, Health Expenditures, and Equity." In *Equity in the Finance and Delivery of Health Care: An International Perspective*, edited by E. van Doorslaer, A. Wagstaff, and F. Rutten. Oxford, England: Oxford Medical Publications.

Dworkin, R. 1981. "What is Equality? Part 2: Equality of Resources." *Philosophy & Public Affairs* 10: 283–345.

Elster, J. 1992. *Local Justice: How Institutions Allocate Scarce Goods and Necessary Burdens*. New York: Russell Sage Foundation.

Evans, R., and G. L. Stoddart. 1990. *Producing Health, Consuming Health Care.* Paper 90-6. Hamilton, Ontario, Canada: Center for Health Economics and Policy Analysis, McMaster University.

Green, R. M. 1976. "Health Care and Justice in Contract Theory Perspective." *Ethics and Health Policy*, edited by R. M. Veatch and R. Branson. Cambridge, MA: Ballinger.

Hahnel, R., and M. Albert. 1990. *Quiet Revolution in Welfare Economics*. Princeton, NJ: Princeton University Press.

Margolis, H. 1982. *Selfishness, Altruism, and Rationality*. Cambridge, England: Cambridge University Press.

Mooney, G. 1994. *Key Issues in Health Economics*. New York: Harvester Wheatsheaf.

———. 1996a. "A Communitarian Critique of Health (Care) Economics." Paper delivered at the inaugural meetings of the International Health Economics Association, Vancouver, British Columbia, 21 May.

———. 1996b. "And Now for Vertical Equity? Some Concerns Arising from Aboriginal Health in Australia." *Health Economics* 5: 99–103.

Mooney, G., J. Hall, C. Donaldson, and K. Gerard. 1991. "Utilisation as a Measure of Equity: Weighing Heat?" *Journal of Health Economics* 10: 475–80.

Nozick, R. 1974. *Anarchy, State, and Utopia*. New York: Basic Books.

Pauly, M. V. 1978. "Is Medical Care Different?" In *Competition in the Health Care Sector: Past, Present, and Future*, edited by W. Greenberg. Washington, DC: Federal Trade Commission.

Rawls, J. 1971. *A Theory of Justice*. Cambridge, MA: The Belknap Press of Harvard University.

Reinhardt, U. E. 1978. "Comment." In *Competition in the Health Care Sector: Past, Present, and Future*, edited by W. Greenberg. Washington, DC: Federal Trade Commission.

Roemer, J. 1995. "Equality and Responsibility." *Boston Review* 20: 3–7.

Sagoff, M. 1986. "Values and Preferences." *Ethics* 96: 301–16.

Sen, A. 1992. *Inequality Revisited.* Cambridge, MA: Harvard University Press.

Stone, D. A. 1996. *Policy Paradox: The Art of Political Decision-Making.* New York: Norton.

Thurow, L. C. 1977. "Government Expenditures: Cash or In-kind Aid?" In *Markets and Morals,* edited by G. Dworkin, G. Bermant, and P. G. Brow. Washington, DC: Hemisphere Publishing.

Tullock, G. 1979. "Objectives of Income Redistribution." In *Sociological Economics,* edited by L. Levy-Garboua. Beverly Hills, CA: Sage.

Wagstaff, A., and E. van Doorslaer. 1992. "Equity in the Finance of Health Care: Some International Comparisons." *Journal of Health Economics* 11: 361–87.

———. 1993. "Equity in Finance and Delivery of Health Care: Concepts and Definitions." In *Equity in the Finance and Delivery of Health Care: An International Perspective,* edited by E. van Doorslaer, A. Wagstaff, and F. Rutten. Oxford, England: Oxford Medical Publications.

Young, H. P. 1994. *Equity in Theory and Practice.* Princeton, NJ: Princeton University Press.

Index

Academic health centers (AHCs),
   151–64
   costs of care in, 156–57, *159*
   government funding for, 13, 152
   and managed care, 155, 157–60,
      158
   mission of, 13, 151–52, 155, 160–63
   pressures on, 81, 162–64
   restructuring in, 158
   revenue for, 152–55, *154*, 157–59,
      160
   and safety net, 127, 132, 322
   and teaching function, 13, 152,
      156, 161
   and uncompensated care, 13, 82,
      92, 153–*54*, *155*, 157, *161*
Accessibility, healthcare, 295–96
   equity in, 5, 8, 11, 19, 90, 400–01
   international, 401–02
   and privatization, 200–01
   as social primary good, 391
   state initiatives for, 110, 297–99
   for uninsured, xii, 36–41, *39*, 43,
      90, 234–35
"Access gap," 378
Accountability:
   internal, 211
   public, 255, 317–19, 348

Acquired immunodeficiency
   syndrome (AIDS), 70, 71, 113, 190,
   193, 200
Acquisitions, 225, 279, 303
   and purposeful avoidance theory,
      226
   See also Mergers
Administration:
   bureaucracy in, 234
   costs of, 331–*32*, 345
   of health services, 328
   of incremental reforms, 253–55,
      320
   program, *68*, 315, 383
Adverse risk selection, 320, 350
Aid to Families with Dependent
   Children (AFDC), 79–80
   eligibility for, 47, 60
   elimination of, 108, 252, 301
   enrollment decrease in, 74, 77, 80,
      290
   and Medicaid, 4, 47, 68, 87, 259
Ambulatory care, 101–02, 111, 224,
   302
American Hospital Association
   (AHA):
   comparative data from, 197–98,
      208, 211, 225

About the Authors

Henry J. Aaron, Ph.D., is currently a Senior Fellow in the Economic Studies Program. Dr. Aaron is a member of the Institute of Medicine, the American Academy of Arts and Sciences, the board of directors of Georgetown University and Abt Associates, Inc., and the advisory committee of the Center for Economic Policy and Stanford University. He holds a Ph.D. in economics from Harvard University.

Karen Davis, Ph.D., is President of The Commonwealth Fund and is a nationally recognized economist, with a distinguished career in public policy and research. A native of Oklahoma, she received her doctoral degree in economics from Rice University. Dr. Davis has published a number of significant books, monographs, and articles on health and social policy issues.

Alain C. Enthoven, Ph.D., is the Marriner S. Eccles Professor of Public and Private Management in the Graduate School of Business at Stanford University and holds degrees in economics from Stanford, Oxford, and the Massachusetts Institute of Technology. Dr. Enthoven is a member of the Institute of Medicine of the National Academy of Science, as well as a member of the Jackson Hole Group. His latest book is *Theory and Practice of Managed Competition in Health Care Finance.*

Judith Feder, Ph.D., is a political scientist and a Professor of Public Policy at Georgetown University's Institute for Health Care Research and Policy. In addition to teaching in the Graduate Public Policy Program, Dr. Feder is conducting health policy research for the Institute. Dr. Feder was a lead official in the Clinton Administration's health reform initiative.

Larry S. Gage has served since 1981 as President of the National Association of Public Hospitals and Health Systems. He is also a partner in the Washington, D.C., office of the Atlanta-based law firm of Powell, Goldstein, Frazer & Murphy LLP, and director of the firm's health practice group. He is a graduate of Harvard College and Columbia Law School.

Darrell J. Gaskin, Ph.D., is an Assistant Professor at Georgetown University Medical Center, Department of Medicine, in the Institute for Health Care Research and Policy. Dr. Gaskin's research interests include the impact of market forces and public policy on hospitals and physicians, access to care for low-income and uninsured populations, and the treatment decisions of patients. Dr. Gaskin earned his Ph.D. in health economics at the Johns Hopkins University School of Hygiene and Public Health.

Bradford H. Gray, Ph.D., is Director of the Division of Health and Science Policy at the New York Academy of Medicine. He is an elected Fellow of the Hastings Center and the New York Academy of Medicine. Dr. Gray has published extensively, and his most recent book is *The Profit Motive and Patient Care: The Changing Accountability of Doctors and Hospitals.* He holds a Ph.D. in sociology from Yale University.

Stuart Guterman has been at the Prospective Payment Assessment Commission since 1988, and has been Deputy Director since 1990. Prior to that, he was Chief of Institutional Studies at the Health Care Financing Administration's Office of Research. Mr. Guterman received an M.A. in economics from Brown University and completed his course work toward a Ph.D. in economics at the State University of New York at Stony Brook.

Daniel R. Hawkins, Jr., is Vice President for Policy Research and Analysis at the National Association of Community Health Centers, Inc. He has written numerous articles on healthcare and health center issues, currently oversees production of several NACHC publications annually, and has provided testimony before numerous congressional committees. He was recently named one of America's 1000 most influential health policymakers.

Robert B. Helms, Ph.D., is Resident Scholar and Director of Health Policy Studies at the American Enterprise Institute. He has written and lectured extensively on health policy, health economics, and pharmaceutical economic issues. Dr. Helms currently participates in the Consensus

Group, an informal task force that is developing market-oriented health reform concepts. He is also the editor of seven American Enterprise Institute publications on health policy.

John F. Holahan, Ph.D., is Director of the Health Policy Research Center at the Urban Institute. He has authored several publications on the Medicaid program and has also published research on the effects of expanding Medicaid on the number of uninsured and the cost to federal and state governments. His other research interests include health system reform, changes in health insurance coverage, and physician payment.

Patricia Seliger Keenan is a Policy Analyst with the Henry J. Kaiser Family Foundation and the Kaiser Commission on the Future of Medicaid, specializing in Medicaid restructuring and health coverage for low-income populations. Previously, she served as a project officer at the Health Care Financing Administration.

Mark V. Pauly, Ph.D., currently holds the positions of the Vice Dean of the Wharton School of Doctoral Programs and Bendheim Professor. He is the Professor of Health Care Systems, Insurance and Risk Management and Public Policy and Management, at the Wharton School, and Professor of Economics in the School of Arts and Sciences at the University of Pennsylvania. Dr. Pauly is an active member of the Institute of Medicine, a commissioner on the Physician Payment Review Commission, and adjunct scholar of the American Enterprise Institute.

James Reuter, Sc.D., is an Associate Professor in the Department of Internal Medicine at Georgetown University, and is Director of the Georgetown Institute for Health Care Research and Policy. He has worked in the healthcare policy and health services research fields for more than twenty years and has held academic positions at the University of Wisconsin–Madison and at Georgetown University.

Thomas Rice, Ph.D., is Professor and Chair of the Department of Health Services, University of California, Los Angeles. Dr. Rice received his Ph.D. in economics at the University of California at Berkeley. His research interests include the effects of competition in healthcare, health insurance, physician payment, and the Medicare program. He is currently editor of *Medical Care Research and Review*.

Trish Riley has served as Executive Director of the National Academy for State Health Policy and President of its Corporate Board since 1989. She codirects the Center for Vulnerable Populations, serves as a member of the Kaiser Commission on the Future of Medicaid, was recently elected to the board of directors of the National Committee on Quality Assurance, and is a member of HCFA's Quality Improvement System for Medicaid and Medicare Managed Care.

Sara Rosenbaum, J.D., is Professor of Health Care Sciences and Director of the Center for Health Policy Research at the George Washington University Medical Center. She also holds appointments in the University's Schools of Business and Law. Ms. Rosenbaum is known nationally for her work in the areas of health law for the poor, healthcare financing, and maternal and child health, and was recently named one of America's 500 most influential health policymakers.

Diane Rowland, Sc.D., is the Executive Vice President of the Henry J. Kaiser Family Foundation and the Executive Director of the Kaiser Commission on the Future of Medicaid. She also serves as Associate Professor in the Department of Health Policy and Management at the School of Hygiene and Public Health of the Johns Hopkins University. She is nationally recognized for her research and publications on health coverage and access to care for low-income and vulnerable populations.

David Schactman is a Senior Research Associate at Brandeis University and the Director of the Council on the Economic Impact of Health Systems Change. Mr. Schactman has authored numerous reports and publications on health market competition and consolidation, and the implications for antitrust and public policy. He has an M.P.A. in health policy from Harvard University's John F. Kennedy School of Government and an M.B.A. in finance from Columbia University.

Raymond C. Scheppach, Ph.D., is the Executive Director of the National Governor's Association. He received his B.A. in business administration from the University of Maine, and his M.A. and his Ph.D. degrees in economics from the University of Connecticut. He has authored and coauthored four books on economics and has written numerous professional articles.

Cathy Schoen is the Director of Research and Evaluation for the Commonwealth Fund, where she also serves as Program Director for the Fund's Health Care Coverage and Quality Program. Ms. Schoen is trained as an economist, specializing in healthcare finance, benefits, and labor issues, and her publications span a range of issues relating to access to care, low-income populations, and the concerns of working families.

Steven A. Schroeder, M.D., has been President of the Robert Wood Johnson Foundation since 1990 and continues to practice general internal medicine on a part-time basis at the Robert Wood Johnson Medical School, where he is clinical professor of medicine. Dr. Schroeder has been a member of many healthcare organizations, and has published widely in the fields of clinical medicine, healthcare organization and financing, manpower, quality of care, and preventive medicine. He graduated from Stanford University and Harvard Medical School.

Thomas A. Scully is President and Chief Executive Officer of the Federation of American Health Systems, the trade association representing the nation's 1,700 investor-owned and -managed hospitals and health systems. He received his bachelor's degree from the University of Virginia and J.D. from Catholic University Law School.

Katherine Swartz, Ph.D., is Associate Professor in the Department of Health Policy and Management at Harvard School of Public Health. In November 1995, she became the editor of *Inquiry,* a journal that focuses on healthcare organization and financing. Dr. Swartz was the 1991 recipient of the David Kershaw Award from the Association for Public Policy Analysis and Management. She has a Ph.D. in economics from the University of Wisconsin.

Gail R. Wilensky, Ph.D., is the John M. Olin Senior Fellow at Project HOPE, where she analyzes and develops policies relating to healthcare reform and to ongoing changes in the medical marketplace. She is currently the chair of the Physician Payment Review Commission and is an elected member of the Institute of Medicine of the National Academy of Sciences and a trustee of the Combined Benefits Fund of the United Mine Workers of America; she also serves as a director for several for-profit and not-for-profit corporations. She has a Ph.D. in economics from the University of Michigan.

About the Editors

Stuart H. Altman, Ph.D., is the Sol C. Chaikin Professor of National Health Policy at the Florence Heller Graduate School for Social Policy, Brandeis University. He is an economist whose research interests are primarily in the area of federal health policy. He was the dean of the Florence Heller Graduate School from 1977 until July 1993. For twelve years, from 1983 to 1996, he was the chairman of the U.S. Prospective Payment Assessment Commission, responsible for advising Congress and the President on appropriate Medicare payment policies to hospitals and other institutional providers.

Dr. Altman is a member of the Institute of Medicine of the National Academy of Sciences and was a member of its Governing Council from 1979 to 1982. He is also a member of the Board of Overseers of Beth Israel Deaconess Medical Center in Boston, Massachusetts, and chairman of the board of the Institute for Health Policy at Brandeis University. He is chair of the Council on the Economic Impact of Health System Change, sponsored by the Robert Wood Johnson Foundation. In addition, Dr. Altman has served on the Board of the Robert Wood Johnson Clinical Scholars Program.

Between 1971 and 1976, Professor Altman was Deputy Assistant Secretary for Planning and Evaluation/Health at the Department of Health, Education, and Welfare. While there, he was one of the principal contributors to the development and advancement of the National Health Insurance Proposal. From 1973 to 1974 he also served as the Deputy Director for Health of the President's Cost-of-Living Council where he was responsible for developing the Council's program on healthcare cost containment.

Professor Altman was also a senior member of the Clinton-Gore Health Policy Transition Team in 1992. He testifies often before various congressional committees, most recently on the implications of the changes in Medicare funding on hospitals and the healthcare system proposed in the 1995 Medicare Reform Act.

Professor Altman has an M.A. and a Ph.D. degree in economics from UCLA and taught at Brown University and the Graduate School of Public Policy at the University of California at Berkeley.

Uwe W. Reinhardt, Ph.D., has taught at Princeton University since 1968, rising through the ranks from assistant professor of economics to his current position, the James Madison Professor of Political Economy. He has taught courses in both micro- and macroeconomic theory and policy, accounting for commercial, private nonprofit, and governmental enterprises.

In 1978, Professor Reinhardt was elected to the Institute of Medicine of the National Academy of Sciences, on whose Governing Council he served from 1979 to 1982. At the Institute, he has served on a number of study panels; currently he sits on the Committee on Technological Innovation in Medicine and on the Committee on the Implications of a Physician Surplus.

From 1987 to 1990, Professor Reinhardt was a member of the National Leadership Commission on Health Care, and he continues to serve on that body's successor, the National Leadership Coalition on Health Care. He is past president of the Association of Health Services Research. From 1978 to 1993, he served on the board of trustees of the Teachers Insurance and Annuity Association, where he was a member of its Mortgage Finance Committee during the same period.

Professor Reinhardt has served on a number of government committees and commissions, among them the National Council on Health Care Technology of the former U.S. Department of Health and Welfare and the Special Advisory Group of the then Veteran's Administration. From 1986 to 1995, he served three consecutive three-year terms as commissioner on the Physician Payment Review Commission. In 1996, he served as a member of the Committee on the U.S. Physician Supply of the Institute of Medicine of the National Academy of Sciences, and that same year he was appointed to the Institution's Board of Health Care Services. He is currently a member of the Council on the Economic Impact of System Change.

Professor Reinhardt received the Bachelor of Commerce degree from the University of Saskatchewan in 1964 and a Ph.D. in economics from Yale University. He has received honorary degrees of Dr.Sci from the Medical College of Pennsylvania and from Mount Sinai School of Medicine, City University of New York.

Alexandra E. Shields, M.A., is a Research Associate at Brandeis University, where she has worked as research staff for the Council on the Economic Impact of Health System Change since January 1994. In addition to coediting this volume, she has coauthored several reports, including studies modeling the impact of federal budget reductions on the number of uninsured, the availability of free care, and hospital revenues. Ms. Shields is also a Doctoral Candidate at the Heller School, Brandeis University. Her dissertation addresses the impact of Medicaid managed care on the clinical process of care and related outcomes for asthma, an important tracer condition for the Medicaid population. Ms. Shields came to Brandeis in 1993 as a Pew Health Policy Fellow. She has received numerous other fellowships and awards, including an AHCPR Health Services Research Training Fellowship, an AHCPR Dissertation award for Health Services Research, as well as research grants from the Caplan Foundation and the Asthma and Allergy Foundation of America.

Prior to her work at Brandeis, Ms. Shields served in Massachusetts state government for six years, first as Regional Director of the Healthy Start Program for the Massachusetts Department of Public Health, a program that provides health insurance for low-income pregnant women, and then as Director of Ambulatory Care for the Massachusetts Rate Setting Commission. At the Commission, Ms. Shields developed reimbursement policy governing 37 different ambulatory health services and directed research on preventable hospitalizations, AIDS services, and access to primary care. Ms. Shields has also worked as an international development consultant in the Philippines and taught in Jamaica. More recently, she has worked as an independent healthcare consultant for the state of Massachusetts establishing statewide, disease-specific quality improvement networks for providers. Ms. Shields has also been active in a number of community organizations, serving as chair of the board of directors for Women, Inc., a nonprofit organization serving women with addictions and their children, for a number of years.

Ms. Shields received her B.A. in sociology and theology from Boston College, where she graduated summa cum laude, Phi Beta Kappa. She was also awarded an M.A. with Distinction from Boston College in the field of systematic theology, where she was the Lonergan Scholar in Theology. She expects to receive her Ph.D. in social welfare policy from Brandeis University in May 1998.